hronic Mental Illness

lume 1
se Management for Mentally Ill Patients: Theory and Practice
ited by Maxine Harris and Helen C. Bergman

lume 2
lping Families Cope with Mental Illness
ited by Harriet P. Lefley and Mona Wasow

dditional volume in preparation

**ouble Jeopardy: Substance Disorders and
evere Mental Illness**
ited by Anthony Lehman and Lisa Dixon

HELPING FAMILIES
WITH MENTAL ILL

Cl

Se
Joh
Ba

Ad

Le
Jef
H.
• F

Vo
Ca
Ec

Vo
He
Ec

Ac

Do
Se
Ec

Th
ma
sh

HELPING FAMILIES COPE
WITH MENTAL ILLNESS

Edited by

Harriet P. Lefley
University of Miami School of Medicine

and

Mona Wasow
University of Wisconsin, Madison

harwood academic publishers
USA ● Switzerland ● Australia ● Belgium ● France ●
Germany ● Great Britain ● India ● Japan ● Malaysia ●
Netherlands ● Russia ● Singapore

Harwood Academic Publishers
Poststrasse 22
7000 Chur, Switzerland

British Library Cataloguing in Publication Data

Lefley, Harriet P.
  Helping Families Cope with Mental
  Illness. - (Chronic Mental Illness Series, ISSN 1066-7407;Vol.2)
  I. Title II. Wasow, Mona III. Marsh, D.
  IV. Series
  362.204

ISBN 3-7186-0580-5

Contents

Contents

Introduction to the Series

This series on chronic mental illness is a result of both the success and failure of our efforts over the past thirty years to provide better treatment, rehabilitation and care for persons suffering from severe and persistent mental illnesses. The failure is obvious to all who walk our cities' streets, use our libraries or pass through our transportation terminals. The success is found in the enormous boost of interest in service to, research on and teaching about treatment, rehabilitation and care of those persons who, in Leona Bachrach's definition, "are, have been, or might have been, but for the deinstitutionalization movement, on the rolls of long-term mental institutions, especially state hospitals."

The first book in our modern era devoted to the subject was that by Richard Lamb in 1976, *Community Survival for Long-Term Patients.* Shortly thereafter, Leona Bachrach's unique study "Deinstitutionalization: An Analytical Review and Sociological Perspective" was published. In 1978, the American Psychiatric Association hosted a meeting on the problem that resulted in the publication *The Chronic Mental Patient.* This effort in turn spawned several texts dealing with increasingly specialized areas: *The Chronic Mentally Ill: Treatment, Programs, Systems* and *Chronic Mental Illness in Children and Adolescents*, both by John Looney; and *The Chronic Mental Patient/II* by Walter Menninger and Gerald Hannah.

Now, however, there are a host of publications devoted to various portions of the problem, e.g., the homeless mentally ill, rehabilitation of the mentally ill, families of the mentally ill, and so on. The amount of research and experience now that can be conveyed to a wide population of caregivers is exponentially greater than it was in 1955, the year that deinstitutionalization began.

This series will cover:

- types of intervention, e.g., psychopharmacology, psychotherapy, case management, social and vocational rehabilitation, and mobile and home treatment;

- settings, e.g., hospitals, ambulatory settings, nursing homes, correctional facilities, and shelters;

- specific populations, e.g., alcohol and drug abusers, the homeless and those dually diagnosed;

— special issues, e.g., family intervention, psychoeducation, policy / financing, non-compliance, forensic, cross-cultural and systems issues.

I am indebted to our hard-working editorial board as well as to our editors and authors, many of whom are involved in both activities.

This second volume is typical of what we will publish; it covers a specific portion of the field, although overlapping with other books in the series; and it deals with experience, research, training, and hands-on service and coping strategies. Its editors are both leaders in the area of family involvement and have the unique ability to bridge the academic and practical worlds.

Future books in this series will cover dual diagnosis, inpatient care, psychiatric rehabilitation, psychopharmacology, the homeless mentally ill, problems with compliance, alcoholism and drug abuse as chronic conditions and the mentally ill in the correctional system. I hope you will look forward to them as eagerly as I do.

John A. Talbott, MD

Introduction

Harriet P. Lefley and Mona Wasow

Serious mental illness can be a devastating stressor in any family, regardless of its strengths and available resources. Major psychiatric disorders such as the schizophrenias, major affective disorders, persistent psychoses, and similarly severe diagnostic conditions often lead to substantial impairment in a person's ability to fulfill an age-appropriate role in life. Persons with these disorders suffer not only from the private terrors of their symptoms, but from the social and psychological sequelae of being mentally ill. For many this means learning to overcome both societal stigma and self-stigmatization because of their enforced dependency on others for treatment and survival. In our culture an adult's prolonged dependency on the family, whether as caregiver or as lifetime support system, has built-in problems for all parties concerned.

Families must develop a range of adaptations to the objective problems posed by serious mental illness in their midst. They must deal with disrupted household routines; time investments in negotiating the mental health, housing, social security, and sometimes the criminal justice systems; impaired relations with an unsympathetic outside world; financial burdens; psychological and career impact on other household members; and difficulties in finding alternatives to hospitalization. The treatment system itself has presented problems. Families of persons with severe and persistent mental illness have reported confusing and sometimes humiliating interactions with service providers, conflicting advice from professionals, histories of costly therapeutic failures, and a lack of guidelines for helping the patient make appropriate treatment decisions.

Families face multiple stressors in dealing with persons whose disorders may make them very difficult to live with. Severe mental illnesses often are manifested in mood swings and unpredictability; demanding, abusive, or even assaultive behaviors; noncompliance with treatment; poor money management; conditions disturbing to household living such as poor personal hygiene, sleep reversal patterns, or fire hazards; and socially embarrassing situations. Families must learn to cope both with the patient's behavior and with their own reactions; to balance the patient's needs against those of other family members; to perceive when expectations are too high and too low; and to know how and when to set limits. They must deal with unwarranted guilt feelings, learn to handle their anger, tolerate the suffering of people they love, and avoid being overwhelmed by empathic pain. Family members must recognize the boundaries of their own rescue fantasies and yet not abandon hope.

Throughout much of history and in most other cultures, families have had to develop their own adaptive strategies in coping with erratic behaviors and in helping their disabled relatives attain some degree of productivity and social acceptance. Paradoxically, it is only in recent centuries, with the isolation of patients in remote institutions, that families began to be separated and later excluded from the treatment process. Initially this was an unintended consequence of social policy that had the simultaneous aim of protecting society from mentally ill persons and protecting mentally ill persons from the pressures and perils of urban life. Later, separation of patients and families was reinforced by theoretical paradigms that viewed a patient's symptoms not as valid presentations of disease, but rather as metaphors of poor parenting or as instrumental behaviors that fulfilled a functional need of the family system. However, clinical interventions based on these theories produced too few successes among persons with severe psychiatric disorders. Many families found themselves depleted of economic resources but with few techniques for dealing with the continuing problems of chronic mental illness in their midst.

Compelling biological research findings, including those that demonstrate genetic factors and/or extrafamilial environmental influences on uterine development, are beginning to contest notions of interpersonal etiology, while new psychopharmacological agents are proving efficacious in some types of symptom control. These research findings, together with studies of the dimensions of family burden, have also impacted clinical training and services. They have been accompanied by new types of supportive interventions that are finally giving families state-of-the-art information and practical illness management techniques.

The era of deinstitutionalization and community care, however, requires a range of helping resources that are targeted to individual family situations and needs. This book is responsive to current trends in the field, including government mandates and agency guidelines that require greater attention to serving the needs of families of deinstitutionalized patients as caregivers, support systems, and as contributors to treatment planning and policy decisions. Most families need basic education on mental illnesses; but beyond this, families' needs will vary as a function of their individual experiences and adaptive strengths. We tap a considerable armamentarium of resources that may be used to help families— various models of clinical intervention, advocacy movement resources, and a rich lode of coping strategies developed by families themselves. We are most grateful to the noted clinicians, educators, and researchers who have agreed to contribute to this endeavor.

In a book of this nature it is almost impossible to avoid redundancy. It is only in recent years that researchers and educators have begun to address family needs and, inevitably, there are common themes and overlapping references to the limited body of research literature that elucidates these themes. However, each chapter deals with a different aspect. Issues ranging from confidentiality to systemic family therapy are addressed from different perspectives or with specific emphases. We are offered a multi-faceted approach to viewing common and pervasive problems of families living with severe mental illness.

Our book begins by taking clinicians and other helpers through the family experience. The first section addresses family burden and coping strategies, and contemporary models of services for families. Families' interactions with professionals are traced in historical perspective, including the movement away from a model of family pathogenesis to a coping/adaptation/competence model of family functioning. Data are presented on what families want from mental health professionals. This section explores the development of the family movement, the National Alliance for the Mentally Ill, and its effects on family-professional relationships and the mental health system generally. Part I concludes with contemporary models of services for families, in which various forms of clinical and nonclinical interventions are compared and contrasted. Generic features of all family-oriented services are highlighted, as well as the therapeutic benefits of active advocacy.

In Part II, current and continuing controversies regarding the family's role in caregiving and treatment are explored. The section begins with an analysis of the family's emerging role in the service delivery system and appropriate relationships of family members, primary consumers, and the professionally staffed service delivery system. We continue with an analytic discussion of the relevance of systems theory, expressed emotion and communication deviance research, and psychodynamic issues in clinical work and nonclinical settings. We describe circumstances in which family therapy may be required in addition to basic psychoeducation, and situations in which the treatment of choice may focus on or combine psychodynamic and systemic elements, including use of larger systems to augment clinical interventions.

Part III focuses on services. Guidelines are offered on the initial interview to determine an appropriate family service plan and to choose from among alternative interventions. Linkages with case managers and other components of the treatment system are discussed. Survey findings of coping strategies developed and tested by families over the years are shared with professionals and other family members. Practical guidelines for illness management are provided, ranging from dealing with threats and suicidal attempts to medication compliance and personal hygiene. The educational and clinical needs of different family members—parents, spouses, siblings, and adult children—are reviewed. Research findings are presented on individual and multi-family intervention models. Service needs of families are discussed in terms of cultural diversity. A detailed analysis focuses on ethical issues in working with patients' families. And some empirical findings are presented on families' assessment of specific categories of services for their loved ones and themselves.

Part IV focuses on training and research. This section articulates goals for professional training and offers a generic curriculum for training graduate students at the levels of exposure, experience, and expertise. A university-based program is described that provides hands-on training in working with families to psychiatric residents and graduate psychology interns. Current issues in family research and fruitful lines of future research are discussed.

In Part V, we end with a perspective on the future of families' relations with consumers, professionals, and the provider system. A consumer's viewpoint stresses the need for a recovery focus in treatment, with families being willing to take risks in order to help their loved ones gain autonomy and self-esteem. The last chapter focuses on ways in which new treatment and rehabilitative approaches can be implemented in a changing service delivery system. We discuss the social policy implications of family and consumer roles, and modes of fulfilling the needs of families and their loved ones in an era of managed care. New cost-effective models, including both consumer-run services and innovative deployment of professional resources, are discussed in terms of fostering more collaborative roles for families and relieving their caregiving burden. We end with suggestions for research, practice, and policy development.

Finally, we want to add a note on the major orientation of this book. In our perspective, families of persons with long-term, serious mental illness are similar in category and in needs to families of persons with other lifetime conditions that pose periodic and sometimes intolerable stress. We subscribe to the systemic viewpoint that the patient's disorder inevitably disturbs the family, in schizophrenia and manic depressive illness just as in Alzheimer's Disease, AIDS, or paraplegia—disabilities that no one claims can be cured nor whose symptoms can be eliminated by family therapy. In contrast to earlier paradigms, families of mentally ill persons are not viewed as instrumental channels for healing the patient—they did not cause these diseases and they cannot cure them— but as valid recipients of aid in dealing with highly adverse life situations. As in other disorders, our work is based on the premise that as family members gain greater understanding of their relatives' experiences and feelings and learn to cope more effectively, both they and the patient will be benefited. The form, extent, and duration of benefit are empirical questions for further research. Meanwhile, the mental health of families living with serious mental illness continues to be a legitimate concern for our attention and help.

Contributors

Kayla F. Bernheim, PhD, Private practice, Lakeville, New York

Agnes B. Hatfield, PhD, Professor Emerita, Department of Human Development, College of Education, Unviersity of Maryland, College Park

Dale L. Johnson, PhD, Professor of Psychology, Department of Psychology, University of Houston, Texas

Kate Judge, MSSW, Research Assistant, School of Social Work, University of Wisconsin, Madison

Stephen M. Kersker, Executive Director, Florida Drop-in-Center Association, St. Petersburg

Harriet P. Lefley, PhD, Professor of Psychiatry, Department of Psychiatry, University of Miami School of Medicine, Florida

Ellen Lukens, MPhil, Director of Research, Department of Social Work, New York State Psychiatric Institute, New York

Diane T. Marsh, PhD, Professor of Psychology, Department of Psychology, University of Pittsburgh at Greensburg, Pennsylvania

Evelyn M. McElroy, RN, PhD, Professor of Nursing, School of Nursing, University of Maryland, Baltimore

Paul D. McElroy, PhD, Associate Professor of Education, School of Education and Urban Studies, Morgan State University, Baltimore, Maryland

William R. McFarlane, MD, Chief of Psychiatry, Maine Medical Center, Portland

Gayle Gubman Riesser, PhD, New Jersey Division of Mental Health and Hospitals, Trenton

Bonnie J. Schorske, MA, New Jersey Division of Mental Health and Hospitals, Trenton

Phyllis Solomon, PhD, Professor and Director, Section of Mental Health Services and Systems Research, Department of Mental Health Sciences, Hahnemann University, Philadelphia, Pennsylvania

LeRoy Spaniol, PhD, Associate Executive Director, Center for Psychiatric Rehabilitation, Boston University, Massachusetts

Nancy J. Warren, PhD, Clinical Associate Professor and Director of Family Transition Program, Department of Psychiatry, Baylor College of Medicine, Houston, Texas

Mona Wasow, ACSW, Clinical Professor of Social Work, School of Social Work, University of Wisconsin, Madison

Anthony M. Zipple, ScD, Vice-President for Mental Health Services, Vinfen Corporation, Boston, Massachusetts

PART I:

FAMILIES AND MENTAL ILLNESS: WHERE HAVE WE COME FROM? WHERE ARE WE NOW?

Chapter 1

RELATIONSHIPS BETWEEN FAMILY CAREGIVERS AND MENTAL HEALTH PROFESSIONALS: THE AMERICAN EXPERIENCE

Gayle Gubman Riesser and Bonnie J. Schorske

INTRODUCTION

A new activism is empowering families of mental health consumers. For the first time since the care and treatment of people with mental illnesses became the domain of governments, social welfare organizations and medical science, families are starting to get the level of support from professionals commensurate with their responsibilities in caring for their ill members (Hatfield, 1987a). Professionals, for their part, are asking about the family's experiences in coping with mental illnesses and validating what the family identifies as its needs in developing a clinical focus (Atwood and Williams, 1978). National policies calling for family involvement in research and planning reflect this greater family role (NIMH, 1991). Especially noticeable are recent family treatment models which provide education and supports to enhance the family's quality of life and competency to cope with a disabling illness. These practices, which encourage collaborative partnerships, provide alternatives to psychodynamic approaches that blame families and create a clinical wedge in the family's relationship with its ill relative and the professional community.

Yet, despite these recent advances, caution remains warranted. Mental health professionals have a long history of, at best, benign neglect of the families of those suffering from mental illnesses. At worst, families have been isolated and stigmatized. Historically, professional attitudes have been most directly affected by prevailing theories regarding the etiology of mental illnesses, advances in treatment, and the extent to

3

which the care of people with mental illnesses was defined as the predominant concern of families, society or the mental health professions.

This chapter examines five major periods in the history of mental
health care and treatment in the United States and discusses their impact
on family and professional interactions. Until the emergence of a family
self-help movement in the 1970's, there was a dearth of published
information regarding how families felt about mental health services in
general and relationships with professionals in particular. Slightly more
is known about professional attitudes toward families. Much must still
be inferred from the historical context. Research based on primary
sources is needed to fill this gap.

THE PURITAN LEGACY OF FAMILY CARE IN THE COMMUNITY

During the colonial period, there were no mental health professionals
per se and family care was focused on behavioral management. Mental
illnesses were seen as disruptions of civic order, demonic possession or
imbalances of humors, and families, in managing their ill members,
related to town officials, ministers and physicians. Because the family
was the basis of community life, disruptive behaviors were their responsibility, a duty complicated by the fact that the labor of every family
member was vital.

Families in straitened circumstances could turn to the courts and town
officials as a last resort. A Massachusetts law enacted in 1676 stated:

> "Whereas, There are distracted persons in some tounes, that
> are unruly, whereby not only the familyes, wherein they are,
> but others suffer much damage by them, it is ordered by this
> Court and the authoritye thereof that the selectmen in all tounes
> where such are are hereby impowred and injoyned to take care
> of all such persons, that they doe not damnify others" (Deutsch,
> 1949:43).

The courts assigned responsibility for care and local officials determined
the community's financial obligation. The family might be paid from
the community treasury to erect a separate dwelling to secure an ill
relative. In many instances, the town paid other community residents
to provide habitation and management (Deutsch, 1949). Certainly, the
practice of indenturing, apprenticing or boarding children, strangers
and other dependents was well-established during this time (Morgan,
1966). Individuals who posed a significant danger to others or the
community were maintained in local jails. However well the community

might address the concrete costs of caregiving, the family's emotional burdens were rarely acknowledged.

The family's need to understand their relative's suffering was hampered by an inability to identify the problem. Symptoms of mental illnesses were frequently indistinguishable from other ailments, e.g., epilepsy, intransigence and religious crises. Primary "professional" guidance came from the community's ministers, who advocated a harsh theology bent on controlling individual impulses. This theology attributed disturbing behaviors and perceptions to a demonic possession that threatened family and community alike. Cotton Mather's dictum to parents, "'Better whipped than Damn'd'" (Morgan, 1966:103) aptly summarized the usual approach to behavioral management (Deutsch, 1949; Grob, 1983).

At the time, there were few practicing physicians and no mental health professionals. In rare instances, communities might send ill and abandoned persons to live with someone who was believed to have medical knowledge (Demos, 1970). The few persons who claimed skills in the medical arts were unaware of the various causes of the mental illnesses, and applied identical treatments to all diseases. Bloodletting was especially popular, perhaps in part because the loss of blood rendered the patient more manageable, if no healthier. St. John's Wort was commonly prescribed, along with herbal purgatives (Deutsch, 1949). Despite claims that these treatments effected rapid cures, "'I have knowne it to cure perfectly to admiration in five dayes'" (Deutsch, 1949:30), there is no evidence that medical treatments were more beneficial than careful observation and management within the family. Behavioral control, through restraint and punishment, was most frequently the only option.

THE EMERGENCE OF THE MENTAL HEALTH PROFESSION

Moral or humanistic treatment first emerged at the end of the Eighteenth Century and was among the first systematic approaches to mental illnesses, differentiating them from other illnesses and mere poverty. Moral treatment's advocates were also the first mental health professionals, the physicians Philippe Pinel in France, William Tuke in England, and Benjamin Rush and Eli Todd in the United States. These physicians viewed mental illnesses as having distinct somatic origins and the victims as human beings, needing humane and dignified environments. Rush and Todd were associated with the first hospitals in the United States for the treatment of persons with mental illnesses and they replaced dank, airless cells with rooms providing adequate heat, light and ventilation. Patients had beds in which to sleep, the sexes were separated to ensure personal dignity, and residents had opportunities for movement and meaningful activity (possible in facilities that accommodated only 40-200 residents) (Deutsch, 1949).

Families must have perceived great benefits from moral treatment for their relatives with mental illnesses. Cure rates at hospitals, which were synonymous with discharges, were purported to exceed 90 percent among persons who had been ill less than a year. The physicians, who were the superintendents at these hospitals, were interested in legitimizing mental health treatment and obtaining public support. In 1844, they founded the Association of Medical Superintendents of American Institutions, a precursor to the American Psychiatric Association, to promote medical treatment for mental illnesses. For families, this new optimism and improved treatment environment were distinct advances in patient care and compassion (Deutsch, 1949; Grob, 1983).

Moral treatment was also a first step toward substituting the authority of mental health professionals for that of clergy, kin and communities (Morrissey and Goldman, 1984). Physicians suggested that the patient's environment, including the family and community, might be an impediment to treatment, and sought a period of separation and respite, even from close relatives (Deutsch, 1949). While an intimate bond between the patient and psychiatrist was seen as central to successful treatment, there was little recognition that the family had a supportive role.

For much of the Nineteenth Century, few families or primary consumers could afford hospital care or moral treatment for mental illnesses. Most families continued to bear the primary burden of care. However, as communities and social dislocation grew in response to waves of immigration and urban migration following the Civil War, families were less able to maintain ill relatives, and the indigent population became more numerous. Communities often dealt with their dependent mentally ill citizens by massing them with the poor and other disabled persons in almshouses (Grob, 1983). This emergent social welfare system did not distinguish among causes of poverty and rarely provided any treatment, let alone humane care, for those with mental illnesses.

If a "distracted" indigent were able-bodied, then the community might entertain "bids" for his labor and maintenance, awarding contracts to the lowest bidder. Those individuals without skills or community ties could receive the early Nineteenth Century equivalent of "Greyhound therapy." They were "warned off" or deposited in a nearby forest or adjoining town (Deutsch, 1948; Demos, 1970). Given the absence of medical treatment and the harsh conditions of indigent care, it is easy to see the appeal of public asylums for the mentally ill. Reformers, most notably Dorothea Dix, brought the abuses of indigent community care to the attention of state legislatures, and called upon states to establish hospitals so that the dependent mentally ill might have decent care and treatment options (Deutsch, 1949).

THE ASYLUM YEARS: 1850-1950

The State Hospitals

The movement toward state hospitals for all dependent persons with mental illnesses was intended to provide the same care and treatment to the needy that were available to those who could afford private asylums. The movement's impact was rapid and dramatic. From 1850 to 1880, the proportion of the general population hospitalized for mental illnesses more than doubled, from .07 to .18 percent (Grob, 1983). By the turn of the century, the hospital was the locus of care for more than 70 percent of the dependent mentally ill in the United States, displacing families and poorhouses (Deutsch, 1949).

The clinical theories of the era encouraged mental health professionals to exclude families. As Emil Kraepelin, one of the first psychiatrists to develop a clear and comprehensive classification of the mental illnesses, noted, "Visits from near relations have a bad effect up to the very end of the illness..." (Kraepelin, 1904:10). Despite early enthusiasm for the asylum movement, both families and the public became disillusioned with treatment outcomes as more and more people had lengthy hospital stays (Deutsch, 1949; Grob, 1983). A primary reason for longer stays was the greater impairment of the patient population as local communities relieved themselves of their most chronically ill residents by committing them to the state hospital. The patient mix included more people with little hope of recovery, including the elderly and those with late stage syphilis. In time, professionals and the public alike came to see the hospitals as long-term custodial settings, rather than acute care facilities. In some hospitals, it was common practice for staff to take monthly collections toward the patients' burial costs (Sclafani, 1993).

Despite professional attitudes, families visited their relatives in increasingly overcrowded and understaffed settings. One hospital held 1,400 patients in facilities designed for only 900 (Grob, 1983). The Association for Medical Superintendents, which had adopted a position that established a maximum census of 250 patients for its hospitals, rapidly had to abandon this principle as some hospitals expanded to anywhere from 600 to several thousand residents (Deutsch, 1949). The difficulties of attracting sufficient custodial staff at low wages led to severe shortages (Deutsch, 1949).

Contributing to the growing sense of hopelessness were prevailing theories, which emphasized the importance of cultural and racial inheritance in the predisposition to mental illnesses. These theories stigmatized families at a time when state hospitals were increasingly made up of new immigrants, African-Americans, and the urban poor, weakening relationships between the largely white, middle-class professional staff and the patient and family (Sicherman, 1967).

By the turn of the century, the professional's expertise concerning mental illnesses was assumed and family compliance with increasingly invasive somatic treatments a given (Stern, 1942). Hospital psychiatrists, claiming scientific justification for their beliefs that mental illnesses resulted from lesions or infections that affected brain function, treated these disorders surgically. Dr. Henry Cotton, the superintendent of Trenton Psychiatric Hospital in New Jersey, performed a range of "corrective" procedures, including appendectomies, tonsillectomies, tooth extractions, hysterectomies, colectomies (removal of the colon), and oophorectomies (removal of the ovaries), with fatalities hovering at 30-40 percent (Timlen, forthcoming). So powerful was Cotton's authority as a physician that he could laconically note, after a woman who had been the recipient of several of his oral and abdominal surgeries succumbed to peritonitis, that her family expressed no complaints regarding her treatment (Timlen, forthcoming). In the absence of a public scandal or investigation, few professionals sought the family's opinions regarding treatment and families probably felt increasingly inadequate to venture an opinion.

The Community

Outside the hospital, however, there continued to be great optimism regarding outcomes from mental health treatment. Environmental theories developed by neurologists and mental hygienists practicing in the community emphasized the importance of the total environment in the breakdown of normal defenses which brought about mental illnesses. The preventive approach of Adolf Meyer and William Alanson White, among later environmentalists, promoted mental health and hygiene through the inculcation by parents and teachers of good character and habits. Personal moderation, self-discipline, and strength of character were pronounced the best prophylactics (Sicherman, 1967). Lay professionals were also expected to promote mental hygiene. Social work, especially, was championed as a means of assessing the family as an aftercare environment (Sicherman, 1967). Professionals became the arbiters of and educators in good parenting skills. Although the literature does not indicate that families were blamed for causing mental illnesses, the fact that they were accountable for prevention during childhood and that their family environment was being assessed, conveyed the implicit message that an illness signaled a failure in parenting, and made it more difficult to publicly acknowledge their problems and seek help. Later family systems theories made this implicit message, explicit, by looking at all mental illnesses as symptomatic of family dysfunction.

DEINSTITUTIONALIZATION

Deinstitutionalization dramatically altered family relationships with mental health professionals. The term denotes the pattern from the 1950's on of eschewing "traditional, institutional settings, particularly state hospitals, for persons with chronic mental disabilities; and the concurrent development and expansion of community based facilities for the care of this population" (Bachrach and Lamb, 1983:142). Deinstitutionalization became possible with the introduction of major neuroleptic medications that greatly reduced behaviors that were difficult to manage in the community.

Deinstitutionalization's most immediate impact was to diversify the locus of care and treatment, giving families more direct responsibility for care and case management, and indirect treatment responsibility in managing the ill relative at home. In 1955, 77 percent of the 1,675,352 episodes of care were in hospitals (Grob, 1991). By 1988, however, most admissions were to outpatient mental health services (3,073,735 episodes or 60.4%) (CMHS and NIMH, 1992). The population in public psychiatric hospitals declined by more than 70 percent (Borus, 1981).

The types of hospital and community settings had also become more varied. By 1988, most inpatient admissions were to general hospitals, with substantial growth in admissions to private and VA hospitals as well (CMHS and NIMH, 1992). Community care included a range of treatments such as day hospitalization, outpatient counseling approaches, medication monitoring and residential services.

The trend away from state hospitals had been building over several decades. The physical plants of state hospitals had deteriorated during the depression and war years, and the lack of funds for new construction and rehabilitation had contributed to overcrowding. The war siphoned off actual and potential staff into the military and higher-paying war-related industries (Grob, 1991). This multi-faceted erosion in hospital resources had an impact on the public image of the asylum.

While hospitals lost prestige, community care gained credibility in treating the mentally ill. During World War II, psychiatrists discovered that stress could precipitate breakdowns in even well-trained and carefully screened soldiers, and that recovery was swifter and more complete the closer the treatment setting was to the individual's combat unit. When translated to peacetime, these findings seemed to confirm the efficacy of community treatment (Grob, 1991).

Not only had hospital resident populations declined, but patients in the hospitals had briefer stays. Some individuals, particularly the more seriously mentally ill, flowed from the hospital to the community and back again. The hospital's "revolving door" was especially hard on families, which were getting their relatives back with greater symptomatology and little preparation and information, only to see them decompensate and return to the hospital again.

Although families were heartened by the introduction of psychopharmacological therapies, beginning with Thorazine's appearance in the 1950's, they were not prepared for the impact of managing their ill relative at home. Few public officials or professionals adequately anticipated the ongoing need for rehabilitation and aftercare services in the community. The Community Mental Health Centers Act of 1963 held out the promise of support for relatives in the commmunity. In reality, few centers were created. By 1989, when 2,400 centers were expected to be in operation, only 768 had been built (Grob, 1991). While federal initiatives failed to provide significant funding for community services through the Community Centers Act or the Alcohol, Drug Abuse and Mental Health Administration's (ADAMHA) block grants to states, the availability of federal Medicaid and Medicare funding for the care of indigents and the elderly in the community initially provided incentives for states to shift costs by discharging patients into fragmented and underfunded community options, particularly nursing homes (Mechanic and Rochefort, 1992). Most discharges ultimately ended up at home.

Effects on Families

The contradiction between the promise and the reality of deinstitutionalization was felt intensely by the families who had to fill the gaps in care and treatment. "Family burden" has come to describe an extensive literature on the felt experience of families in coping with the acute and long-term responsibilities associated with an inadequate system of community care and treatment (Grad and Sainsbury, 1963; Hoenig and Hamilton, 1966; Kreisman and Joy, 1974; Hatfield, 1978; Thompson and Doll, 1982; Lefley, 1987a). Burdens included specific behaviors disruptive to daily family living, such as a relative being active in the home late at night or failing to eat regularly and wear appropriate clothing. Burden was experienced as worry and a sense of loss, as well as tangible costs in savings spent, time lost, and social isolation. It was further affected by the family life cycle, particularly caregiver aging (Lefley, 1987a; Marsh, 1992); by peer influences on young adults with serious mental illnesses, e.g., alcohol and drugs (Pepper, Kirshner, and Ryglewicz, 1981); and by cultural perspectives on the illness (Lefley, 1987b).

Deinstitutionalization contributed to these burdens by inappropriately separating care from treatment. Mental health professionals claimed exclusive authority concerning treatment, but did not provide continuity in the caregiving setting. Many residential treatment options which might have provided alternatives for families and their ill relatives, e.g., foster care and supervised residences, were inadequate to meet the need and only accommodated a minority of the mentally ill (Grob, 1991). As a result, families became the de facto caregivers for their relatives with mental illnesses. Fully two-thirds of those discharged from hospitals, returned to their families, primarily families of origin (Goldman, 1982; Minkoff, 1978; Talbott, 1978).

Families were additionally burdened by clinical theories which stigmatized them. Many community professionals were trained in an etiology that blamed families for the illnesses (Beels and McFarlane, 1982; Hatfield, 1987a; Lefley, 1989). Psychoanalysis had always looked to early childhood development in its explanations for emotional disturbance.

In the postwar era, theories of psychotherapy began to emphasize intrapsychic, rather than interpersonal theories of the etiology of even the serious mental illnesses. In the late 1950's and early sixties, a group of family therapists began to focus on the whole family as the treatment unit. Taking their cue from group therapy, these therapists viewed the family as a natural group with an observable structure and rules governing the conduct of individual members. In their view, schizophrenia was an "adaptation" to dysfunctions in the parents. Although family theory claimed to avoid issues of etiology, this focus on the whole family as the treatment unit led to considerable blaming of parents for a child's illness.

Under the auspices of these new radical environmental approaches to family therapy, the very fabric of family life and structure was scrutinized for deviations from normative patterns. Role theories assumed that the conventional nuclear family, with a balance and clear role differentiation between the father and mother, was the only healthy pattern. Variations were identified as causes of schizophrenia. Lidz and his co-workers spoke of "marital schism" in which the mother undercut the father and both sought to elicit support from their daughter(s), thus violating generational norms and producing schizophrenia in daughters, and "marital skew," which was characterized by a dominant mother and passive father, departing from gender expectations of paternal authority and presumably affecting the mental health of sons (Lidz et al., 1957; Mishler and Waxler, 1965).

Other therapists focused on patterns of family communication, looking for contradictory messages or rules, such as parents requesting that the child exercise more independent initiative, but expressing anger when the child does so without consulting them. Illness emerged as the child sought a solution for the "double bind" that would simultaneously preserve the child's good standing in the family and the family's structural integrity. Bateson emphasized the significance of the mother-child dyad in producing the double bind (Bateson et al., 1956). Haley, Bowen, Palazzoli and others elaborated these theories to include a larger number of family members and more complex subsystems (Haley et al., 1962; Bowen, 1966; Palazzoli et al., 1978).

Radical environmental approaches to family therapy had a powerful and unfortunate impact. Stigmatizing families and adding the burden of guilt to family members' efforts to cope with the impact of mental illnesses in their lives, environmentally oriented therapies offered little practical assistance. As a result, such approaches increased the schism between families and professionals as families perceived therapy as adding to, rather than reducing, their burdens.

A final source of burden came from an activist legal profession which, in securing patient rights, also affected the family's ability to cope. Profoundly affecting family caregivers were legal decisions which gave patients the right to refuse treatment, which made dangerousness, rather than need for treatment the criterion for commitment, and which advocated for strict confidentiality of information and records. In interviews with family members, Tessler et al. (Tessler, et al., 1987) found numerous instances in which the ill relative was acting out in ways that to the family signaled potential danger or imminent decompensation, and yet the only resource available to deal with the situation was not mental health professionals, but the police. Families have an obligation to be alert to adverse medication effects and assist in medication monitoring, but psychiatrists and other professionals were often unwilling to communicate with the family about the medication the relative was taking (Zipple et al., 1990).

POST-DEINSTITUTIONALIZATION: THE EMERGENCE OF NEW MODELS

Recent models for family and professional relationships offer alternatives to early approaches to family therapy and attempt to breach the schism of distrust which grew during the postwar and deinstitutionalization periods. An example of the dramatic shift in perceptions can be found in Bernheim and Lehman's *Working with Families of the Mentally Ill* (Bernheim and Lehman, 1985: dust jacket), which offers "practical advice for integrating educational, behavioral and supportive techniques to assist families in helping ill relatives as well as themselves." Such words reveal much about a radical change in clinical perspective, which underscores the role of families in the care of their ill relative; acknowledges the burdens that mental illness places on families, who have to balance their own needs with those of their ill relatives; and redefines the role of the professional as offering concrete help and consultation to empower families to help themselves. Especially noticeable in how Bernheim and Lehman's book is summarized is the absence of the word "therapy."

Up until the late 1970's, families endured the burdens of care and blame, alone and in silence. It was natural, with other self-help groups forming, that families of people with mental illnesses would discover one another (Hatfield, 1981) and modify their relationships with mental health professionals and their ill relatives. While there were other self-help organizations prior to the 1980's, the formation of the National Alliance for the Mentally Ill (NAMI) in 1979 marked the beginning of a national movement (Hatfield, 1987b; McLean, 1990). At its inception, when several local self-help groups came together in Madison, Wisconsin, the organization had 284 members. By early 1989, membership had grown to over 65,000 (McLean, 1990), and currently stands at 140,000 with 1,000 state and local affiliates (NAMI, 1993).

NAMI was unified around several guiding principles (Hatfield, 1987). Partially as a consequence of the sometimes dramatic benefits obtained with neuroleptic medications and proliferating biological and genetic research findings, the organization became committed to the disease model of the mental illnesses and opposed to the radical environmental theories that had been inappropriately applied to schizophrenia and the affective disorders (Hatfield, 1987b; Johnson, 1989). More recently, the organization's efforts have improved funding for medical research and provided a forum in which families can keep abreast of current developments in pharmacological therapies and brain research.

Another organizational principle is that the best help is self-help, an implicit criticism of professionalism generally (Hatfield, 1987b). Not only is NAMI an advocacy organization, but most of its local affiliates sponsor groups in which families can meet, exchange information about mental health and generic services and discuss personal experiences, receiving support, concrete assistance, and feedback. If professionals are involved, it is only by invitation and usually to provide expert information. In contrast to many family therapies which produced anxiety in families or seemed irrelevant to their needs, self-help groups imparted useful information and inspired greater confidence in the ability of families to cope (Holden and Lewine, 1982; Terkelsen, 1983; Drake and Sederer, 1986; Grunebaum and Friedman, 1988).

Family experiences of mental illness and the mental health services system have become valid topics of inquiry, largely in response to the heightened awareness brought about by family advocates. Radical environmental theories ascribing etiology of mental illnesses to family dysfunction were increasingly discredited as lacking empirical support and conveying contradictory messages regarding family competency (Goldstein and Rodnick, 1975; Hirsch and Leff, 1975; Beels and McFarlane, 1982; Terkelsen and Cole, 1984; Marsh, 1992). Most mental health services were shown to have minimal value to families (Hatfield, 1978; Holden and Lewine, 1982; Johnson, 1990; Grella and Grusky, 1988; Spaniol and Zipple, 1988; Hanson and Rapp, 1992), and studies found little relationship between a family's priorities and the focus of its family therapy (Hatfield, 1979). Despite the widespread evidence for family dissatisfaction, comparisons of family and professional attitudes indicated that professionals viewed families as more satisfied than they really were (Spaniol et al., 1987). While one study showed that professionals are taking a more positive view of families, with 85 percent identifying families as allies in the treatment process, progress among professional disciplines has been uneven (Bernheim and Switalski, 1988). Even when families were satisfied with the quality of the treatment their ill relative had received, the families' burdens did not diminish (Test and Stein, 1980; Reynolds and Hoult, 1984). Clearly something else was needed from the professional community to address the expressed needs of families (Goldstein, 1981).

Surveys to determine what families wanted from mental health professionals came to similar conclusions (Hatfield, 1979; Holden and Lewine, 1982; Hanson and Rapp, 1992; Herman, 1992). Families wanted: better residential options for their ill members; to be appropriately involved in treatment decisions; information about mental illnesses, including diagnosis, symptoms and treatment options; an understanding of medications and their side effects; concrete suggestions on how to manage troublesome behaviors; interactions with people who had had similar experiences; understanding and support from friends, relatives and professionals; help during crisis situations and long-term in the form of respite, financial assistance and future planning.

Concerns have been raised that surveys of family attitudes and beliefs were conducted primarily of NAMI members, who are largely white, educated, older, middle-class parents of schizophrenics (Bernheim and Lehman, 1985; Johnson, 1987). NAMI membership is not the issue. A few surveys of predominantly white, non-NAMI families show similar hierarchies of need (Reinhard, 1990; Gubman, Minsky and Schorske, 1991). However, the scant research describing how minority families view and cope with mental illnesses indicated sufficient differences in perceived burden, satisfaction with mental health services and concept of the ill member's problem to warrant caution in generalizing from non-representative surveys to all families and cultural groups (Lefley, 1987b; Lefley, 1990; Guarnaccia and Parra, 1991).

The response of the professional community to the obvious need to lend assistance to families developed partly from the growing body of research on schizophrenia and affective disorders. This research validated bioneurological theories on the constitutional vulnerability of some people to develop these illnesses, and demonstrated that relapse rates for schizophrenia were, in conjunction with medication, amenable to environmental manipulation (Brown et al., 1972; Vaughn and Leff, 1976; Goldberg et al., 1977; Bernheim and Lewine, 1979; Heinrichs and Carpenter, 1983; Marsh, 1992). These new environmental approaches rejected earlier ones which identified pathological patterns in family structure and communication as causes of mental illness. Advocates of these diathesis-stress theories accepted the notion of a biological vulnerability to stress in people with mental illnesses and looked at ways the environment could be altered to reduce crises.

Diathesis-stress theories (Brown et al., 1972; Zubin and Spring, 1977; Leff and Vaughn, 1981) suggested that families could learn new ways of communicating with their ill relatives that were low in expressed emotional involvement and conveyed thoughts one at a time and clearly. These theories were based on research which compared the frequency of critical comments and those indicating emotional overinvolvement among families with relatives diagnosed with schizophrenia. This research, consistently showed that relapse rates were 50-60% among ill relatives who had families high in expressed emotion and 9-17% among those living with families low in expressed emotion (Brown et al., 1972; Goldstein and Doane, 1982; Vaughn et al., 1984).

Diathesis-stress studies also looked at the level of environmental stimulation and its relation to relapse rates and symptomatology (Wing and Brown; 1970; Bernheim and Lewine, 1979; Heinrichs and Carpenter, 1983). Overstimulation, such as a highly active social life at home, was associated with higher rates of relapse, while understimulation, such as watching television all day, was associated with an exacerbation of negative symptoms, e.g., lack of motivation, poor self care, and social withdrawal. It was inferred from this research that persons who live with and care for people with mental illnesses should adapt their communication patterns to be simple and respectful of interpersonal distance, and provide environments which are moderately stimulating and highly structured.

Psychoeducation Approaches

Psychoeducational programs were initially designed to educate families about schizophrenia and help them manipulate their environment and alter normal communication patterns to minimize symptomatology and risk of relapse. These programs achieved these objectives by forging alliances between professionals and families in which mental health practitioners became consultants to the family and, in turn, families became extensions of the mental health profession providing specific information about ill relatives, e.g., signs of progress or decompensation and evidence of medication compliance.

The first psychoeducational approaches (Ryglewicz, 1984) varied in professional involvement, duration, group membership and specific program objectives. Some programs were focused on brief crisis intervention. For example, Goldstein and Kopeikin's program (Goldstein and Kopeikin, 1981) consisted of six sessions in which the goals were to identify key precipitants to psychotic episodes and develop effective strategies to deal with them. Other approaches were more long-term. Berkowitz, Kuipers, Eberlein-Fries and Leff (Berkowitz et al., 1981) used a three-part intervention that included ongoing bimonthly family groups. The intervention goals were to reduce patient-family contact, lower expressed emotion, focus communication, and provide encouragement, information and support to families. Falloon, Boyd, McGill, Strang and Moss (Falloon et al., 1981) implemented a home-based approach with weekly sessions for the first three months, biweekly sessions for the next six months, and monthly meetings thereafter for an additional fifteen months. Objectives were to use behavioral, educational and supportive strategies to improve family communication and problem-solving skills. Some programs included the ill relative, while others did not. A four phase program in survival skills developed by Anderson, Hogarty and Reiss (Anderson et al., 1980) offered individual family sessions without the patient soon after a hospitalization or psychotic episode, followed by family sessions with the relative continuing for six months to a year.

Although models varied significantly, psychoeducational programs generally shared the following treatment goals and objectives: support for the family and grief counseling; emphasis on medication compliance; information about the illness; positive and negative symptom management; reduction of relapse or rehospitalization; crisis intervention; stress reduction; adjustment of family expectations; clarification of the role of the mental health system; increased networks of social support; and strategies for the future (McGill and Lee, 1986). The combination of educational, supportive, and behavioral techniques had a positive impact on patient relapse in all program approaches.

Limitations of early diathesis-stress models of family psychoeducation have been noted by Hatfield and others (Hatfield et al., 1987c; Marsh, 1992). Criticisms include the models' exclusive focus on the ill relative and insufficient consideration of family outcomes. It has also been pointed out that new environmental approaches place an added burden on families to change their normal patterns of communication and household activity. Labeling families as "high" in expressed emotion may lead to negative or stigmatizing views of the family, and interfere with recognizing family competency in adapting and coping with serious mental illnesses (Hatfield et al., 1987c; Marsh, 1992).

Psychoeducation programs also tend to be costly, because of numerous single-family sessions. As a result, William McFarlane and his colleagues at the New York State Psychiatric Institute (McFarlane, 1990) questioned the feasibility of replicating these models within the public sector. They piloted several multi-family group approaches, and with the support of the New York State Office of Mental Health and the State Alliance for the Mentally Ill, began a comparison of multi-family and single-family psychoeducation (McFarlane et al., 1993). More extensive information on McFarlane's work is found in Chapter 10 of this book.

Other Support Programs

Other supportive approaches were developed that looked at both client and family outcomes. "Supportive family counseling" (Bernheim, 1982) included the tasks of counseling families on creating low stress environments to minimize relapse, but went further in addressing the family's concrete needs and burden. Professionals aligned themselves with family members and through support and information empowered families to make informed decisions, successfully negotiate the mental health system, and balance responsibilities to the ill relative with their individual needs.

Recently, family support programs are being offered as part of the public mental health system. Studies indicate that families may benefit from a menu of service and setting options from which to choose, including agency and home-based consultation, psychoeducation, support groups, respite care, and referral and linkage. In New Jersey's public mental health system, multiple service use showed greater reductions in family burden and improved satisfaction with mental health services than use of any one service alone (Gubman et al., 1991). These recent studies are also unique in emphasizing family outcomes as well as showing dramatic benefits for ill relatives, including reductions in crisis service use and hospitalizations (Gubman et al., 1991; Reinhard et al., 1992; Reinhard, forthcoming). Within the family, members have unique needs in relating to professionals. In one study, spouses and children preferred agency-based professional contacts, while parents preferred that professionals come to the home (Gubman, Minsky and Schorske, 1991). Another study (Horwitz, 1993) has suggested that siblings also have unique needs in relating to professionals.

With their growing expertise, families are now developing new models for family education and support. NAMI, with 32 family education specialists in 29 states (Hatfield, 1993), has developed an educational curriculum intended for peer or professional leadership. Groups meet for a specified duration, cover topics of demonstrated importance to families (e.g., medication, how to assist in recovery), allow the exchange of ideas, and provide support and individual feedback (Hatfield, 1991). Group discussions include concerns the family may want to raise with mental health professionals, such as the sharing of non-confidential information or the availability of professional help in a crisis situation.

The Journey of Hope program, which has been implemented in 15 states, is a family-to-family model that combines education with support, offering a twelve week in-depth curriculum presented by a two-person family team (Burland, 1992) and ongoing family support groups based on principles of self-acceptance and acceptance of the illness (L'AMI-Baton Rouge, LA, 1993). The model provides linkages between education and advocacy, and for an over-burdened mental health system, offers a model for collaboration which establishes family expertise and addresses many of their expressed needs.

In addition to answering many of their own educational and support needs, families are also becoming important resources for quality improvement within the mental health system. In some states, they are participating in state hospital review processes (Reiter and Plotkin, 1985). In New Jersey, they are participating in site reviews of community fee-for-service programs. At the federal level, mental health block grant distributions to the states now require family involvement in oversight and planning (P.L. 99-660, 1987; P.L. 100-690, 1988). Many family organizations are engaged in service development and operation, particularly in the area of housing resources, long considered inadequate by families (Grosser and Vine, 1991). Families are also developing Planned Lifetime Assistance Networks to coordinate services and provide continuity and social support for their ill relatives after they are gone. Thus, the past few years have seen considerable diversification in the ways that families can collaborate with professionals.

CONCLUSION

Families are becoming full partners in their interactions with mental health professionals. This new role marks a dramatic advance from the universal family stigmatization of only a few decades ago. The family-professional relationship is still dynamic, occurring in a new context of family competency rather than pathology (Marsh, 1992) and affected by a changing mental health system, which recognizes the need for systems coordination even as its direction is increasingly shaped by cost considerations.

The past decades have also seen enormous changes in the nature and meaning of family caregiving. Families are becoming ever smaller and more mobile, with more varied composition, and a greater likelihood that the traditional caregivers, women, will be in the labor force rather than at home. The impact of these changes have yet to be studied.

Leaving aside the social policy question of whether or not it is appropriate for families to bear so much of the responsibility of primary care, the family today has many more professional resources at its disposal than its Puritan ancestors. Family care as it has evolved has been able to benefit from heightened advocacy, psychopharmacologic advances and a broadened etiologic view that encompasses biological and environmental factors. For their part, professional interventions which acknowledge and are responsive to family needs promise new effectiveness.

REFERENCES

Anderson, C.M. Hogarty, G.E. and Reiss, D.J. "Family treatment of adult schizophrenic patients: A psycho-educational approach." *Schizophrenia Bulletin.* 6:490-505, 1980.

Atwood, N. and Williams, M.E.D. "Group support for the families of the mentally ill." *Schizophrenia Bulletin.* 4:415-426, 1978.

Bachrach, L.L. and Lamb, H.R. "Conceptual issues in the evaluation of the deinstitutionalization movement." *Innovative Approaches to Mental Health Evaluation.* Edited by G.J. Stahler and W.R. Tash. New York: Academic Press, 1983.

Bateson, G. Jackson, D., Haley, J., and Weakland, J. "Toward a theory of schizophrenia." *Behavioral Science* 1:251-264, 1956.

Beels, C. and McFarlane, W. "Family treatments of schizophrenia: Background and state of the art." *Hospital and Community Psychiatry.* 33:541-550, 1982.

Berkowitz, R., Kuipers, E., Eberlein-Vries, R. and Leff, J. "Lowering expressed emotion in relatives of schizophrenics." *New Developments in Interventions with Families of Schizophrenics.* Edited by M.J. Goldstein. San Francisco: Jossey-Bass, 1981.

Bernheim, K.F. "Principles of professional and family collaboration." *Hospital and Community Psychiatry.* 41:1353-1355, 1990.

Bernheim, K.F. and Lehman, A.F. *Working with Families of the Mentally Ill.* New York: Norton, 1985.

Bernheim, K.F. and Lewine, R.R.J. *Schizophrenia: Symptoms, Causes, Treatments.* New York: W.W. Norton & Company, 1979.

Bernheim, K.F. and Switalski, T. "Mental health staff and patient's relatives: How they view each other." *Hospital and Community Psychiatry.* 39:63-68, 1988.

Borus, J.F. "Deinstitutionalization of the chronically mentally ill." *New England Journal of Medicine.* 305:330-342, 1981.

Bowen, M. "The use of family theory in clinical practice." *Comprehensive Psychiatry.* 7:345-374, 1966.

Brown, G.W., Birley, J.L.T., and Wing, J.K. "Influence of family life on the course of schizophrenic disorders." *British Journal of Psychiatry.* 121:241-258, 1972.

Burland, J. *AMI-VT Family Education Course.* Brattleboro, VT: AMI-VT, 1992.

Center for Mental Health Services and National Institute of Mental Health. *Mental Health, United States, 1992*. Edited by R.W. Manderscheid and Sonnenschein, M.A. DHHS Pub. No. (SMA) 92-1942. Washington, D.C. Supt. of Docs., U.S. Government Printing Off., 1992.

Demos, J. *A Little Commonwealth: Family Life in Plymouth Colony*. London: Oxford University Press, 1970.

Deutsch, A. *The Mentally Ill in America: A History of their Care and Treatment from Colonial Times*. Second edition. New York: Columbia University Press, 1949.

Drake, R.E. and Sederer, L.I. "The adverse effects of intensive treatment of chronic schizophrenia." *Comprehensive Psychiatry*. 27:313-326, 1986.

Falloon, I.R.H., Boyd, J.L. and McGill, C.W. *Family Care of Schizophrenia*. New York: The Guilford Press, 1984.

Falloon, I.R.H. Boyd, J.L., McGill, C.W., Strang, J.S. and Moss, H.B. "Family management training in the community care of schizophrenia." *New Developments in Interventions with Families of Schizophrenics*. Edited by M.J. Goldstein. San Francisco: Jossey-Bass, 1981.

Goldberg, S.C., Schooler, N.R., Hogarty, G.E., and Roper, M. "Prediction of relapse in schizophrenic outpatients treated by drug and social therapy." *Archives of General Psychiatry*. 34: 171-184, 1977.

Goldman H. "Mental illness and family burden: A public health perspective." *Hospital and Community Psychiatry*. 33:557-560, 1982.

Goldstein, E.G. "Promoting competence in families of psychiatric patients." *Promoting Competence in Clients: A Newfold Approach to Social Work Practice*. Edited by A.N. Maluccio. New York: The Free Press, 1981.

Goldstein, M.J. and Doane, J.A. "Family factors in the onset, course, and treatment of schizophrenic spectrum disorders." *Journal of Nervous and Mental Disease*. 170:692-700. 1982.

Goldstein, M.J. and Kopeikin, H.S. "Short- and long-term effects of combining drug and family therapy." *New Developments in Interventions with Families of Schizophrenics*. Edited by M.J. Goldstein. San Francisco: Jossey-Bass, 1981.

Goldstein, M.J. and Rodnick, E.H. "The family's contribution to the etiology of schizophrenia: Current status." *Schizophrenia Bulletin*. 14:48-63, 1975.

Grad, J. and Sainsbury, P. "Mental illness in the family." *Lancet*. 1:544-547, 1963.

Grella, C.E. and Grusky, O. "Families of the seriously mentally ill and their satisfaction with services." *Hospital and Community Psychiatry.* 40:831-835, 1989.

Grob, G.N. *Mental Illness and American Society: 1875-1940.* Princeton, NJ: Princeton University Press, 1983.

Grob, G.N. *From Asylum to Community: Mental Health Policy in Modern America.* Princeton, NJ: Princeton University Press, 1991.

Grosser, R.C. and Vine, P. "Families as advocates for the mentally ill: A survey of characteristics and service needs." *American Journal of Orthopsychiatry.* 61:282-290, 1991.

Grunebaum, H. and Friedman, H. "Building collaborative relationships with families of the mentally ill." *Hospital and Community Psychiatry.* 39:1183-1187, 1988.

Guarnaccia, P. and Parra, P. The Impact of Minority Status on Family and Agency Interaction in the Care of the Seriously Mentally Ill. Unpublished manuscript. Institute for Health, Health Care Policy and Aging Research. Rutgers University, New Brunswick, NJ., 1991.

Gubman, G., Minsky, S. and Schorske, B. "Intensive family support services: A cooperative evaluation." *Bureau of Research & Evaluation Report.* New Jersey Division of Mental Health and Hospitals, 1991.

Haley, J. "Family experiments: A new type of experimentation." *Family Process.* 1: 265-293, 1962.

Hanson, J.G. and Rapp, C.A. "Families' perceptions of community mental health programs for their relatives with a severe mental illness." *Community Mental Health Journal.* 28:181-196, 1992.

Hatfield, A.B. "Psychological costs of schizophrenia to the family." *Social Work.* 23:355-359, 1978.

Hatfield, A.B. "The family as partner in the treatment of mental illness." *Hospital and Community Psychiatry.* 30:338-340, 1979.

Hatfield, A.B. "Self-help groups for families of the mentally ill." *Social Work.* 26:408-413, 1981.

Hatfield, A.B. "Families as caregivers: A historical perspective." *Families of the Mentally Ill: Coping and Adaptation.* Edited by A.B. Hatfield and H.P. Lefley. New York: The Guilford Press, 1987a.

Hatfield, A.B. "The National Alliance for the Mentally Ill: The meaning of a movement." *Mental Health.* 15:79-93 1987b.

Hatfield, A.B., Spaniol, L. and Zipple, A.M. "Expressed emotion: A family perspective." *Schizophrenia Bulletin.* 13:221-226, 1987c.

Hatfield, A.B. *Coping with Mental Illness: A Family Guide.* NAMI Book No. 6. National Alliance for the Mentally Ill, 1991.

Hatfield, A.B. Family Education Specialist, NAMI. Personal communication, 1993.

Heinrichs, D.W. and Carpenter, W.J. "The coordination of family therapy with other treatment modalities for schizophrenia." *Family Therapy in Schizophrenia.* Edited by W.R. McFarlane. New York: The Guilford Press, 1983.

Herman, S. "Needs of people with mental illness: Consumer and family perspectives." *NASMHPD Research Institute, Inc. Second Annual Conference on State Mental Health Agency Services Research, 1991.* Alexandria, VA: NASMHPD Research Institute, Inc., 1992.

Hirsch, S.R. and Leff, J.P. *Abnormalities in Parents of Schizophrenics.* Maudsley Monographs No. 22. London: Oxford University Press, 1975.

Hoenig, J. and Hamilton, M.W. "The schizophrenia patient in the community and his effect on the household." *International Journal of Social Psychiatry.* 12:165-176, 1966.

Holden, D.F. and Lewine, R.R.J. "How families evaluate mental health professionals, resources, and effects of illness." *Schizophrenia Bulletin.* 8:626-633, 1982.

Horwitz, A.V. Siblings as caregivers for the seriously mentally ill." forthcoming in *The Milbank Quarterly,* 1993.

Johnson, D.L. "Schizophrenia as a brain disease: Implications for psychologists and families." *American Psychologist.* 44:553-555. 1989.

Johnson, D.L. "The family's experience of living with mental illness." *Families as Allies in Treatment of the Mentally Ill: New Directions for Mental Health Professionals.* Edited by H.P. Lefley and D.L. Johnson. Washington, D.C.: American Psychiatric Press, 1990.

Kraepelin, E. *Lectures on Clinical Psychiatry.* London: Balliere, 1904.

Kreisman, D.E. and Joy, V.D. "Family response to the mental illness of a relative: A review of the literature." *Schizophrenia Bulletin.* 10:34-54, 1974.

LA-AMI. *Journey of Hope: Family Education and Family Support.* Baton Rouge, LA: LA-AMI, 1993.

Leff, J. and Vaughn, C. "The role of maintenance therapy and relatives' expressed emotion in relapse of schizophrenia: A two-year follow-up." *British Journal of Psychiatry.* 139:102-104, 1981.

Lefley, H.P. "Aging parents as caregivers of mentally ill adult children: An emerging social problem." *Hospital and Community Psychiatry.* 38:1063-1070, 1987a.

Lefley, H.P. "Culture and mental illness: The family role." *Families of the Mentally Ill: Coping and Adaptation*. Edited by A.B. Hatfield and H.P. Lefley. New York: The Guilford Press, 1987b.

Lefley, H.P. "Family burden and family stigma in major mental illness." *American Psychologist*. 44:556-560, 1989.

Lefley, H.P. "Research directions for a new conceptualization of families." *Families as Allies in Treatment of the Mentally Ill*. Edited by H.P. Lefley and D.L. Johnson. Washington, D.C.: American Psychiatric Press, 1990.

Lidz, T., Cornelison, A., Fleck, S. and Terry, D. "The intrafamilial environment of schizophrenic patients: II. Marital schism and marital skew." *American Journal of Psychiatry*. 114:241-248, 1957.

Marsh, D.T. *Families and Mental Illness: New Directions in Professional Practice*. New York: Praeger, 1992.

McFarlane, W.R. "Multiple family groups and the treatment of schizophrenia." *Handbook of Schizophrenia, Volume 4: Psychosocial Treatment of Schizophrenia*. Edited by M.I. Herz, S.J. Keith, and J.P. Docherty. New York: Elsevier Science Publishers, 1990.

McFarlane, W.R. and Dunne, E. "Family psychoeducation and multifamily groups in the treatment of schizophrenia." *Directions in Psychiatry*. Vol. 11, Lesson 20, 1991.

McFarlane, W.R., Dunne, E., Lukens, E., McLaughlin-Toran, J., Deakins, S. and Horen, B. "From research to clinical practice: Dissemination of New York State's Family Psychoeducation Project." *Hospital and Community Psychiatry*. 44:265-270, 1993.

McGill, C. and Lee, E. "Family psychoeducational intervention in the treatment of schizophrenia. *Bulletin of the Menninger Clinic*. May:269-286, 1986.

McLean, A. "Contradictions in the social production of clinical knowledge: The case of schizophrenia." *Social Science Medicine*. 30:969-985, 1990.

Mechanic, D. and Rochefort, D.A. "Toward a policy of inclusion for the mentally ill." *Health Affairs*. 11:128-150, 1992.

Minkoff, K. "A map of the chronic mental patient." *The Chronic Mental Patient*. Edited by J.A. Talbott. Washington, D.C.: American Psychiatric Association, 1978.

Mishler, E.G. and Waxler, N.E. "Family interaction processes and schizophrenia: A review of current theories." *Merrill-Palmer Quarterly of Behavior and Development*. 11: 269-315, 1965.

Morgan, E.S. *The Puritan Family: Religion and Domestic Relations in Seventeenth Century New England*. New York: Harper & Row, Publishers, 1966.

Morrissey, J.P. and Goldman, H.H. "Cycles of reform in the care of the chronically mentally ill." *Hospital and Community Psychiatry*. 35:785-793, 1984.

NAMI Central Office. Personal communication, 1993.

National Institute of Mental Health. *Caring for P eople with Severe Mental Disorders: A National Plan of Research to Improve Services*. DHHS Pub. No. (ADM) 91-1762. Washington, D.C.: Supt. of Docs., U.S. Govt. Print. Off., 1991.

Neill, J. "Whatever became of the schizophrenogenic mother?" *American Journal of Psychotherapy*. 44:499-505, 1990.

Palazzoli, M.S., Boscolo, L., Checchin, G., and Prata, G. *Paradox and Counterparadox*. New York: Jason Aronson, 1978.

Pepper, B., Kirshner, M.C., and Ryglewicz, H. "The young adult chronic patient: Overview of a population." *Hospital and Community Psychiatry*. 32:463-469, 1981.

Public Law 99-660 (The Public Health Service Act), 1987.

Public Law 100-690 (Anti-Drug Abuse Act), 1988.

Reinhard, S. "Families and professionals: Help-seeking among families with seriously mentally ill members." Paper presented at the 40th Annual Meeting of the Society for the Study of Social Problems. Washington, D.C., 1990.

Reinhard, S.C. "Living with mental illness: Effects of professional support and personal control on caregiver burden." Forthcoming in *Research in Nursing & Health*.

Reinhard, S., Gubman, G., Horwitz, A.V. and Minsky, S. *Burden assessment scale for families of the seriously mentally ill*. Forthcoming in *Evaluation and Program Planning*.

Reiter, M. and Plotkin, A. "Family members as monitors in a state mental hospital." *Hospital and Community Psychiatry*. 36:393-395, 1985.

Reynolds, I. and Hoult, J.E. "The relatives of the mentally ill." *Journal of Nervous and Mental Disease*. 172:480-489, 1984.

Ryglewicz, H. "An agenda for family intervention: Issues, models, and practice." *Advances in Training the Young Adult Chronic Patient. New Directions for Mental Health Services, No. 21*. Edited by B. Pepper and H. Ryglewicz. San Francisco: Jossey-Bass, 1984.

Sclafani, M. Assistant Director, Office of Specialty Hospitals and Special Populations. New Jersey Division of Mental Health and Hospitals. Personal communication, 1993.

Sicherman, B. *The Quest for Mental Health in America: 1880-1917.* Ph.D. dissertation. Columbia University, 1967.

Spaniol, L., Jung, H., Zipple, A.M., and Fitzgerald, S. "Families as a resource in the rehabilitation of the severely psychiatrically disabled." *Families of the Mentally Ill: Coping and Adaptation.* Edited by A.B. Hatfield and H.P. Lefley. New York: The Guilford Press, 1987.

Spaniol, L. and Zipple, A.M. "Family and professional perceptions of family needs and coping strengths." *Rehabilitation Psychology.* 33:37-45, 1988.

Stern, E.M. *Mental Illness: A Guide for the Family.* New York: Harper & Row, Publishers, 1942.

Talbott, J. *The Death of the Asylum.* New York: Grune & Stratton, 1978.

Terkelsen, K.G. "Schizophrenia and the family: II. Adverse effects of family therapy." *Family Process.* 22:191-200, 1983.

Terkelsen, K.G. and Cole, S.A. "Methodological flaws in the schizophrenic hypothesis: Implications for psychiatric education." Unpublished manuscript cited in Bernheim, K.B. and Lehman, A.F. *Working with Families of the Mentally Ill.* New York: Norton, 1985.

Tessler, R.C., Killian, L.M., and Gubman, G.D. "Stages in family response to mental illness: An ideal type." *Psychosocial Rehabilitation Journal.* 10:3-16, 1987.

Test, M.A. and Stein, L.I. "Alternative to mental hospital treatment. III. Social cost." *Archives of General Psychiatry.* 37:409-412, 1980.

Thompson, E. and Doll, W. "The burden of families coping with the mentally ill: An invisible crisis." *Family Relations.* 31:379-388, 1982.

Timlen, W. Article on Dr. Henry A. Cotton. Forthcoming in *American Heritage.*

Vaughn, C.E. and Leff, J.P. "The influence of family and social factors on the course of psychiatric illness: A comparison of schizophrenic and depressed neurotic patients." *British Journal of Psychiatry.* 129:125-137, 1976.

Vaughn, C.E., Snyder, K.S., Jones, S., Freeman, W.B., and Falloon, I.R.H. "Family factors in schizophrenic relapse." *Archives of General Psychiatry.* 41:1169-1177, 1984.

Wing, J.K. and Brown, G.W. *Institutionalism and Schizophrenia.* London: Cambridge University Press, 1970.

Zipple, A.M., Langle, S., Spaniol, L., and Fisher, H. "Client confidentiality and the family's need to know: Strategies for resolving the conflict." *Community Mental Health Journal.* 26:533-545, 1990.

Zubin, J. and Spring, B. "Vulnerability: A new view of schizophrenia." *Journal of Abnormal Psychology.* 96:103-126, 1977.

Chapter 2

PROFESSIONAL AND PARENTAL PERSPECTIVES

Mona Wasow

> I cradled him close and rocked him, singing to him as if he were a small child, singing inside my fear as well as his, singing sweetness to the sour of his breath, singing softness to the sores on his body, singing love and life into his whole being, and willing, with all my heart, with all my mind and with all my strength that I would keep him safe from harm. But deep inside I already knew that I had failed.
>
> *Anne Deveson, 1991*

There is no winning in this battle with mental illness. A stalemate sometimes, or a little stability now and then, a flicker of hope, maybe even coming to terms with it—but you can't win. This may be the only statement I can make that seems to apply to all families, and at that, there are undoubtedly some exceptions.

"The Family Experience"—whose family? Are they the families of the deeply religious or the atheist; the rich or poor; the family with 8 children or 1 child; the highly educated or uneducated; people with high coping abilities or the dysfunctional family....? The list is infinite. I start with this cautionary note because obviously all of the above, and more, is going to make a big difference in the family experience. Also, whatever it is we do know about families is based on a biased sample of those family members who have been willing to talk. We do not know about the experiences of those who are still in the closet, of those we have not reached, and most certainly we know nothing about the families who, for whatever reasons, have dropped away from their ill members and no longer have any contact.

27

Now, to proceed with what we *do* know.

Catastrophe

McCubbin and Figley (1983:143) define catastrophic stress as "...sudden, unexpected, and frightening experiences that are often accompanied by a sense of helplessness, destruction, disruption, and loss." What distinguishes this loss from "normal" loss is: little time to prepare for it, no previous experience, no guidance, feeling isolated, remaining in crises for a long period of time, lack of control, disruption and destruction, and high emotional impact. By this description, serious mental illness (SMI) surely fits the definition of catastrophic stress. Additionally, because many families feel shame and stigma, they do not talk about mental illness, so we do not know the extent to which it exists in the world.

In all the research done on SMI and family stress there is one consistent finding; SMI is a catastrophic event for families (Marsh, 1992; Terkelsen, 1987). Terkelsen calls it a "disaster in which all are victims of the event and its sequelae." The reports from family members are equally consistent on this subject: "We parents of the mentally ill are a tongue-tied, self-castigating, silently grieving subculture" (Garson, 1987:10). Parents describe the frequent crises with emergency services, police, hospitals, jails, involuntary commitments that tear families apart, the terror of waiting for the next catastrophe, occasional flares of violence, and so on.

Lefley, both a researcher and family member adds another dimension to the picture when she points out: "Perhaps the most devastating stressor for families, however, is learning how to cope with the patient's own anguish over an impoverished life." (Lefley, 1989:557). So we have the phenomenon of catastrophe for the family, and an additional agony for the suffering and catastrophe families sense their relatives with severe mental illness feel.

Burdens

Family burdens are many, and fall into several categories. There are objective, practical burdens such as money, housing, finding reliable health care professionals, getting the legal and mental health systems to work and trying to hold a family together. These objective burdens are enormous, and will remain so as long as our systems of community care remains so inhumanely inadequate.

There are behavior management problems that never seem to get better. For reasons no one seems to entirely understand, many people with mental illness do not seem to learn from experience. You can ask someone to shower and change his clothes, and he may do it willingly. Chances are, however, that you will have to make this request anew every single time. Behavioral problems permeate all aspects of the lives of persons with mental illness. Hallucinations and delusions cause bizarre actions beyond our comprehension. Other problematic behaviors are mood swings, unpredictability, emotional and social withdrawal, sleep and appetite disturbances, poor hygiene, pacing, aggression, no motivation, and so on. The list is endless, almost entirely negative, and very hard to experience.

A recent sample of 1,401 NAMI members (1992:29) were asked what behaviors they found most problematic in their SMI relative. 79.40% listed difficulties in concentrating; 73.9% said impaired judgment; 60.1% said emotional withdrawal; 56% said verbal abuse; 32.7% embarrassing public behavior; and 17.9% listed alcohol and drug abuse. When you add to this the fact that 71% of this sample of SMI people had little or no activity beyond watching TV, smoking, and drinking coffee (46% absolutely no activity; 25% no activity "most of the time"), it is easy to understand why these behaviors are a burden for all concerned.

Then there are the nebulous burdens of grief, fear, and sadness, that have no resolution. These are the subjective burdens.

> "How can you adjust to seeing someone you love so crushed
> and destroyed? You never get over it. Death would be easier."
> *A parent, 1992.*

Although human beings have struggled with loss and grief from the dawn of history, interestingly enough it is only within the last fifty years or so that scientists have done any systematic research on grieving. This may be symptomatic of why our culture tends to handle grief poorly.

In the substantial research on psychological recovery there is a consistency to the finding of the importance of social supports. People that we are close to play a crucial role in our adaptation to loss and grief. When people have positive social support it helps them to feel cared for and validated and offers an avenue for expressing feelings. Unfortunately, the responses of our culture to people with serious mental illnesses are stigmatizing and hostile. As a result, social isolation often occurs.

Intense grief may go on for an average of two years. Varying forms of *chronic* grief and sorrow may go on forever. Unrealistic expectations about grieving add on to grief, burdens of feeling anxious, neurotic, afraid, and self-doubting. Those whom we have loved and those with whom we have unfinished business often remain with us forever in vivid ways. One of the most difficult aspects of grief involves the loss of potential, and this is one of the agonies of remembering what loved ones were like prior to their illness.

Cycles of exacerbation and remission, which are typical in mental illnesses, cause patterns of hope and despair in family members. During periods of remission, shades of the once well person may be seen, only to be followed by incomprehensible changes. "He was doing so well," a friend said, "We had fallen in love with him all over again." The following week he killed himself.

Adaptation

By what means, and how well or how poorly a family manages to survive living with SMI will of course, vary with every family. An important concept to keep in mind is that adaptation to SMI usually results in compromise, rather than success. To repeat the opening sentence of this chapter, "There is no winning in this battle"—battle, an interesting choice of words. What are some of the other adjectives often employed to describe the struggles surrounding SMI? We talk about "strategic retreats, delay, regrouping of forces, abandoning untenable positions, giving up, holding the line, winning the war with mental illness..." It does sound like combat, and it is.

The process of adaptation is never ending. Zipple and Spaniol (1987) identify four main stages in adaptation: 1. Denial, 2. Recognizing and labeling the illness, 3. On-going coping and adjusting, and 4. Advocacy. Not all families go through these stages. Some never move beyond denial, it may be a minority that reach advocacy, and many families wander back and forth in the process of adaptation. "Few parents reach an emotional promised land; most have good days and bad days." (Marsh, 1992:147)

Various researchers (Figley, MCubbin, Marsh, 1992; Lefley & Johnson, 1990, Zipple and Spaniol, 1987) have looked at the components that are found in families that cope well with SMI and seem to function comparatively well. They are characterized by an ability to identify their problems; to solve problems within the family; high tolerance and respect for each other; high levels of affection; clear communication; role flexibility; effective use of community resources; and a lack of substance abuse. It also helps to have adequate money, good health, and a lot of knowledge about serious mental illness.

A great deal will also depend on the family member with mental illness. The severity of their illness, their pre-illness relationships within the family, their personality, whether or not violence plays a role, and how they presently relate to individuals within the family—all of these factors play a role in adaptation. A friend complimented my eldest child about her consistent kindness to her ill brother. She responded "How could one be otherwise with him? He's so sweet and kind himself."

A word about resilience is appropriate. When catastrophic events pile up, one upon the other, with no rest and no solution, families can be exhausted and beaten into the ground. The end result can be the destruction of the family as a unit, as well as the individuals within. In contrast, when catastrophic events serve as catalysts for the emergence of strengthened lives, some families feel stronger. They have a positive response and take satisfaction in having survived. This is called resilience, and gets a lot of approval in our culture.

It is not only the mental illness that disintegrates families, nor even all the extraneous circumstances in which families find themselves. How much they know about the illnesses, whether or not they blame themselves, and the ways in which they react to the illness and to each other, all will play vital roles in adaptation.

Dickman and Gordon (1993, revised) have a chapter called "Part of Your Life, Not All of it. How Not to Become a Handicapped Family." They write about the "rights of parents," and list the rights to: cry, be angry, not ashamed, not guilty, to feel you're doing the best you can, to make your own decisions, to respect, to get help, to have and be a family, to go on living, to be human and only human, to laugh, and to believe in miracles. It is a sweet list, and one I agree with. I would also add: the right to feel unremittingly sad at times, and not believe in miracles.

Before leaving this topic, an interesting thought: to date there has been very little research on the possible positive aspects of family experiences in living with SMI. Research by Greenberg, Greenley, Benedict and Goldman (1993) indicated that some individuals with serious mental illness have provided practical help and companionship to their families. A great deal more exploration is needed in this important area.

Coping and Controllability

It is a particularly North American phenomenon to think that people should be able to manage negative feelings and be happy most of the time. Most cultures in this world accept the fact that life is often a struggle and our expectation that it should be otherwise probably compounds our troubles.

As an example of how this expectation that life should go smoothly makes things worse, look at what we know about the Christmas holidays in the U.S. The five weeks between Thanksgiving and New Year's has the highest rates in the entire year for suicide, depression, and general violence. There is a cultural belief that we should all be having a holiday season full of joy and love. Since this is not the norm for many, the discrepancy is enormous, and the resulting pain makes for increased violence and depression.

Along with the notion that life should be good if we just do things right (i.e., children will turn out fine if we raise them right), is the belief that we have control over our destiny. It is hard for us to accept the fact that "Bad things happen to good people." Avery Weisman, an elderly psychoanalyst, wrote an excellent book, *The Coping Capacity*, (1984). In it he emphasized the foolishness of leading people to believe that if they could "just get it all together," their lives would be smooth and happy. Life is full of unpredictable events entirely outside of our control: everything from earthquakes and hurricanes and getting hit by drunk drivers, to schizophrenia and holes in the ozone. We do *not* have control over much that happens in our lives, and therefore, says Weisman, our aim should be to increase our coping capacity, rather than a futile attempt to control that over which we have no control. This notion is quite applicable to coping with the stresses of mental illness in the family.

Having things outside of our control, forces people to face the existential crises of unpredictability and meaninglessness. Most of us have trouble dealing with the arbitrariness of bad luck. Human beings have struggled with this from times immemorial. We live in a "fix it" society, but strong feelings cannot be "fixed," as fixing a broken window pane.

After experiencing a shattering loss that cannot be fixed, like the death of a loved one, a mental illness, Chernobyl, etc., people learn just how vulnerable they are, and that they are capable of profound suffering. After that, the world never feels entirely safe again. It might be more helpful if we had a better understanding and acceptance of our lack of control. Then we could redirect our energy towards increasing our coping capacity.

Dealing with Shattered Beliefs

How do people come to grips with severe trauma or loss? Most people have a need to believe in a just world in which they get what they deserve, and are therefore deeply threatened by random, negative events. One of the ways we try to hold on to our basic assumptions, is to blame ourselves, i.e., if we had just raised our children right, this would not have happened. Such an attitude can be seen as neurotic and dysfunctional. But it can also be viewed as a healthy attempt to hang on to our beliefs about the world as a safe and predictable place. In other words, if we are to blame, then the world is a safe place, we just did not do it right.

In the mid 1970's Bulman and Wortman conducted a study on the reactions of paralyzed survivors of accidents and came up with a surprising finding: self-blame was associated with high levels of coping! This was the case even though the people who had been involved in freak accidents were not at fault. "Self-blame reflects the struggle of survivors to make sense of their victimization, to understand 'Why me?' and minimize the possibility of randomness in their world." (Bulman, 1992:125) Survivors of car accidents are not necessarily the same as survivors of losing a loved one to severe mental illness. But it is interesting to consider the possibility that, in both cases, self-blame can be seen as a way of maintaining equilibrium in the face of shattered beliefs about one's world.

People use a variety of strategies to cope with and rebuild shattered beliefs; to somehow integrate the old (the world is safe) and the new (tragedy can strike any time). One time honored method is to make appraisals based upon comparisons with others, particularly other victims. If misery loves company, it loves even more, miserable company! "It could have been worse..." Another strategy is to examine and interpret one"s role in the tragedy. Here most people run the gamut from "If only I had..." (self-blame), to a realization that mental illnesses are brain diseases that can and do strike anywhere, and therefore they play no role in the disease.

Many people cope by re-evaluating the experience in terms of benefits and purpose. Surely the mental illness serves no benefit to the sufferer, but many family members say things like: "This has made me a more tolerant person; or stronger, kinder, wiser..." As Bulman said (Bulman, 1992:118): "Survivors' reappraisals locate and create evidence of benevolence, meaning, and self-worth in the events that first challenged and shattered their illusions."

Victor Frankel made this point eloquently in 1946, when he survived the horrors of a Nazi Concentration camp.

> "We must never forget that we may also find meaning in life when confronted with a hopeless situation, when facing a fate that cannot be changed. [People have the ability to] ...transform a personal tragedy into a triumph, to turn one's predicament

into a human achievement."

(Frankel:135)

Avery Weisman also commented: "Our obligation to cope well enough to make survival significant is about all we can be sure about." (Weisman, 1984:157).

We cannot change the fact that mental illnesses exist. They do, and they are horrendous illnesses. Nothing is gained by denying their catastrophic effects on the family. On the other hand, nothing is gained by wallowing in the misery of it either. So what alternatives are left?

Exploring Other Cultures

There are other cultures and systems of thought that give quite different meanings to illness and suffering. Many cultures, for example, emphasize distancing oneself from pain; or believe strongly in acceptance and resignation. Less emphasis is placed on striving to fix things, or control one's destiny.

Just to give an example of this: Valles (Valles,1988) went on extensive retreats in India, with a spiritual leader, Anthony De Mello. He then wrote a book about *Mastering Sadhana*. Sadhana is a Sanskrit word meaning "Spirituality." In this book he emphasized:

> "Don't fret about things. Things are what they are, and life is what it is... If you rebel and protest, you are the loser. You are hitting your head against a wall, you are hurting yourself with the hard rock of reality. But if you understand and accept reality as it is, you get in tune with life, you enter the current, you ride the storm..."

We are carrying in our heads a model of reality that was developed by our traditions, training, and culture, and our individual families. This model, in some sense, is arbitrary—nowhere is it written in stone. Some of our upset then, comes from our inner conditioning that tells us that we must do something to alleviate the suffering and to make things better. DeMello (1988) exemplifies this notion by pointing out that a married man in India would be very upset if a guest in his house slept with his wife, but an Eskimo man might invite a guest to do so. The point to this example is that part of our upset comes not from outside causes (i.e., the mental illness of our loved one), but rather from inside—our brains that have been conditioned to view the mental illness as catastrophic. To paraphrase it in the words of Sadhana: "Nobody upsets you; you upset yourself."

Perhaps some families can change or modify that part of the conditioning that causes some of the pain. We may benefit from exploring the coping strategies used by eastern civilizations, different American Indian tribes...and so on. This is a big world we live in; *all* human beings have struggled with tragedy, and coping. There are many systems of thought other than the ones mentioned in this chapter. We need to broaden our coping repertoire to include meaning in our lives, even when events seem catastrophic.

Summary

When talking about "The Family Experience" it is important to acknowledge that we have only heard from a limited number of families. Even within our limited sample, there are so many variables that play a role: health, money, support systems, community care, age, religion, inborn characteristics, the degree of illness and personality of the person with mental illness, social class, race, size of family, cultural background—ad infinitum.

We need to know something about the families who no longer have contact with their ill relative; about families with great variety of different backgrounds; and we also do not know anything about families who are in contact with their ill relatives, but not with the people who are writing about them. Then there are families that are still in "the closet," and we do not know about them either.

On the positive side of family experiences there are also gaps in our knowledge. What about the families that get increased self-esteem from having survived, and from giving to their loved ones? We think that some families develop a philosophy of life that adds meaning to all that they do, and that living with severe mental illness has had something to do with that. We need to know more about the families that say their relative with severe mental illness has contributed to their lives.

Having reminded us of what we do not yet know, we can summarize what the families we have talked to have been saying. Living with SMI has catastrophic affects on them. The burdens are enormous, the process of adaptation is never ending, and the grieving both for oneself and for the ill relative is very intense.

Families of mentally ill people have not been singled out for suffering. Many families have members who are severely disabled in one way or another. We need to develop a philosophy of life that works for us and helps us to find meaning. People who can think flexibly and reshape ideas and feelings from multiple perspectives, have an advantage over people who are rigid in their thinking. We also need to increase our coping capacities just as much as we can. But paradoxically, it is equally as important to accept our human limitations.

It is very important to move on from: "If only I had..." and to accept the inevitability of sadness, anger, and grief, without inflicting upon ourselves the additional burden that we should not have negative feelings. Dealing with mental illness is a part of our lives, but we do not need to let it take over.

In order to come to terms with strong feelings, people need to find some balance between knowing the world is neither safe and predictable, nor entirely dangerous. Events that happen can still make sense, but not always; we are decent and competent people, but helplessness occurs too.

For the survivor who recovers from grief, trauma is sometimes seen as a potential source of strength and a personal sense of victory, if not over the event, at least over the self to have survived it. How often we hear people say with pride: "I survived!" Many people speak of a renewed appreciation of the good in life, after they know how bad things can be. Now they know what is important. Wisdom of maturity replaces the ignorance of naiveté. The survivor emerges somewhat sadder, but considerably wiser.

And in the end families hope for the best. This acknowledges real possibilities, both good and bad, of disasters and triumphs, in spite of our human limitations to control.

REFERENCES

Bick, B. "Love and Resentment" N.Y. Times Magazine, March 25, 1990, pp. 26-28.

Borden, W. (1992). "Narrative Perspectives in Psychosocial Intervention Following Adverse Life Events." *Social Work*, 3/92, Vol. 37, No. 2, pp. 135-141.

Bulman, R.J.., Wortman, C. (1992). *Shattered Assumptions*. The Free Press, N.Y., p. 125.

"Clinical Services Research," *Schiz. Bulletin*, Vol. 18, No. 4, 1992, p. 577.

Deveson, A. *Tell Me I'm Here*, Penguin Books, Australia, 1991, pp. 255-256.

Dickman, I. and Gordon, S. *One Miracle at a time*. A Fireside Book, Simon and Schuster, rev. 1993.

Figley, C.R., McCubbin, H.I. (Eds.) "Catastrophes: An Overview of Family Reactions" Stress and the Family, Vol. II, Coping With Catastrophe, N.Y., Brunner/Mazel, 1983, pp. 3-20.

Frankl, V. (1946). *Man's Search for Meaning.* Washington Squre Press, N.Y.

Garson, S. "The Sound and Fury of Mania" Newsweek, April 13, 1987, p. 10

Greenberg, Goldman, Greenley, and Benedict. "Contributions of Persons with Serious Mental Illness to Family Life." Unpublished paper, 1993.

Greenley, J., McKee, D., Stein, L., Griffin-Francell, C., Greenberg, J. (1989, Aug.). "Families Coping With Schizophrenia: Stress and Distress." Paper presented at the meeting of the society for the Study of Social Problems, Berkeley, CA.

Keillor, G. (1987). "Prairie Home Companion." Radio Show, St. Paul, Minnesota.

Lefley, H. P. "Families of the Mentally Ill in Cross-Cultural Perspective" *Psychosocial Rehabilitation Journal,* pp. 56-73. Vol. VIII, No. 4, April, 1985.

Lefley, H. P. "Family Burden and Family Stigma in Major Mental Illness" *American Psychologist,* March, 1989, Vol. 44, No. 3, pp. 556-560.

Lefley, H. P. "Aging Parents as Caregivers of Mentally Ill Adult Children; An emerging Social Problem" *H & CP,* Oct., 1987, Vol. 38, No. 10, pp. 1063-1070.

Lefley, Harriet, Ph.D. & Johnson, Dale, Ph.d., Eds. Families as Allies in Treatment of the Mentally Ill. *APA Press,* Inc. 1400 K. St., N.W. Washington, D.C. 20005. 1990.

Marsh, D. T. *Families and Mental Illness: New Directions in Professional Practice.* Praeger, 1992.

Skinner, E.A., Steinwachs, D.M., Kapwe, J.. "Family Perspectives on the Service Needs of People with Serious and Persistent Mental Illness; Part I: Characteristics of Families and Consumers" pp. 23-30 (1992), *Innovations and Research,* Vol. 3, 1992. Published by NAMI and The Center for Psychiatric Rehabilitation, Boston Univ., Boston.

Stears, A.K. (1984). *Living Through Personal Crises.* The Thomas More Press, Chicago, Illinois.

Valles, S. J. C. (1988) *Mastering Sadhana, On Retreat With Anthony DeMello.* Doubleday, Garden City, N. Y.

Weisman, A. (1984) *The Coping Capacity.* Human Sciences Press, Inc. N.Y.

Zipple, A.M., and Spaniol L., "Families that Include a Person With a Mental Illness: What They Need and How to Provide It." *Trainer*

Manual. Boston: Boston Univ. Center for Psychiatric Rehabilitation. 1987.

Chapter 3

SERVICES FOR FAMILIES: NEW MODES, MODELS, AND INTERVENTION STRATEGIES

Diane T. Marsh

The current era has witnessed significant change in theory, research, and practice concerned with families of people with serious mental illness. There are new modes of family-professional relationships, new models for professional practice with families, and new nonclinical and clinical intervention strategies for meeting their needs.

NEW MODES AND MODELS

The new modes of service delivery are essentially collaborative partnerships designed to build on the strengths and expertise of all parties; to respect the needs, desires, concerns, and priorities of families; to enable families to play an active role in decisions that affect them; and to establish mutual goals for treatment and rehabilitation. There is increasing recognition of the value of an institutional alliance with families that is designed to meet the meets of all family members (Grunebaum & Friedman, 1988), and of family-professional collaboration (e.g, Lefley & Johnson, 1990; Marsh, 1992a; Peternelj-Taylor & Hartley, 1993).

There are also new models of service delivery that emphasize the strengths, resources, and competencies of families, which have traditionally received little acknowledgement from professionals. Two such models will be discussed: a competence paradigm for professional practice and a coping and adaptation framework.

A Competence Paradigm

A competence paradigm for professional practice with families offers a constructive alternative to the pathology paradigm that has often guided clinical practice in the past. As indicated in Table 1, competence and pathology paradigms differ in many fundamental ways. In contrast to a pathology paradigm, for example, a competence paradigm offers a developmental model that views families as competent or potentially competent; that emphasizes their positive characteristics; that views

---

A Paradigm Shift in Professional Practice With Families

PATHOLOGY PARADIGM   COMPETENCE PARADIGM

NATURE OF PARADIGM
Disease-based medical model   Health-based developmental model

FAMILIES VIEWED AS
Pathologic, pathogenic,   Competent or
or dysfunctional   potentially competent

EMPHASIS ON
Weaknesses, liabilities   Strengths, resources
and illness   and wellness

ROLE OF PROFESSIONALS
Practitioners   Enabling agents

ROLE OF FAMILIES
Clients or patients   Collaborators

ASSESSMENT BASED ON
Clinical typologies   Competencies and
                                              competence deficits

GOAL OF INTERVENTION
Treatment of family   Enablement and
pathology or dysfunction   empowerment

MODUS OPERANDI
Provision of   Enhancement of
psychotherapy   coping effectiveness

SYSTEMIC PERSPECTIVE
Family systems   Ecological systems

Table 1 Adapted from Marsh (1992b)

professionals as enabling agents and families as collaborators; that has as its goal the enablement and empowerment of families; that assumes an ecological systems framework; and that employs an educational services model. A competence paradigm provides a comprehensive framework that subsumes some elements of a pathology paradigm. For instance, a competence paradigm recognizes the possible presence of competence deficits, as well as the value of professional intervention designed to help families correct these deficits.

A competence paradigm offers many advantages for professional practice (e.g., Marsh, 1992a; Masterpasqua, 1989). A competence paradigm is likely to foster the development of alliances between between families and professionals; to facilitate the identification, assessment, and enhancement of the competencies that are relevant to coping with serious mental illness; to encourage more precise theory and research concerned with families; to provide a blueprint for designing, implementing, and evaluating professional services; to improve the service system for people with mental illness; and to promote the empowerment of families.

A Coping and Adaptation Framework

In addition to a competence paradigm, there are other conceptual models that can facilitate the design, implementation, and evaluation of services for families. A coping and adaptation model also focuses on the strengths, resources, and adaptive capacities of families (e.g., Hatfield & Lefley, 1987). The serious mental illness of a relative is a catastrophic event for families. As in the case of other catastrophic stressors, such as serious physical illness or developmental disability, families who are coping with serious mental illness undergo a process of adaptation.

This adaptation process can be viewed productively in terms of Hill's (1949) ABCX model of family stress; more recently, the Double ABCX model has been formulated to reflect the family's adaptation through time (see Figley, 1989).

Wikler (1986) has provided an overview of the ABCX model, as well as its application to the familial experience of disability. The ABCX schema contains four components: A, family life events; B, family resources; C, family appraisal of the event; and X, family adaptation. The model reflects an assumption that familial adaptation to a member's disability is a complex process that is influenced by family life events, resources, and appraisal. The application of the ABCX model to the familial experience of serious mental illness is presented in Figure 1.

The ABCX Model

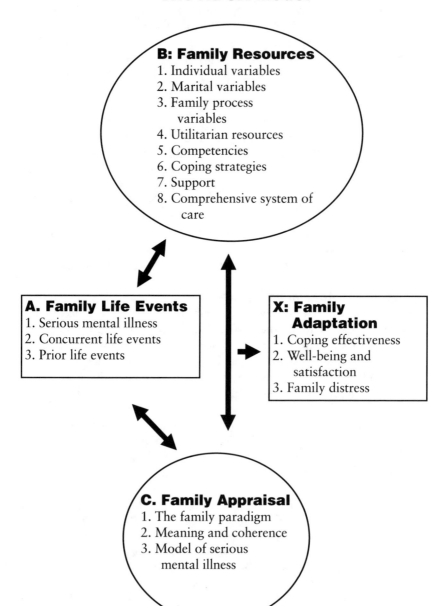

Figure 1: Familial adaptation to serious mental illness: An application of the ABCX model.

The model incorporates research concerned with coping and adaptation (e.g., Kessler et al., 1985; Matheny et al., 1986); with familial stress (e.g., Figley, 1989); with the familial experience of developmental disability (e.g., Frey et al., 1989); and with the familial experience of serious emotional disturbance (Marsh, in press). Although the model has a number of limitations (e.g., Walker, 1985), there is empirical support for the value of the ABCX model in conceptualizing the process of family adaptation to stress and in enhancing the coping effectiveness of families (e.g., Orr et al., 1991). Each of the four components of the ABCX model will be discussed.

A: Family life events. When applied to families of people with mental illness, the first component of the ABCX model is family life events, which include: (a) the serious mental illness itself; (b) other concurrent life events; and (c) prior life events. Family life events are those present and past events that are potential stressors for family members. There is much evidence that the mental illness of a family member has a devastating impact on the entire family. As Lefley (1989) has discussed, such families experience a subjective burden consisting of the emotional consequences of the illness for other family members, and an objective burden consisting of the reality demands associated with the illness, such as those related to ongoing caregiving. The overall context of familial stress also includes concurrent life events that may increase the family burden, as well as prior events that may have depleted family resources.

B: Family resources. The second component is family resources, which include: (a) individual variables (wellness, self-esteem, self-efficacy, beliefs, commitments); (b) marital variables (status, satisfaction, roles, consensus); (c) family process variables (boundaries, hierarchical organization, family homeostasis, information processing, differentiation, emotional climate); (d) utilitarian resources (educational level, family income); (e) competencies (cognitive, behavioral, affective, social); (f) coping strategies; (g) support (informal, formal); and (h) a comprehensive system of care. There is an extensive literature concerned with many of these variables (see Marsh, in press). For example, there is valuable work concerned with the familial process of coping and adaptation (e.g., Hatfield & Lefley, 1987; Zipple & Spaniol, 1987b).

C: Family appraisal. The third component is family appraisal: the collective set of beliefs about the stressor that may or may not make it traumatizing for a particular family (Figley, 1989). As depicted in the transactional model of stress, a life event becomes stressful only after it has been appraised as threatening (Singer & Davidson, 1991). Family appraisal can be delineated in terms of the following variables: (a) the family paradigm, which consists of the underlying assumptions about reality that are shared by all family members and that guide their construction of reality (Reiss & Klein, 1987); (b) meaning and coherence, which is the family's sense of significance in the event (see Thompson & Janigian, 1988); and (c) model of serious mental illness (e.g., interpersonal, biological, diathesis-stress).

As Terkelsen (1987) has discussed, many variables can influence the familial process of appraisal in the case of serious mental illness, including the extent of involvement in primary caregiving; the models of causation, symptoms, and outcomes assumed by family members; and the particular circumstances and attributes of individual family members. Family appraisal also affects many other dimensions of the family experience. For example, the family's model of serious mental illness has an impact on elements of the subjective burden experienced by the family, such as their feelings of guilt and helplessness (Terkelsen, 1987), as well as on parental attitudes and caregiving patterns (Chesla, 1989).

X: Family adaptation. The final category is family adaptation, which includes: (a) coping effectiveness (with the serious mental illness, with other adaptive demands); (b) sense of well-being and satisfaction; and (c) level of family distress.

Implications for services. The ABCX model provides an excellent framework for conceptualizing family-oriented services, with the goal of improving family adaptation. Family adaptation is likely to be fostered by services that increase resource availability and utilization (e.g., coping skills workshops, a support group, improved services for their relative), or that alter family appraisal in constructive ways (e.g., by educating families about serious mental illness). In essence, intervention strategies that improve family resources and appraisal are also likely to have a positive impact on family adaptation. Measures of many of these variables are available (see Marsh, in press), thus facilitating the evaluation of services designed to enhance family adaptation.

SERVICES FOR FAMILIES: GENERAL CONSIDERATIONS

There are a number of general considerations in designing services for families of people with serious mental illness. First, consistent with the new modes and models of professional practice that have been discussed, the central objective of professional practice is to empower families in achieving mastery and control over the circumstances of their lives, including the mental illness of their relative. Accordingly, services must be delivered in a manner that acknowledges the strengths, resources, and expertise of families, that provides opportunities for them to strengthen family functioning, and that promotes a sense of intrafamilial mastery and control (see Dunst et al., 1988).

Second, family consultation can assist families in making an informed choice regarding their use of available services. As explicated by Bernheim (1989; also see Chapter 8), family consultants offer expertise and advice to family members, who have responsibility for determining their own goals. Decisions about service utilization need to take into account the family's agenda, as well as professional recommendations. Open, direct, and respectful communication will ensure that professionals are aware of the goals and priorities of families, and that families are aware of the rationale underlying professional recommendations.

Third, the objective of family consultation is to provide an optimal match between the needs, desires, and resources of particular family members and the services that are available. Thus, consideration should be given the potential benefits, risks, and costs of all services. A full continuum of family-oriented services includes nonclinical services designed primarily to offer education and support, and clinical services designed to offer treatment.

Fourth, a more differentiated approach to family-oriented services is needed. Shifting from the family system to family subsystems, it is important to offer services not only to parents of people with mental illness, but also to spouses, siblings, and children. The experiences, needs, and coping resources of family members may differ significantly as a function of their role in the family (e.g., Marsh et al., 1993; also see Chapter 10). For example, there is some evidence that family members find nonclinical intervention, such as educational programs and support groups more beneficial than clinical intervention, such as individual or family therapy (e.g., Lefley, 1987). In contrast, in a national survey of adult siblings and children of people with serious mental illness (Marsh et al., 1993), over three-fourths (77%) of respondents reported that they had received psychotherapy (primarily individual therapy); 63% rated the therapy as very or extremely helpful.

Fifth, once families have made an informed choice regarding their use of services, professionals should make appropriate referrals. Families may decide to decline services or defer their use of services; to receive a single service offered in a clinical setting or in the community; or to pursue complementary services, such as an educational or psychoeducational program led by professionals and a family-facilitated support group in the community. Following the initial decision regarding service utilization, professionals should remain available to families, since their needs and desires may change. Furthermore, some families may benefit from services on an as-needed basis, particularly during crises or periods of inpatient treatment.

Finally, effective and responsive services are dependent upon an understanding of family experiences and needs. Increasingly, family members have become providers of educational and support services to other families (e.g., Burland, 1991). There are also many excellent resources available for professionals who wish to offer services for family members, including training manuals (e.g., Bisbee, 1991; Meisel & Mannion; 1989; Zipple & Spaniol, 1987b); books (e.g., Bernheim & Lehman, 1985; Hatfield, 1990; Lefley & Johnson, 1990; Marsh, 1992a); and chapters and articles (e.g., Bentley & Harrison, 1989; Ferris & Marshall, 1987; Gingerich et al., 1992; Kuipers, 1991; Lam, 1991; McFarlane et al., 1993; Zastowny et al., 1992).

NONCLINICAL SERVICES FOR FAMILIES

Families who are coping with the serious mental illness of a relative have a number of essential needs, including their needs for information about mental illness and community resources; for skills to cope with the illness and its consequences for the family; and for support for themselves. As Zipple and Spaniol (1987a) have discussed, nonclinical programs may be primarily educational, skills-oriented, or supportive; in addition, a multimodal program can be designed to fulfill all of these functions. Educational programs and support groups are two effective nonclinical strategies that have evolved to address the expressed needs of families.

Educational Programs

The professional literature offers many descriptions of educational programs for families (e.g., Moller & Wer, 1989), as well as empirical evidence for the value of such programs (e.g., Abramowitz & Coursey, 1989). Family-oriented educational programs should cover a range of topics, as indicated in the ten-week educational program outlined in Table 2. Such a program might be beneficial for families of people who have been hospitalized with a diagnosis of serious mental illness. The general structure of the program can be modified to meet the needs of specific providers and populations, such as children and adolescents with serious emotional disturbance (see Marsh, in press). Weekly topics include: (a) nature and purpose of program; (b) family-professional relationships; (c) serious mental illness (two weeks); (d) managing symptoms and problems; (e) the family experience; (f) stress, coping, and

Ten-Week Educational Program for Families

Week 1. Nature and Purpose of Program
Introductions; overview of agency program; written survey of family needs and requests

Week 2. Family-Professional Relationships
Establishing collaborative partnerships; roles and responsibilities; communication

Week 3. Serious Mental Illness I
Diagnosis; etiology; prognosis; treatment

Week 4. Serious Mental Illness I
Symptoms; medication; diathesis-stress model; recent research

Week 5. Managing Symptoms and Problems
Positive symptoms; negative symptoms; specific problems

Week 6. The Family Experience
Family burden and needs; life span perspectives; family system and subsystem issues

Week 7. Stress, Coping, and Adaptation
Dealing with a catastrophic stressor; enhancing coping effectiveness

Week 8. Enhancing Personal and Family Effectiveness I
Behavior management; conflict resolution; communication; problem solving

Week 9. Enhancing Personal and Family Effectiveness II
Stress management; assertiveness; meeting personal and family needs

Week 10. Community Resources
Consumer-advocacy movement; community support system; appropriate referrals

Table 2 Adapted from Marsh (1992a)

adaptation; (g) enhancing personal and family effectiveness (two weeks); and (h) community resources.

Educational programs can also be offered by family members (e.g., Burland, 1991), or by a family-professional team (e.g., Mannion & Meisel, 1989). There are many resources available for professionals and family members who wish to offer an educational program for family members (e.g., Hatfield, 1990; Zipple & Spaniol, 1987b).

Support Groups

Families who are coping with serious mental illness often feel stigmatized by the larger society and alienated from their usual channels of social support. There is strong evidence for the value of support groups for families under these circumstances (e.g., Hatfield & Lefley, 1987; also see Chapter 11 for multifamily vs. individual family interventions). Support groups can offer families opportunities to mobilize resources and resolve their emotional burden in a protected and nurturing environment; to obtain information about mental illness, coping strategies, and community resources; and to move into roles as effective advocates. As is the case for educational programs, there are many resources available for professionals and family members who wish to offer support groups for families (e.g., Donner & Fine, 1987). When support groups are offered in clinical settings, professionals can serve as facilitators or as cofacilitators with family members. In addition, professionals can assist families by making referrals to family-facilitated support groups in their communities. They may also wish to visit a local support group and to offer consultation and programs on specific topics.

Guidelines for Nonclinical Services

In addition to educational programs and support groups, there are many other nonclinical services that may benefit families of people with serious mental illness, including educational seminars focusing on specific topics, skills-oriented workshops, a crisis group, a drop-in center, an advocacy group, written materials, a newsletter, multifamily groups, and forums that utilize professional and community resources. To ensure the usefulness of nonclinical programs, the input of family members should be solicited as such programs are designed and implemented. Furthermore, many programs can benefit from the involvement of family members as consultants, as presenters, and as facilitators or cofacilitators with professionals.

A comprehensive program of nonclinical services should include the following: (a) a didactic component that provides information about

serious mental illness and the mental health system; (b) a skills component that offers training in communication, conflict resolution, problem
solving, assertiveness, behavioral management, and stress management;
(c) an emotional component that provides opportunities for grieving,
sharing, and mobilizing resources; (d) a family process component that
focuses on the impact of mental illness on the family unit and on
individual family members; and (e) a social component that increases
utilization of informal and formal support networks.

Family-Facilitated Services

All of the nonclinical services discussed previously can be offered by
professionals, by a family-professional team, or by family members.
Family-facilitated services are now available in most communities,
largely as a result of the growth of the National Alliance for the Mentally
Ill (NAMI), whose local affiliates frequently offer a multimodal approach to family services, including support groups, educational programs, coping skills workshops, and advocacy activities. Family-facilitated services have a number of advantages. Such programs are likely
to be relatively inexpensive, since they are usually offered by volunteers;
to be responsive to the needs of families, since they are family-driven;
and to enhance the sense of family empowerment, since such groups
often have a strong advocacy component. Family-facilitated interventions can benefit from professional expertise through professional consultation and programs on specific topics.

CLINICAL SERVICES FOR FAMILIES

Clinical intervention also offers a valuable resource for some family
members, who may benefit from psychotherapy designed to assist them
in resolving problems that are reactive to their relative's mental illness
or in addressing other mental health problems that may have been
precipitated or exacerbated by current stress. More generally, psychotherapy offers the potential for improvements in interpersonal functioning, in self-esteem and self-confidence, in satisfaction, in mastery and
competency, and in level of distress (Strupp, 1989).

Consistent with more general changes in family-professional relationships, clinical services should be offered in a manner that fosters family-professional collaboration and family empowerment (e.g., Combrinck-Graham, 1990; Hoffman, 1990; Kuipers, 1991; Simon et al.,
1991; Taylor, 1987). Once a family member has chosen to pursue a
course of psychotherapy, the family consultant can employ a process of
differential therapeutics to ensure selection of the most efficacious treatment.

In their discussion of differential therapeutics, Clarkin and his associates (1992) distinguish between two levels of treatment planning: the macro level, which includes five dimensions (setting, format, strategies and techniques, duration and frequency, and medication); and the micro level, which involves the adjustments of therapeutic strategies within the treatment process itself in light of the client's problem complexity, coping style, and reactance level. The authors also distinguish between the final goals of therapy, which are to alleviate the symptoms and conflicts for which assistance was sought, and the mediating goals of therapy, which are hypothesized to be related to the the initial symptoms and conflicts.

In discussing the treatment of depression, for example, Clarkin and his colleagues note that the choice of mediating goals is based on such factors as phase and severity of depressive symptoms; presumed causes leading to their development and maintenance; and individual assets, liabilities, stressors, and social supports. Mediating goals of treatment might include symptom improvement, cognitive changes, interpersonal changes, and personality/dynamic changes. Similarly, in the case of families of people with serious mental illness, the final goal is the alleviation of the presenting symptoms and conflicts; mediating goals will reflect the unique problems, attributes, and circumstances of particular family members.

Differential Therapeutics with Families

Based on the discussion of Clarkin and his colleagues (1992), the process of differential therapeutics will be applied to professional practice with families of people who have serious mental illness. The following topics will be discussed: format, strategies and techniques, duration and frequency, and no treatment as the prescription of choice.

Format. The choice of treatment format determines the number of individuals who will be present and defines the interpersonal context of the intervention. Alternative formats include individual, marital, family, heterogeneous group, and homogeneous group treatment. Given the diversity among families, each of these formats has potential value. For example, individual intervention is likely to be beneficial when psychological issues are most prominent, and group intervention when there are pressing needs for social support (Toseland et al., 1990).

Clarkin and his colleagues (1992; Frances et al., 1984) have discussed the relative indications and contraindications of individual, marital/family, and group formats. In working with families of people with mental illness, individual treatment may be appropriate for a family member who desires the privacy and intimacy of a dyadic relationship; who is having difficult resolving the emotional burden associated with the mental illness of a relative; who is experiencing intrapsychic conflict (see Chapter 6); or whose striving for autonomy is undermined by familial circumstances (e.g., separation difficulties in an adolescent sibling). On the other hand, individual treatment may result in distortion, isolation, scapegoating, and infantilization, as well as failure to address important marital or family problems.

Family or marital therapy may be indicated when preexisting family or marital problems have been exacerbated by current circumstances (e.g., difficulties in communication, problem solving, or conflict resolution); the family is unable to cope adequately with the mental illness of the family member; or successful treatment of an individual requires the involvement of other family members. Potential risks of marital or family therapy include reduced autonomy, increased family disruption, loss of privacy, undermining of internal boundaries of family subsystems, and deflection from individual problems and concerns. There are additional risks associated with general prescriptions of family therapy that are based on assumptions of family dysfunction or pathogenesis and that do not take into account the needs, desires, and resources of particular family members (see Marsh, 1992a, 1992b).

Homogeneous group treatment is a relatively economical format that focuses on the common needs of families of people with serious mental illness. Sometimes called multiple family therapy, this group format can address the needs of families for information, skills, and support. However, the narrow focus of a group format may deflect attention from important individual, marital, or familial issues.

Strategies and techniques. Strategies and techniques are the technical interventions used by the therapist to induce change. As Clarkin and his colleagues (1992) point out, the current era has witnessed a proliferation of treatment strategies and techniques, as well as the availability of treatment manuals written from the perspective of various schools (e.g., psychodynamic, behavioral, cognitive). Based on their review of existing treatment manuals, the authors discuss the strategies and techniques common to the various schools of therapy: establishing and fostering a therapeutic alliance, managing patient resistance, structuring the treatment, focusing the treatment, and terminating the treatment. They also examine the specific strategies and techniques that might be appropriate in particular cases. Depending on the mediating goals of treatment, for instance, psychodynamic techniques might be used to promote insight and conflict resolution; behavioral techniques to encourage specific behavioral changes; cognitive techniques to alter conscious thought processes; and experiential-humanistic techniques to increase awareness.

From the perspective of differential therapeutics, the selection of specific strategies and techniques is guided primarily by empirical evidence regarding their effectiveness in treating particular populations or disorders. Norcross and Newman (1992) note that such an approach is often referred to as technical eclecticism, whose proponents use procedures drawn from different sources without necessarily subscribing to the theories that spawned them. Indeed, as the authors discuss, there is much interest in psychotherapy integration, which is intended to increase therapeutic efficacy, efficiency, and applicability by looking beyond specific theories and the techniques traditionally associated with those theories.

In spite of these transtheoretical efforts, the orientations of practitioners continue to influence developments in theory, research, and practice. There are numerous biological, psychological, systems, and multidimensional models. Biological models emphasize the biological substrate of serious mental illness, including genetics, neurochemistry, neurophysiology, and neuroanatomy (see Andreasen, 1991). Psychological models are largely concerned with the understanding and treatment of individuals. These models include the psychodynamic model, which underscores the role of early childhood experience and intrapsychic conflict in personality development and psychopathology (see Chapter 6); the cognitive behavioral model, which focuses on present cognitions and behaviors and on the strategies that can modify maladaptive patterns of thinking and behaving; and the existential-humanistic model, which emphasizes the innate potential of human beings for growth and self-actualization.

Systems models conceive of phenomena as complex systems that are characterized by such qualities as wholeness, organization, differentiation, integration, and teleology (see Kanfer & Schefft, 1988). There are many models of family systems therapy, including psychoanalytic, contextual, symbolic-experiential, structural, strategic, behavioral, Bowenian, Ericksonian, focal, systemic, and psychoeducational (Gurman & Kniskern, 1991; also see Chapter 5).

Multidimensional models are designed to integrate impressive advances in the social, behavioral, and biological sciences, and to offer a comprehensive framework for treatment and rehabilitation. For example, McDaniel and her associates (1992) have developed medical family therapy, a biopsychosocial approach to families with health problems.

Similarly, in the area of serious mental illness, the diathesis-stress model assumes the presence of a predisposing factor, such as a biological vulnerability, that interacts with a range of environmental events that may precipitate, exacerbate, or ameliorate the disorder (e.g., Liberman et al., 1986). Two family variables that have received attention within this model are communication deviance and expressed emotion. As is the case for several other models, the diathesis-stress model has generated intervention strategies designed for families (see the discussion of psychoeducational programs later in this section).

From the perspective of professional practice with families of people with serious mental illness, at the macro level of treatment planning, clinicians should employ the strategies and techniques likely to address the expressed needs of such families, including their needs for information about mental illness and its treatment, for effective coping skills, and for support for themselves. At the micro level, treatment planning should be adapted to the complexity, coping style, and reactance level of individual family members. Technical eclecticism, with its emphasis on the the potential value of the full range of strategies and techniques, offers a data-based approach that can increase therapeutic efficacy with families. All of the models that have been mentioned have potential value for families members. For example, systems and multidimensional models provide a conceptual framework for working with the family system or with the larger social system, and for integrating research across multiple domains (see Chapter 5).

The psychological models also offer a range of technical interventions. Psychodynamic strategies are likely to be helpful in addressing issues of loss and mourning, in working through issues pertaining to earlier losses that have been resurrected, and in resolving conflicts pertaining to the family of origin. Cognitive behavioral strategies furnish an effective means of meeting the informational and skills needs of families, and of treating the depression that is often a central component of the subjective burden. The experiential-humanistic orientation emphasizes the establishment of a supportive and validating therapeutic milieu, and employs the techniques of abreaction, empathy, sharing, identification, reframing, clarification, and reassurance. In light of the anguish experienced by many family members, this orientation also has potential value for this population.

Duration and frequency. Duration and frequency pertain to the way the treatment is embedded in time. Clarkin and his colleagues (1992) discuss three treatment forms that vary along these dimensions. The first is crisis intervention, which is an intense, timely, brief, and goal-di-

rected treatment designed to resolve a crisis of major and urgent proportions and of recent onset. Indications for crisis intervention may
include the presence of severe symptoms, distress, and risk factors that
warrant urgent and intense attention; evidence for a major precipitating
stressor; and relatively recent onset of symptoms.

The second form is brief therapy. The authors note that most therapy
has always been brief; a very high percentage of individuals seeking
clinic outpatient therapy remain in treatment for fewer than 12 sessions.
What is new in the present era, however, is the notion of time-limited
therapy by design. There is much variability in brief therapies, which
may differ in goals, techniques, strategies, format, setting, and selection
criteria, although there are several essential features, including an established time limit, clear and limited treatment goals, and an active
therapist. The following are indications for brief therapy: (a) a definite
focus, precipitating event, or intervention target; (b) sufficient (if limited)
motivation and goals for brief treatment; (c) capacity for separation
from treatment; (d) adequate level of functioning; (e) limited financial
or time resources; and (f) a desire to avoid secondary gain, negative
therapeutic reactions, unmanageable therapeutic attachments, or other
iatrogenic effects.

Long-term psychotherapy is appropriate for problems that are ingrained, complex, and extensive. The extended treatment permits the
dissection and resolution of problems and the assimilation and application of new solutions into daily life. As Clarkin and his associates
(1992) note, long-term psychotherapy is expensive and only weakly
supported by empirical evidence. Accordingly, it should be recommended only after a careful assessment of indications, contraindications,
and enabling factors. Patient factors associated with treatment of longer
duration include the presence of serious mental illness, multiple problems areas, few enabling factors for treatment, relatively poor premorbid
functioning, and an unsatisfactory response to brief treatment.

From the perspective of professional practice with family members,
a course of brief therapy would be suggested by satisfactory prior functioning, the presence of precipitating stress, the relatively poor match
between the expressed needs of families and ambitious treatment goals,
and the likelihood of poor motivation for extended therapy among
families who are coping with a catastrophic event. On the other hand,
a recommendation of long-term psychotherapy is appropriate for family
members who have serious mental illness themselves, who are experiencing severe problems in several areas of their lives, or who have chosen
to pursue psychoanalysis.

No treatment. Clarkin and his colleagues also discuss no treatment as the prescription of choice. They distinguish among three groups who might be considered for no treatment: (a) those likely to improve without treatment (e.g., those suffering from acute stress, but with a history of effective functioning and coping); (b) those who are at risk for a negative response to the treatment itself (e.g., due to the nature of the treatment or the disorder) ; and (c) those who are at risk for failing to respond to treatment (e.g., due to poor motivation).

Clearly, a recommendation of no treatment should be considered in the case of many family members, particularly those who are have a history of effective functioning and are likely to improve on their own (or with nonclinical intervention). A recommendation of no treatment also avoids the risks of negative treatment effects among families who do not see themselves as needing or wanting therapy, and of low motivation for psychotherapy among families whose resources are depleted by the recurrent crises and continuing reality demands associated with serious mental illness.

Psychoeducational Programs

The orientations or models espoused by professionals often serve as a guide to theory, research, and practice. For example, research from the perspective of the diathesis-stress model has generated psychoeducational programs for families. Although the terms education and psychoeducation are sometimes used interchangeably, there are important differences between the two approaches. As discussed previously, educational programs are a nonclinical form of intervention designed to meet the needs of families for information about mental illness and its treatment, about caregiving and management issues, about the mental health system and community resources, and about family coping and adaptation.

In contrast, psychoeducational programs have most often been offered as a form of clinical intervention designed to enhance the family's ability to cope with the schizophrenia of a family member and to reduce the risk of relapse. There is now a substantial literature concerned with psychoeducational programs (e.g., Anderson et al., 1986; Brooker, 1990; Falloon et al., 1984; Kavanagh, 1992; Kuipers et al., 1992; Lam, 1991; Tarrier & Barrowclough, 1990). Researchers have found a greater risk of relapse among individuals with schizophrenia who return to family environments characterized by a high level of expressed emotion, which is operationalized as critical comments, hostility, and emotional overinvolvement. There is also evidence of reduced risk or delay of relapse following psychoeducational programs designed to lower an initially high level of expressed emotion in families. Following her review of the relevant literature, Lefley (1992) has concluded that although research concerned with expressed emotion has a number of limitations, the findings are important in highlighting the adverse impact of over-stimulating or high-demand environments for individuals who have the core information-processing deficits of schizophrenia.

Family components of psychoeducational programs generally include the following: (a) an empathic, validating, nonblaming, task-oriented alliance with the family; (b) comprehensive family assessment (e.g., the Camberwell Family Interview); (c) education about schizophrenia and its management; (d) training in specific skills and competencies (e.g., problem solving, communication); (e) family treatment designed to lower expressed emotion; and (f) contact with other families. In addition, psychoeducation programs generally include consumer components, such as education about schizophrenia and its management, emphasis on medication compliance, and training in social skills.

From the perspective of services for families, psychoeducational programs are in many respects a constructive development, since such programs are designed to foster collaborative family-professional relationships and to meet many essential family needs (e.g., Fox, 1992). On the other hand, psychoeducational programs pose a number of problems. For example, such programs are generally offered as an adjunct to the treatment of the relative who has schizophrenia, with the goals of reducing relapse and of improving the family's ability to cope with the illness. As a result, psychoeducational programs may not meet the needs of particular families, including those who are low in expressed emotion or who do not function as primary caregivers. In addition, such programs are typically viewed as a form of treatment, with emphasis on the adverse impact of high expressed emotion on the course of schizophrenia; there is often a pejorative quality to the term "high-EE family" that recalls the earlier phrase "schizophrenogenic mother." Furthermore, psychoeducational programs sometimes ignore the strengths, resources, and expertise of families, and such programs often neglect the larger sociocultural context, including the need for a comprehensive system of community-based care.

Guidelines for Clinical Services

There are a number of general guidelines for offering clinical services to family members. First, consistent with the ethical principle of informed consent, professional consultants should inform family members of the nature and purpose of specific nonclinical and clinical services; of the potential benefits, risks, and costs of these services; of the risks of forgoing the services; and of the available alternatives.

Second, the risk of negative treatment effects should be minimized (see Marsh, 1992a, 1992b). There are risks of adverse effects when family therapists inappropriately assume that families are pathogenic or dysfunctional (e.g., Carr, 1990; Drake & Sederer, 1986; Terkelsen, 1983). There are also risks when family therapy is mandated as a condition for treating the relative who has mental illness, since families may not see themselves as needing or wanting treatment (Grunebaum & Friedman, 1988), and may object to being treated as the "unidentified patient" (Bernheim, 1989). Such mandatory therapy is also in conflict with the ethical principle of informed consent and with the process of differential therapeutics.

Third, a number of treatment goals are appropriate for family members who have chosen psychotherapy, including provision of support, enhancement of coping effectiveness, reframing of personal and familial experience, and expression and resolution of the emotional burden. At the macro level of treatment planning, Bernheim's (1982) supportive family counseling is an example of a clinical approach that is likely to be beneficial to many family members. In addition, clinicians should be sensitive to the unique experiences and needs of individual family members, such as young family members.

Finally, consistent with the general psychotherapy literature, the overarching consideration is the quality of the therapeutic alliance that is formed with families. A constructive therapeutic alliance is likely to be fostered by a respectful and empathic attitude toward families, an understanding of their phenomenological reality, an effort to meet their expressed needs, and a goal of family empowerment.

REFERENCES

Abramowitz, I. A., & Coursey, R. D. (1989). Impact of an educational support group on family participants who take care of their schizophrenic relatives. *Journal of Consulting and Clinical Psychology, 57,* 232-236.

Anderson, C. M. et al. (1986). *Schizophrenia and the family.* New York: Guilford.

Andreasen, N. C. (1991). *Introductory textbook of psychiatry.* Washington, DC: American Psychiatric Press.

Bentley, K. J., & Harrison, D. F. (1989). Behavioral, psychoeducational, and skills training approaches to family management of schizophrenia. In B. A. Thyer (Ed.), *Behavioral family therapy* (pp. 147-168). Springfield, IL: Charles C. Thomas.

Bernheim, K. F. (1982). Supportive family counseling. *Schizophrenia Bulletin, 8,* 634-641.

Bernheim, K. F. (1989). Psychologists and families of the severely mentally ill: The role of family consultation. *American Psychologist, 44,* 561-564.

Bernheim, K. F., & Lehman, A. F. (1985) *Working with families of the mentally ill.* New York: Norton.

Bisbee, C. (1991). *Educating patients and families about mental illness: A practical guide.* Gaithersburg, MD: Aspen.

Brooker, C. (1990). Expressed emotion and psychosocial intervention: A review. *International Journal of Nursing Studies, 27,* 267-276.

Burland, J. (1991). *The Journey of Hope Family Education Course.* Poultney, VT: Alliance for the Mentally Ill of Vermont.

Carr, A. (1990). Failures in family therapy: A catalogue of engagement mistakes. *Journal of Family Therapy, 12,* 371-386.

Chesla, C. A. (1989). Parents' illness models of schizophrenia. *Archives of Psychiatric Nursing, 3,* 218-225.

Clarkin, J. F. et al. (1992). Differential therapeutics: Macro and micro levels of treatment planning. In J. C. Norcross & M. R. Goldfried (Eds.), *Handbook of psychotherapy integration* (pp. 463-502). New York: Basic Books.

Combrinck-Graham, L. (1990). Developments in family systems theory and research. *Journal of the American Academy of Child and Adolescent Psychiatry, 29,* 501-512.

Donner, R., & Fine, G. Z. (1987). *A guide for developing self-help/advocacy groups for parents of children with serious emotional problems.* Washington, DC: Georgetown University Child Development Center.

Drake, R. E., & Sederer, L. I. (1986). The adverse effects of intensive treatment of chronic schizophrenia. *Comprehensive Psychiatry, 27,* 313-326.

Dunst, C. J. et al. (1988). *Enabling and empowering families: Principles and guidelines for practice.* Cambridge, MA: Brookline.

Falloon, I. R. H. et al. (1984). *Family care of schizophrenia.* New York: Guilford.

Ferris, P. A., & Marshall, C. A. (1987). A model project for families of the chronically mentally ill. *Social Work, 32,* 110-114.

Figley, C. R. (1989). *Helping traumatized families.* San Francisco: Jossey-Bass.

Fox, P. (1992). Implications for expressed emotion therapy within a family therapeutic context. *Health & Social Work, 17,* 207-213.

Frances, A. et al. (1984). *Differential therapeutics in psychiatry: The art and science of treatment selection.* New York: Brunner/Mazel.

Frey, K. S. et al. (1989). Stress and coping among parents of handicapped children: A multidimensional approach. *American Journal on Mental Retardation, 94,* 240-249.

Gingerich, E. et al. (1992). The therapist as psychoeducator. *Hospital and Community Psychiatry, 43,* 928-930.

Grunebaum, H., & Friedman, H. (1988). Building collaborative relationships with families of the mentally ill. *Hospital and Community Psychiatry, 29,* 1183-1187.

Gurman, A. S., & Kniskern, D. P. (Eds.). (1991). *Handbook of family therapy. Vols. I and II.* New York: Brunner/Mazel.

Hatfield, A. B. (1990). *Family education in mental illness.* New York: Guilford.

Hatfield, A. B., & Lefley, H. P. (Eds.). (1987). *Families of the mentally ill: Coping and adaptation.* New York: Guilford.

Hill, R. (1949). *Families under stress.* New York: Harper & Row.

Hoffman, L. (1990). Constructing realities: An art of lenses. *Family Process, 29,* 1-12.

Kanfer, F. H., & Schefft, B. K. (1988). *Guiding the process of therapeutic change.* Champaign, IL: Research Press.

Kavanagh, D. J. (1992). Recent developments in expressed emotion in schizophrenia. *British Journal of Psychiatry, 160,* 601-620.

Kessler, R. C. et al. (1985). Social factors in psychopathology: Stress, social support, and coping processes. *Annual Review of Psychology, 36,* 531-572.

Kuipers, L. (1991). Schizophrenia and the family. *International Review of Psychiatry, 3,* 105-117.

Kuipers, L. et al. (1992). Psychosocial family intervention in schizophrenia: A review of empirical studies. *British Journal of Psychiatry, 160,* 272-275.

Lam, D. H. (1991). Psychosocial family intervention in schizophrenia: A review of empirical studies. *Psychological Medicine, 21,* 423-441.

Lefley, H. P. (1987). Impact of mental illness in families of mental health professionals. *Journal of Nervous and Mental Disease, 175,* 613-619.

Lefley, H. P. (1989). Family burden and family stigma in major mental illness. *American Psychologist, 44,* 556-560.

Lefley, H. P. (1992). Expressed emotion: Conceptual, clinical, and social policy issues. *Hospital and Community Psychiatry, 43,* 591-598.

Lefley, H. P., & Johnson, D. L. (Eds.). (1990). *Families as allies in treatment of the mentally ill.* Washington, DC: American Psychiatric Press.

Liberman, R. P. et al. (1986). New methods for rehabilitating chronic mental patients. In J. A. Talbott (Ed.), *Our patients' future in a changing world* (pp. 99-129). Washington, DC: American Psychiatric Press.

Marsh, D. T. (1992a). *Families and mental illness: New directions in professional practice.* New York: Praeger.

Marsh, D. T. (1992b). Working with families of people with serious mental illness. In L. VandeCreek, S. Knapp, & T. L. Jackson (Eds.), *Innovations in clinical practice: A source book* (Vol. 11, pp. 389-402). Sarasota, FL: Professional Resource Press.

Marsh, D. T. (in press). Families of children and adolescents with serious emotional disturbance: Innovations in theory, research, and practice. In C. A. Heflinger (Ed.), *Families and mental health services: Policy, services, and research.* Newbury Park, CA: Sage.

Marsh, D. T. et al. (1993). Troubled journey: Siblings and children of people with mental illness. *Innovations & Research, 2*(2), 17-28.

Masterpasqua, F. (1989). A competence paradigm for psychological practice. *American Psychologist, 44,* 1366-1371.

Matheny, K. B. et al. (1986). Stress coping: A qualitative and quantitative synthesis with implications for treatment. *Counseling Psychologist, 14,* 499-549.

McDaniel, S. H. et al. (1992). *Medical family therapy: A biopsychosocial approach to families with health problems.* New York: Basic Books.

McFarlane, W. R. et al. (1993). From research to clinical practice: Dissemination of New York State's family psychoeducation project. *Hospital and Community Psychiatry, 44,* 265-270.

Meisel, M., & Mannion, E., (1989). *Teaching manual for coping skills workshops* (rev. ed.). Philadelphia: Mental Health Association of Southeastern Pennsylvania/The T.E.C. Network.

Moller, M. D., & Wer, J. E. (1989). Simultaneous patient/family eduction regarding schizophrenia: The Nebraska model. *Archives of Psychiatric Nursing, 3,* 332-337.

Norcross, J. C., & Newman, C. F. (1992). Psychotherapy integration: Setting the context. In J. C. Norcross & M. R. Goldfried (Eds.), *Handbook of psychotherapy integration* (pp. 3-45). New York: Basic Books.

Orr, R. R. et al. (1991). Coping with stress in families with children who have mental retardation: An evaluation of the Double ABCX model. *American Journal on Mental Retardation, 95,* 444-450.

Peternelj-Taylor, C. A., & Hartley, V. L. (1993). Living with mental illness: Professional/family collaboration. *Journal of Psychosocial Nursing, 31,* 23-28.

Reiss, D., & Klein, D. (1987). Paradigm and pathogenesis: A family-centered approach to problems of etiology and treatment of psychiatric disorders. In T. Jacobs (Ed.), *Family interaction and psychopathology* (pp. 203-255). New York: Plenum.

Simon, C. E. et al. (1991). The family and schizophrenia: Toward a psychoeducational approach. *Families in Society, 72,* 323-333.

Singer, J. E., & Davidson, L. M. (1991). Specificity and stress research. In A. Monat & R. S. Lazarus (Eds.), *Stress and coping: An anthology* (3rd ed., pp. 36-47). New York: Columbia University Press.

Strupp, H. H. (1989). Psychotherapy: Can the practitioner learn from the researcher. *American Psychologist, 44,* 717-724.

Tarrier, N., & Barrowclough, C. (1990). Family interventions for schizophrenia. *Behavior Modification, 14,* 408-440.

Taylor, E. H. (1987). The biological basis of schizophrenia. *Social Work, 32,* 115-121.

Terkelsen, K. G. (1983). Schizophrenia and the family. II. Adverse effects of family therapy. *Family Process, 22,* 191-200.

Terkelsen, K. G. (1987). The meaning of mental illness to the family. In A. B. Hatfield and H. P. Lefley (Eds.), *Families of the mentally ill: Coping and adaptation* (pp. 128-150). New York: Guilford.

Thompson, S. C., & Janigian, A. S. (1988). Life schemes: A framework for understanding the search for meaning. *Journal of Social and Clinical Psychology, 7,* 260-280.

Toseland, R. W. et al. (1990). Comparative effectiveness of individual and group interventions to support family caregivers. *Social Work, 35,* 209-217.

Walker, A. J. (1985). Reconceptualizing family stress. *Journal of Marriage and the Family, 47,* 827-837.

Wikler, L. M. (1986). Family stress theory and research on families of children with mental retardation. In J. J. Gallagher & P. M. Vietze (Eds.), *Families of handicapped persons: Research, programs, and policy issues* (pp. 167-195). Baltimore: Brookes.

Zipple, A. M., & Spaniol, L. (1987a). Current educational and supportive models of family intervention. In A. B. Hatfield & L. P. Lefley

(Eds.), *Families of the mentally ill: Coping and adaptation* (pp. 261-277). New York: Guilford.

Zipple, A. M., & Spaniol, L. (1987b). *Families that include a person with a mental illness: What they need and how to provide it. Trainer Manual.* Boston: Boston University Center for Psychiatric Rehabilitation.

Zastowny, T. R. et al. (1992). Family management of schizophrenia: A comparison of behavioral and supportive family treatment. *Psychiatric Quarterly, 63,* 159-186.

PART II

CURRENT CONTROVERSIES

Chapter 4

THE FAMILY'S ROLE IN CAREGIVING AND SERVICE DELIVERY

Agnes B. Hatfield

Unanticipated in the moverment toward the community care of people with psychiatric illnesses were the many roles that families would play in caregiving and service delivery. The development of these roles, however, has rarely been a matter of concerted discussion and planning in either the family movement or the service delivery system across the country. Rather, various forms of involvement have happened as groups of families sought inclusion and interested providers have tried to respond to these demands and/or the needs of the system for utilizing families.

Since family involvement in caregiving, service provision, education, and policy making has developed in such an unplanned way during the past few years, issues are now arising as to the appropriate role of families in these various endeavors. The goal of this chapter is to address some of these issues and to make recommendations in regard to appropriate roles for families.

THE ROLE OF THE FAMILY IN CAREGIVING

In spite of the strong emphasis of consumer and family advocates in the past decade for more community-based housing, studies show that families are still the primary caregivers of persons with mental illnesses. For example, in a recent study of the National Alliance for the Mentally Ill (NAMI) (Steinwachs, Kasper, Skinner 1992) , 42% of the families reported that their ill relatives were living with them and only 12% had supported housing in the community. The rest were either living alone, or were in a variety of settings such as hospitals, jails, or in the street.

While the major role of families in caregiving is now generally recognized, there is lack of agreement as to whether this is a desirable situation. Some providers and families may feel that families are the most appropriate caregivers, and while others may not agree, they accept the inevitability of the situation given present fiscal restraints. Other families however, are unyielding in their position, that adult mentally ill offspring like other young adults should live outside the family home (Howe, 1985:15 20).

The response of three hundred and eight families to a questionnaire circulated at the 1986 NAMI Convention (Hatfield, 1990) indicated that a preponderance of members in attendance (97%) felt their relative should live outside the family home. Torrey (1983) says that where a patient should live is complex but the majority do better living away from the family home. Dincin (1975) concurs, saying that living together is too stressful for both family and patient.

Lefley (1987) makes a convincing argument that we will soon face a serious social problem in our excessive reliance on elderly parents to provide housing for their adult mentally ill children. She cites several studies which indicate that families do not feel home care is in the interests of the person with mental illness nor the rest of the family. Lefley notes profound changes in household routines, altered relationships with friends and relatives. curtailment of social relationships, excessive commitment of time, and neglect of other family members as reasons for aging parents favoring separation.

Patients are faced with dependency roles that generate anger and frustrations They may see their parents as stumbling blocks to their independence and normal adulthood. If conflict is high, serious breaches in relationship with other family members may occur with patients eventually losing the only irreplaceable social support they have, that of their natural family.

Almost without exception parents will predecease their mentally ill offspring. This is a matter of great concern to most families and especially to those who still have their relative living at home. The difficulty of shifting their relative from the family home after he or she has lived there for many years is indicated in a recent study of families in Maryland (Hatfield. 1992). The separation process is anxiety-ridden for both parent and offspring and they both need considerable support in the process. A gradual separation is recommended which can best be accomplished while parents are still alive and vigorous.

This is not to say that there are no situations in which people with serious mental illnesses can be accommodated in parental homes. Sometimes they can find a productive role in the family that compensates for the extra burden entailed. In some subcultures family care of a disabled family member is expected and other solutions cannot easily be entertained. Such caregiving probably works best when there is an extended family to share some of the burden.

Ideally families should have a choice as to whether they wish to be direct caregivers. Whether they are caregivers by choice or necessity, however, families should have access to supportive services to lessen the burden. This might take the form of support groups, classes and workshops, or psychoeducational groups of which there are now many models from which to choose. Respite care for family members in a form that is appropriate to people with psychiatric disorders is badly needed. For family care to work effectively, providers who work with the ill person must be trained to work with the family as well. If rules of confidentiality get in the way of families being properly informed, families may have an untenable situation and may be encouraged to consider having the person move to other quarters.

ROLE OF THE FAMILY IN SERVICE DELIVERY

It is now generally recognized that relationships with families must be addressed in all service settings—hospitals, residential and rehabilitation services, crisis services, case management, and the like. The ability of families to cope effectively and the progress of the person with mental illness depend on the adequacy of these relationships. Studies show that there are still significant difficulties to overcome in this area.

How Families View Relationships with Professionals

Earlier studies indicated that families were rather consistently negative about their relationships with service providers (Hatfield, 1978, 1979. 1983; Holden & Lewine, 1979; Johnson, 1984). Apparently some professionals were unaware of the degree of dissatisfaction families were experiencing. For example, Hatfield (1983) found essentially no relationship between the kinds of help families sought and the issues that were addressed by the professionals they consulted. McElroy (1987) found significant discrepancies between families' and nurses' perceptions of difficulties faced and educational needs. Spaniol, Jung et al. (1987) surveyed families to determine their satisfaction with services and mental health professionals to determine their perception of family satisfaction. They reported that 82% of professionals thought families were satisfied with services whereas only 45% expressed overall satisfaction with services.

More recent studies suggest reasons for dissatisfaction. For example, Bernheim and Switalski (1988) surveyed inpatient and outpatient staff and families and found generally favorable attitudes toward each other and about the role of the family in the patient's treatment. Staff felt that families should be meaningfully involved, but 61% said they spent less than one hour per week in contact with the family. Staff said that conflict among themselves about the role of the family and lack of time as the greatest impediments to including families. These findings suggest that current problems are less attitudinal ones and more practical matters of knowing what role to expect from families.

Professionals are urged to "involve families" in treatment and rehabilitation, but because no basis guidelines have been forthcoming, many well motivated staff may be baffled as to how to go about this. The purpose of this section is to offer some preliminary suggestions.

Collaborative Approaches to Families

The word "collaboration" is frequently used to suggest family and provider relationships, but the word is not always used with a uniform meaning and requires definition. It is based on the fundamental democratic principle that everyone affected by a decision should have a part in making it. Collaboration means shared problem definition, shared decision making, and shared responsibility with final decisions reflecting a balance of the needs of all those involved. It means working with people rather than doing things to them.

The idea of collaboration represents a departure from traditional hierarchical relationship in which professionals maintained the balance of power and families played a more passive role. Collaboration requires a shift from therapeutic models of viewing families in which pathology or deficits are the primary concerns to competence models which focus on strengths, Finally the idea of collaboration calls for new skills in communication, problem solving. and consensus building.

Roles and Responsibilities of Families

As noted earlier, providers say that one of the barriers to involving families is their inability to agree on appropriate roles for families, In an earlier work, we have suggested four major roles for families: (1) Serving as the most important source of support for their relative with mental illness; (2) providing information about their relative; (3) monitoring services and providing feedback to providers: and (4) advocating for services.

Providers of services should be respected for the professional knowledge they possess and for the accumulated experiences of their professional lives. It is their responsibility to stay full informed about new knowledge and current research and to apply it to their respective situations. They must be able to translate their professional knowledge into a form that lay people can understand so that families can become effective participants in their relative's support and treatment planning.

Relationships between families and providers usually work best if the role of each is clearly established. Providers are hired to develop and implement programs for people with mental illnesses. Their work may be hampered if individual families become highly intrusive in program development. Providers must be the experts on program development and families the experts on their own member. Families should have input in several ways. They should help staff understand their relative, monitor his or her progress and provide feedback. Families should also serve on the advisory boards of agencies and help determine over all policy and program for the agency.

Meeting the Developmental Needs of Families

Verbal commitment to involving families is growing, but actual policy and program to carry out this commitment is generally lacking. More common are isolated efforts of well meaning providers generating an occasional activity in their agencies to address family concerns. While these sporadic efforts are to be commended they do not serve the needs of families for regularly scheduled services on which families can depend. There are duplications of efforts in some places and significant gaps in others, resulting in poor use of scarce resources.

We believe that it is time now for states to give consideration to developing a comprehensive plan for integrating the concept of family involvement in all facilities and agencies of the state. Such an effort would require an agreed upon philosophy about relating to families and a generic set of guidelines for interacting with families in all institutions and agencies. In addition there would be more specific guidelines for working with families in the various agencies in the system. These guidelines should be a collaborative effort of representatives from family groups and from staff. The focus in these agencies to a large extent would be the developmental issues families are facing at the time their relative is receiving services. Some examples might be:

Hospitals. Most families have their first contact with the mental health system in the hospital. This is usually a time of crisis and great emotional upheaval. Staff need to be fully prepared to offer the appropriate kinds of support in these circumstances. They need to be ready to respond to myriad anxious questions that families might raise: Why is my loved one behaving this way? What kind of treatment will he get? What is the prognosis? Since patient stays now tend to be brief, there must be a careful selection of information given to meet immediate needs. Families should be routinely referred to regularly scheduled classes and support groups in their local areas for further help. Of course they should be fully involved with the treatment team and in the process of discharge planning.

Community Mental Health Centers. Ideally at least one regularly scheduled family class, providing an understanding of mental illness and coping strategies, would be available each year in a local jurisdiction. For those who still feel overwhelmed by the difficulties in their families small problem solving groups might be offered for a limited time.

Case Management Service. To the degree that the consumer and his or her family prefer, families should be involved in planning for services for their relative. Since there is potential for disagreement as to what is best, the professional needs to be a skillful negotiator or consensus builder.

Residential Services. The transition from home care to residential services may entail considerable anxiety on the part of both the parent and the consumer. This marks the beginning of shifting dependence from parents to provider and learning to trust someone new. It means a changed relationship between parent and offspring with all the unknowns it entails.

Psychiatric Rehabilitation Services. When this service is being used, families are concerned about the productive side of their relative's life. Paid employment is on the minds of many parents and they need to have considerable dialogue with staff about their relatives' prospects for work and what is being done to help them. For those whose likelihood of work is limited, other productive day activities must be found.

It is not our purpose to fully describe what should be occurring in each facility and agency in regard to families, but rather to suggest that what they do may be different according to the developmental stage of the family.

THE ROLE OF FAMILIES IN RESOURCE DEVELOPMENT

The National Alliance for the Mentally Ill (NAMI) appeared on the scene a little more than a decade ago with its basic mission rather unchanged since its inception. Its major goals are clearly stated in many of their publications: Support, Education, Advocacy, and Research. Resource development has not been a stated priority. This differs from the early experiences of other kinds of parent organized groups, such as the families of retarded members, who became involved in creating housing, training facilities, and respite care.

Several arguments have been advanced by NAMI leaders as to why they deem it unwise for affiliates to invest themselves heavily in resource development. Operating a service is very time consuming and drains the energy of members that is needed to carry out major NAMI goals. They feel that it is the public sector's responsibility to provide services for the disabled and that citizen groups must work continuously to see that governmental agencies fulfill their obligations. When families see providers they may run into conflict of interest between their provider role and their advocacy function. They may find themselves beholden to the source of money for their projects—usually government on some level—and their capacity for vigorous advocacy is compromised.

When groups of families try to establish and manage a resource such as housing or a business for the mentally ill they sometimes run into serious conflicts among themselves. Families who initiate such activities often do this for the sake of their own relatives who badly need these services. However it sometimes happens that some of these relatives eventually display such disruptive behaviors that others want them leave the program. This may set up so much discord among famines that the project ultimately fails.

Nevertheless some NAMI affiliates have developed resources for people with mental illnesses without meeting major difficulties. The experience of the Alliance for the Mentally Ill of Montgomery County in Maryland is a case in point. They have operated the Threshold Thrift Shop for over ten years to raise money for their affiliate and to provide training for consumers. A second project called the Upscale/Retail Store has more recently been initiated to provide job training for people with psychiatric disabilities. There is little evidence is the experience of this group that these projects interfere with the advocacy function of the organization: People who volunteer in these shops prefer to make their contribution to AMI in this way: it gives them a stake in the organization they might not otherwise have. It is important to note that AMI of Montgomery County is a large organization with over 600 members which can have some of their members involved in service provision and still carry out the major NAMI objectives.

AMI of Montgomery County has also undertaken several housing initiatives. However, realizing the potential for conflict of interest when using public funds, they have started these projects and later incorporated them separately from their affiliates. While undertaking such projects takes time and energy, the organization gains recognition from the community and approval from some members who want concrete evidence that their organization "is doing something".

Clearly the decision to develop a service for people with mental illness should not be undertaken lightly. It is not to be recommended for all affiliates because it can absorb the energies of its members, cause conflict within the group, and compromise its ability to advocate freely. Still in some groups limited service provision may work to the advantage of the clients who need them and to the organization by providing another outlet for the interests and talents of members.

THE ROLE OF FAMILIES IN EDUCATION

Education is a stated objective of NAMI and educational activities have taken many directions. From the beginning members of NAMI have committed themselves to being as fully educated about mental illness and its treatment as possible. In earlier years some professionals expressed doubt that families could guide their own education, but few such doubts now remain. The quality of NAMI programs and materials and those on the state and local levels insure a high level of education for every interested member.

Much family education occurs in local support groups. While few question the value of support groups. there is disagreement as to whether they ought to be led by families or professionals. Initially there was a strong feeling that only families could understand the pain and suffering as well as the needs of other families and therefore a family member made the best leader. In a large part this was also due to the alienation families then felt toward professionals (Hatfield, 1981). In more recent years as professionals have gained a better understanding of families and the value of mutual support, many of them now lead support groups which families find very helpful. Nevertheless support groups continue to be a central activity of most AMI affiliates and most families in the organization get their supports there. The debate as to who should lead support groups has now largely abated.

Other educational activities such as classes and workshops are developing at a rapid rate throughout the country. Some of them are an outgrowth of the Family Education Specialist program sponsored by NAMI. The central idea of this program is to train an AMI member selected by each state affiliate to take the leadership in initiating family education programs and in training others to be family educators in their states. Family education specialists from this program are now developing their own training models of which the Journey of Hope program developed by the state affiliates of Vermont and Louisiana is a leading example (NAMI Advocate, 1993:6)

In addition to the NAMI effort in family education, professionally led programs are available in many parts of the country. For example, there is the Family Education program of Maryland (Hatfield, 1990); Coping Skills Workshop in Philadelphia (Mannion and Meisel 1989); and the Supportive Family training in New York (1989). These programs are similar in many ways, but vary somewhat in length of program and topics emphasized. There is no comparative data to suggest the adequacy of one of these models over others.

Although educational programs are relatively inexpensive compared to other approaches to working with families, it is difficult in some areas to support them. Whether given by AMI members or providers, these efforts take time and effort and need financial support by some agency to sustain them. Unfortunately this kind at service is not covered by insurance, whereas the more expensive and sometimes less acceptable individual and family therapies are billable.

THE ROLE OF THE FAMILY IN ADVOCACY AND POLICY MAKING

Few have questioned the important role that families have played in advocating for services for people with mental illnesses. The legislative agenda for NAMI develops within the organization and represents the needs of families and consumers as families perceive them. Often the organization works in coalition with other advocacy groups and with professional groups who share a similar goal. NAMI has been seen as a strong player in many major legislative achievements in the past few years—the Americans with Disabilities Act, the increase in federal research dollars for mental illness, and the return of the National Institute of Mental Health to the National Institutes of Health, to name a few of the most significant ones. It is generally granted that families can be more effective than professionals in influencing legislators because providers of services are seen to have a financial stake in the outcome.

While few question the effectiveness of NAMI on the national level and its affiliates on the state and local levels, some take issue with the position it takes on many important issues. Currently the burning issue in the changing insurance picture is how people with serious mental illnesses are to be appropriately covered. It is NAMI's position that the serious mental illnesses should be covered like any other physical illness because that is, in fact, what these illnesses are. The contrary position is that all mental health problems should have equal coverage with the serious mental illnesses. NAMI's concern is that if insurance companies are required to cover such a wide range of problems, none of them, including the serious mental illnesses, will get adequate coverage. Some question whether adjustment disorders and personal unhappiness, while they may be painful, are really illnesses and should come under the rubric of "health" problems at all. This issue will certainly become more heated as the federal government brings forth its reform package.

Roles and Relationships with Providers

From the beginning NAMI has been adamant about maintaining its autonomy from any other group that has an interest in the way services are provided. This has been particularly true of governmental agencies on all levels and of professionals who earn their living in service provision. Members of NAMI argue that the stakes of each interest group differs at least in part. AMI members may work in coalition with other groups but only after it has carefully defined its own position.

While this approach seems clear enough and should put the issue to rest, in fact, there is considerable concern that members of the organization may be coopted by service providers or governmental authorities and that they will find themselves serving an agenda other than their own. Some affiliates find they have difficulty maintaining their autonomy when they receive public money or receive support from professional organizations. Others may find themselves so warmly supported by providers that they avoid any disagreement with them lest they jeopardize this comfortable relationship. The challenge to AMI advocates is clear: they must be able to sort out their self interests from those of other interest groups and learn to make effective alliances when it is politically important for them to do so.

Roles and Relationships with Consumers

Difficult as it is for families to define appropriate relationships with providers in their advocacy work, relationships with consumer organizations are infinitely more complex. From the beginning of the NAMI movement, some consumers have raised questions as to whether families of the mentally ill should be in the business of advocacy for consumers at all. They argue that only people who have had mental illnesses are in a position of really understanding what is needed.

Family advocates offer a number of arguments as to why families should have an important roles in advocacy. They point out that only a small subset of people with serious psychiatric disabilities are well enough, or choose to be vigorously involved in advocacy. Many of the most vocal consumer advocates do not have contact with the most seriously disabled people and the positions they take on issues only reflect the interests of those who have made substantial recovery. Families, it is argued, are in contact with the full range of persons with mental illness, including those with the most serious disabilities, and are the best spokespersons for them. In addition. unlike families, consumers have failed to get involved with the more difficult issues of the mentally ill with substance abuse problems and those in jails and prisons. Finally family advocates point out there is frequent dissension within and between consumer groups. Until consumers can develop a consensus among themselves it is impossible to know what consumer positions are.

It has been emotionally troublesome for family advocates to find themselves in conflict with consumer advocates. While they acknowledge that it is the consumer who suffers most with these devastating disorders, they feel families, also, are greatly affected by them. As long as families provide the bulk of caregiving, they feel they must insist on power in decision making so that taking this responsibility is tenable for them. They also feel that consumers have not marshaled enough strength on major issues yet to suggest that they can carry the ball without the family movement.

Undoubtedly the debate between the family and consumer movement will continue. It is unlikely that either group will disappear. It is probably important to have these various perceptions represented even though it frustrates policy makers who feel that all consumer groups should speak with one voice. Increasingly consumers are joining NAMI so many issues will be threshed out within the confines of that organization. Other issues will be worked out through negotiation as various groups become more adept at consensus building, and on still other issues they will agree to disagree and, it is hoped, without acrimony.

SUMMARY AND CONCLUSIONS

The family advocacy movement is a relatively recent development in the field of mental illness. No comparable family organization nor such a high degree of family empowerment has been known before. This has raised many new issues about appropriate roles for families and how they might differ from other interest groups—service providers, policy makers, and consumers—who also have important stakes in the mental health system. We have identified a number of issues which present a profound challenge to the family movement: What should be the family role in direct caregiving? What kinds of relationships with professionals are most productive? What role should families play in providing services? Who should lead support groups and provide the education to families? What are the appropriate roles of families, providers, and consumers in advocacy? This chapter presents some of the arguments that are being advanced, but does not attempt to resolve them here. Conflict is healthy and inevitable in social movements; those presented here will be with us for a long time.

REFERENCES

Bernheim, E. & Switalski, T. Mental health staff and patients' relatives: how they view each other. Hospital and Community Psychiatry, 39, 63-68.

Dincin, J. (1975) Psychiatric rehabilitation. Schizophrenia bulletin, 15, 131-147.

Hatfield. A. (1978) Psychological costs of schizophrenia to the family. Social Work, 23, 355-359.

Hatfield, A. (1979) Help-seeking behavior in families of schizophrenia. American Journal of Community Psychology, 7, 563-569.

Hatfield, A. (1983) What families want of family therapy. In W. McFarlane (ed.) Family therapy in schizophrenia. New York: Guilford.

Hatfield, A. (1990) Family education in mental illness. New York: Guilford.

Hatfield, A. (1992) Leaving home: separation issues in psychiatric illnesses. Psychosocial Rehabilitation Journal, 15, 37-48.

Holden, D. & Lewine, R. (1982) How families evaluate mental health professionals. Schizophrenia Bulletin. 8, 628-633.

Howe, J. (1985) National Alliance for the Mentally Ill perspective. Psychosocial Rehabilitation Journal, 8, 15-18.

Johnson, D. (1984) The needs of the chronically mentally ill: As seen by the consumers. In M. Mirabi (ed.) The chronically mentally ill: Research and services. New York: Spectrum. pp. 45-56.

Lefley, H. (1987) Aging parents as caregivers of mentally ill adult children: An emerging social problem. Hospital & Community Psychiatry. 38, 1063-1070.

Le Gacy, S. (1989, July) Supportive family training: A model for family work. TIE-Lines, pp. 5-6.

Mannion, E. & Meisel, M. (1989. July) Psychoeducation: a new way of working with families. TIE-Lines. pp. 4-5.

McElroy, E. (1987) The beat of a different drummer. In A. Hatfield and H Lefley (eds.) Families of the mentally ill: Coping and adaptation.

Spaniol, L., Jung, H., & Fitzgerald, S. (1987): Families as a resource in the rehabilitation o the severely mentally ill. In A. Hatfield and H. Lefley (eds.) Families of the mentally ill: Coping and Adaptation. New York: Guilford.

Steinwachs, D., Kasper, J., & Skinner, E. (1992) Family Perspectives on Meeting the Needs for Care of Severely Mentally Ill Relatives: A National Survey. Baltimore: Johns Hopkins University, School of Hygiene and Public Health.

Torrey, E.F. (1983) Surviving schizophrenia: A family manual. New York: Harper & Row.

Chapter 5

SYSTEMS THEORY REVISITED: RESEARCH ON FAMILY EXPRESSED EMOTION AND COMMUNICATION DEVIANCE

William R. McFarlane and Ellen Lukens

Early theorists had posited several family interactional factors that appeared to them to be associated uniquely and ubiquitously with schizophrenia. The underlying assumption was that family interaction, especially in the marital pair, was disordered and that family integrity was maintained by the expression of schizophrenic symptoms in one member. This version of a systems theory of schizophrenia explicitly placed the origin of the patient's disorder in the family and its processes over time—sometimes even across generations. This had its clearest exposition in Haley and Madanes' writings (Madanes, 1983). The present chapter reviews the current literature within what we hope is a more comprehensive version of systems theory. We propose that a systems perspective demands the inclusion of variables from all relevant levels of a system before a conclusion is reached about causality.

The fundamental error of early family systems notions was that other levels were excluded from consideration, sometimes from an ideological commitment to a family-dynamic and/or psychodynamic orientation, and sometimes from a lack of awareness of research that proceeded from different assumptions, especially that dealing with the contribution of social network and other variables loosely subsumed under "societal" influences. Not considered at all were the mass of data that has documented the primary role of biological factors in the etiology and course of the illness. The perspective presented here owes much to a critical but largely ignored work by Albert Scheflen that proposed the same general viewpoint, but that was published during the height of the family systems interest in schizophrenia (Scheflen, 1981). In particular, we examine current knowledge about communication deviance and expressed emotion. These two family interactional factors have emerged as predictors of outcome and correlates of presence of schizophrenia. That makes them candidates for causative factors in the course and even onset of the disorder. However, we conclude from the available data that only a much more complex and circular model, involving mutual influence of patient symptom and behavioral factors with family behavior and communication factors, presently fits that data.

There are several areas that must be included in any discussion of family influences on the course of schizophrenia, but that we are choosing to assume a priori in the discussion that follows. In particular, a large literature has developed that documents the effects on families of stigma, burden and social isolation, all of which appear to be mainly secondary to the presence and evolution of a major psychotic disorder in a member of the family. Our view of that accumulated and remarkably unambiguous knowledge is that families are devastated by the onset of schizophrenia in their midst, forced to re-reorganize their life around the illness, suffer a significant degree of secondary stigma, usually become isolated from sources of casual, instrumental and emotional support and frequently are actually made poorer and/or physically and mentally sicker themselves by the prolonged caretaking and case managing responsibilities that most families choose to assume. This reality needs to be kept constantly in mind as one assesses the data that suggest that family interaction may influence the illness, because the opposite direction of causal influence has been extensively documented. Earlier chapters in this volume make this case, as have previous volumes and reviews (Johnson, 1990; Hatfield, 1983; Hatfield and Lefley, 1987).

COMMUNICATION DEVIANCE

An Historical Context

It was in the historical and conceptual context of the family systems movement that Margaret Singer and Lyman Wynne began reporting increasingly convincing evidence that at least one aspect of family life was disordered when schizophrenia was present. They consistently observed that interaction, or more precisely conversation, between parents of patients with schizophrenia was more likely to be "fragmented" or "amorphous" than in families without schizophrenia (Wynne, et al., 1977; Singer and Wynne, 1985). They developed a set of factors, which they termed communication deviance (CD), that described aspects of verbal interaction and, by implication, thinking processes in relatives. Analysis revealed seven factors: referent problems, commitment (e.g., to an idea or argument) problems, language anomalies, contradictory or arbitrary sequences in reasoning, and disruptions. These factors emerged from scoring of responses to presentation of Rorschach cards to parents who were asked to develop a consensus description of the various images. Clearly, this was a very different type of test than the usual Rorschach procedure; it tested the ability of the couple to acknowledge unique perspectives in the partner, communicate them clearly, resolve their differences, and integrate their individual perceptions.

From these studies, it was clear that conversation in the families in which CD was present was likely to be somewhat more fragmented and difficult to follow than in those lacking CD; they had difficulties in establishing and maintaining a shared focus of attention. Further, the consensus Rorschach procedure was a test of the family's capacity for the simultaneous validation and resolution of difference. High CD ratings implied that one or both capacities might be diminished. For instance, one type of CD involved the ignoring of actual differences and the creation of pseudo-consensus, as if the acknowledgement of differences would force the issue of the difficulty of resolution, which for a particular family might be too anxiety-provoking or simply too difficult cognitively. Another type of high-CD family might acknowledge differences, but veer into a series of non-sequiturs that prevented the sifting of possible areas of agreement and the eventual creation of consensus.

Although there was some overlap between CD and actual psychopathology, the CD variable correlated more strongly with the diagnostic category than did classic psychiatric symptoms, leading to the conclusion that CD was specific to schizophrenia and independent of psychopathology in the parents. In these families, the interactional process had many of the hallmarks of thought disorder, especially of tangential thinking, at the individual or psychological level. Implicitly, there was the possibility that this type of interaction was a risk factor, because it could conceivably prevent one or another of the offspring in the family from developing a number of specific cognitive capacities. In particular, these were capacities that involve sequencing of thought and conversation and the testing of mental constructs against external reality, especially against the opinions of others. This type of family interaction might model for children inefficient mental problem-solving, particularly when that involved other members of a natural social group.

Thus, CD was not like other family systems ideas. Singer and Wynne, unlike family theorists of their time, remained circumspect in their interpretation of these findings. First, the authors refused to assume that it was the sole factor in the development of the disorder, and secondly, if it was, it was not really a family systems process. In fact it was more precisely a simple linear cause and effect model, or a risk factor among others. The fact that there was a remarkable similarity between family CD and patient thought disorder implied another logical possibility: perhaps both phenomena were the result of inherited defects in information processing. That is, there could be genetically mediated deficiencies in, for example, attentional functioning that could be expressed in a subclinical form as CD in relatives and as full-blown thought disorder in patients with schizophrenia. That concept was at the opposite end of the intellectual spectrum from family systems ideas, because it implied that all members of the family were victims of their own genetic constitution. It also implied that during development, the offspring were in a situation of cognitive double jeopardy: a subtle form of brain dysfunction might predispose them to a variety of attentional and cognitive difficulties, while the conversational milieu in which they were learning methods of information processing included tendencies for poor closure, vagueness and tangentiality.

Also, the genetic vulnerability concept was distinguished from family systems theories because it lent itself to testing, using relatively conventional methods, even available tests of cognitive functioning. One criticism of the theory that symptoms are stabilizing a more pervasively dysfunctional family interactional system has been the difficulty in validly and rigorously testing the hypothesis. The genetic vulnerability concept was also more attractive to clinicians who spent a great deal of time with families, because it fit better their observations that most families with a schizophrenic member do not appear to be grossly dysfunctional and often improve interactionally as the patient's symptoms and general functioning improve. Those clinical insights have been confirmed by recent experience in studies of family educational and training strategies (see Chapter 11). Families have responded not only with improvements in family emotional climate and gratitude for the support and education, but also for the symptomatic and functional improvement that they observe in their affected relatives. Oddly, the best confirmation of earlier theories would have been the systematic failure of attempts to help families manage and adapt to schizophrenia.

The Present State of Knowledge

Although the questions of the genetic basis for CD and its possible role as a risk factor are far from resolved, much progress in our empirical understanding has occurred in the intervening years. The existing literature has confirmed that CD is indeed a characteristic of a significant proportion of families with a schizophrenic member. In the following section, that literature is reviewed with regard to several other key questions. The first is whether it can be found before the onset of the illness, as a control for the possibility that CD is induced in family interaction by the presence of an individual family member with schizophrenia. The second is whether its presence predicts later emergence of schizophrenic or other psychiatric or functional disorders. The third is whether CD is found in families with younger children and, if present, what clinical phenomena are associated with it. The fourth issue is whether CD can be found in other syndromes and in other cultures, a key to resolving whether it or any family characteristic is uniquely associated with schizophrenia and thereby a candidate for a specific and unitary etiologic factor. The fifth is whether CD is associated with cognitive and attentional dysfunction, with the implication that it is indeed related to biologically-based and probably inherited brain abnormalities in both patients and relatives. The sixth issue relates to the diagnostic subtype specificity of CD: does a family interactional factor correlate with any particular type of schizophrenia? Finally, we examine the relationship of CD to other family interactional factors, especially expressed emotion.

1. Is CD present before the onset of psychosis? The clearest evidence that parental CD is not simply the result of overt psychotic symptoms in a child is the UCLA High-Risk Project, conducted by Goldstein and colleagues. This ambitious study followed 54 of 64 recruited and eligible index offspring from adolescence well into the age of risk for onset of schizophrenia (mean age = 30), having assessed parents and the index adolescents for family CD, expressed emotion (EE) and the study's measure of family emotional interaction, affective style (AS). AS differed from EE primarily in the test format: in AS assessments, the family members were asked to discuss a controversial subject for that family with the index adolescent present, whereas in EE assessment, the patient was absent and the relatives were asked to describe and discuss the index person. The adolescents were recruited from a population of 16-year-olds presenting for treatment at a psychiatric clinic for typical behavioral and symptomatic disorders. However, all those presenting with psychosis were excluded from the study. The adolescents' behavioral profiles were assessed and categorized. The original hypothesis was that psychopathology at follow-up would prove to be a function of the form of the adolescent's original problem and the parental attributes; that is, CD, AS and EE.

2. Does CD predict the onset of psychosis? At follow-up, at five and 15 years later, only the second element of the hypothesis was confirmed: family interaction predicted emergence of schizophrenia in the index offspring, but the adolescents' behavioral and symptomatic profile at baseline did not. More precisely, a construct that included CD, AS and EE predicted the emergence of schizophrenia *spectrum* disorders in *any* offspring in a given family (Goldstein, 1985; 1987). Further, the same construct predicted poor quality of intimate relationships in adulthood, independently of the emergence of psychotic symptoms, but it did not predict other dimensions of adult social functioning (Doane, et al., 1982; Doane and Mintz, 1987). None of the three family interactional factors predicted outcome alone. This carefully conducted study demonstrates that some characteristics of family interaction predate the onset of an acute and initial episode of schizophrenia. In so doing, these results satisfy one of the criteria for concluding that CD, EE or AS plays a causative role in the development of a disorder. However, they also leave ambiguous the more crucial issue: the influence of these factors on the development of the behavioral/symptomatic profile and dysfunctions with which these adolescents presented prior to the assessment of parental interaction. That is, it is possible that the development of difficulties in the index offspring was either the cause or the result of the family interaction. In fact, it is possible that the relationship was bi-directional or circular: the behavioral/symptomatic profile led to deterioration in family interaction, which in turn precipitated further exacerbation of the offspring's dysfunction. Of course, a rigorous and conclusive resolution of this conundrum would require a follow-along study that began, ideally, prior to conception and went to the end of the onset-risk period. Such a forbidding undertaking is unlikely to occur in the near future. Therefore, we turn to more recent research to attempt to fill in some of the intervening gaps in knowledge.

3. Is CD found in families of younger children? One implicit question is whether CD appears in the families of younger children prior to the onset of even non-psychotic behavioral disorders. Doane and her colleagues measured CD in three different settings in the parents of boys aged seven to ten (Doane, et al., 1982). When mothers manifested CD across two or three settings their sons were functioning poorly as judged by teachers, peers and parents. Importantly, one of the settings was an individual Rorschach procedure, in which CD and parental thought disorder become difficult to distinguish. In a similar study, Fisher and Jones (1980) examined school competence of 65 children. They found that the social-emotional domain was correlated linearly and only with parental CD, whereas problem-solving was related to three factors: CD, non-acknowledgement and clear communication, all parental variables. Ditton and Green (1987) studied the relationship of parental CD and learning disability. They compared 30 learning-disabled children to 30 average students, after their parents were scored for CD on an interactional task. CD scores correlated highly significantly to the presence or absence of learning disability. More recently, Asarnow, Goldstein and Ben-Meir (1988) found that parental CD was significantly higher in parents of childhood-onset schizophrenia and schizotypal disorder than in parents of children with major depression and dysthymic disorders. Within the schizophrenia-spectrum children, there was a correlation between parental CD scores and both severity of impairment and attentional functioning. Few of the schizophrenia-spectrum children had low CD parents. Greenwald (1989) found correlations between parental CD and adaptive functioning and IQ three years later, in children at risk for psychiatric disorder by virtue of parental prior psychiatric hospitalization. Here again, parental CD predicted social-emotional and cognitive functioning in the offspring at risk. These studies rather conclusively demonstrate that CD occurs in the families of young children. Further, they provide evidence that CD is associated with poor social functioning and cognitive dysfunction, especially in the children of psychiatric patients, and is more severe in families in which there are children with early-onset schizophrenia-spectrum disorders.

4. *Is CD found in other disorders and other cultures?* Until recently, CD has been associated only with schizophrenia. That relationship appeared to establish this factor as the only potential candidate for a specific etiologic or risk factor. However, a study of CD in schizophrenia and mania (Miklowitz et al., 1991) demonstrated that there was no difference between parents of patients with either psychotic disorder. Instances of odd word usage were actually higher in the families of manic patients. There were more ambiguous references made by parents of schizophrenic patients. Furthermore, CD is apparently not culture-bound. Mexican-American parents of schizophrenic patients had nearly identical levels of CD to those of a carefully matched sample of English-speaking Americans. Factor sub-scores also did not distinguish the two cultural and language cohorts.

5. *and 6. Is CD associated with any specific subtype of schizophrenia and cognitive dysfunction?* One study supporting the hypothesis that CD is a heritable cognitive disorder determined that non-paranoid patients manifested cognitive disturbance, while paranoid patients did not (Rund and Blakar, 1986). The non-paranoid patients had parents with

more CD than the parents of the paranoid patients. The cognitive impairments were primarily attentional dysfunctions. Similarly, Sass and colleagues (1984) found a correlation between high parental CD and high levels of formal thought disorder in schizophrenic offspring. They also noted that paranoid patients without thought disorder had parents whose CD scores were in the same range as normals' parents. Wagener and colleagues (1986) directly addressed the relationship of parental cognitive functioning. They gave the subjects and their mothers the Continuous Performance Test and the Span of Apprehension Task to assess attention and information processing capacity. Performance by the patient on the SAT was significantly related to both the mother's SAT performance and CD factor scores. Mothers' CD scores were associated with their performance on both CPT and SAT. Patients' CPT scores were not related to maternal CPT or interactional factors. The SAT findings support the assumption that attentional difficulties might underlie both parental CD and patient thought disorder in schizophrenia, and that the connection is rooted in a common genetic substrate.

Whether or not that is the case, there is now abundant evidence that parental CD seems to be associated with and even predicts learning disabilities, formal thought disorder and attentional dysfunction in children and adults across some diagnostic categories. However, the correlational studies need replication and more longitudinal studies are needed to determine whether the inter-generational relationships are causal at the interactional level, or whether CD and attentional measures are in fact assessing the same cognitive deficits. The double-jeopardy hypothesis—that interaction that is vague and/or fragmented is more likely to occur in families in which there is a child who has significant impairment in cognitive function, leading to a multiplicative risk for attentional dysfunction and thought disorder—remains a distinct possibility.

7. Is CD related to expressed emotion? The final question is the relationship between CD and expressed emotion, the latter being a well-researched factor, reviewed extensively later in this chapter, that has predicted relapse in patients with schizophrenia. The data are sparse, but a study by Miklowitz and colleagues (1986) found that there was a strong association between high CD scores and the emotional over-involvement component of EE, as measured by the Camberwell Family Interview. The investigators saw the overlap as possibly being secondary to the stressful effects of living with a relative who is highly symptomatic and/or recently psychotic. Here again, one can posit a circular causal process in which symptoms in the patient induce in other family members stress and anxiety, which then leads to more fragmented or ambiguous communication and induces more parental preoccupation and hyper-vigilance. These rather natural parental reactions could readily induce further clinical deterioration in the schizophrenic member, and a spiralling, deteriorating process could ensue. From the perspective of the parent, it is likely that the prospect of a deteriorating adult child could be expected to lead to confusion, anxiety and ambiguous responses and attitudes. The fact that some studies show that these kinds of processes occur in childhood suggests that they can persist over long periods and may constitute a risk factor for both patients and family members. The fact that 30% of the sample were low on total EE ratings and that only 16% of the entire sample manifested the combination of high emotional overinvolvement and high CD suggests that this process can only worsen the course of schizophrenia and not induce it by itself. It is far from being as ubiquitous as would be necessary to ascribe to it a sole-causal influence.

EXPRESSED EMOTION AND ITS INFLUENCE ON THE COURSE OF ILLNESS

The Original Research Work and Refinement of the Construct

In 1958, Brown and Rutter, a sociologist and psychiatrist, respectively, collaborating in London, England, began to focus extensively on the course of mental illness, particularly schizophrenia. They hypothesized that differing social environments would affect relapse rates among patients released from the hospital, and found that those who returned to live with parents or in large boarding homes had worse outcomes than those who lived elsewhere. The question as to why this should be remained open.

In 1962, Brown conducted a similar study with a group of adult males suffering from schizophrenia. His hypotheses were first, that patients would deteriorate and relapse if they returned to a home setting where there was strongly expressed emotion of any kind; and second, that even if the patient returned home, relapse could be avoided if the amount of contact with family members was kept low. For the purpose of this and subsequent work Brown defined relapse as either the reappearance of the positive symptoms of schizophrenia in a patient free of them at discharge from index admission, or a marked exacerbation of persistent psychotic symptoms (Brown et al., 1972). To measure the kind of relationship between family member and patient, Brown used five measures, including amount of emotion, hostility, and dominant or directive behavior by the relative toward the patient, and emotion and hostility expressed by the patient toward his or her relative.

Brown and his colleagues (Brown & Rutter, 1966; Rutter & Brown, 1966) subsequently refined the measures for the components of expressed emotion, dropping those reflecting patient attitudes because of lack of findings and retaining those which have been measured in many subsequent studies and described in this chapter (i.e. criticism, overinvolvement, and warmth). They defined the social environment of the family in terms of this so-called "showering of affect". This refined construct was comprised of eight scales including a) number of critical comments toward the patient, b) severity of criticism, c) hostility, d) dissatisfaction, e) warmth, f) number of positive comments, g) emotional overinvolvement, and h) an overall index of relative's expressed emotion. The ratings for criticism were based on both an actual count of statements judged to be critical because of tone of voice *and/or* content (i.e. a clear statement of either resentment, disapproval, or dislike), as well as an overall measure of harshness of content. Hostility was rated as either present or absent and included rejecting statements regarding the individual as a person. Dissatisfaction included a series of four point scales and an overall index measuring eight areas of family life such as irritability, quarreling, leisure activity, and communication within the household. Warmth was represented in terms of a six point scale which included sympathy and concern, interest and appreciation of the individual as a person, and shared enjoyment in mutual activities. Overinvolvement was also rated on a six-point scale and reflected a combined measure of overprotection, intrusiveness, control, and general anxiety regarding the patient. The overall index for expressed emotion reflected a high count on critical comments (i.e. seven or more), or a high score on overinvolvement, or the presence of high levels of hostility. These scales were measured by a series of common sense signs and observable behaviors which included tone of voice and manner of presentation, reported behavior, observed behavior, and content of speech. Information was gathered during a lengthy (five or six hour) interview which has become known as the Camberwell Family Interview (CFI). The main goal in this semi-structured interview was to encourage the respondent to express him or herself in ways that represented inner feelings and attitudes regarding the patient in the three months prior to interview.

Brown made the assumption throughout that expressed emotion was an indirect way of assessing the emotional climate of a family over time. However he was careful to state that "the measure reflects a quality of relationship with a particular person (the patient), not a general tendency to react to everyone in a similar way" (Brown, 1972, p 246).

The results were noteworthy. Levels of expressed emotion and hostility of key family members were both related to the likelihood of relapse during the follow-up period. Moreover, the patients who did most poorly had family members who were most expressive in terms of affect. The patient's own level of expressed emotion and hostility toward the family was not related to relapse.

In 1972, Brown, Birley and Wing modified this study somewhat, interviewing only key family members in what was still a five or six hour interview. They wanted to test the hypothesis that a high degree of expressed emotion among relatives would cause relapse among patients, independent of length of illness, type of symptoms, or kind of behavior during the year prior to index admission (i.e. work impairment, aggressive or delinquent behavior, or social withdrawal). They used a prospective design in which past behaviors, emotional response among relatives, and relapse were measured independently.

Not surprisingly, Brown and his colleagues found that hostility and criticism were highly related to each other and negatively related to warmth, that overinvolvement was positively related to warmth, that only about half of those described as warm were also described as overinvolved and that those rated either markedly high or low on overinvolvement tended to be more critical or hostile.

In these early studies, the authors focussed on relapse among first episode as well as chronic patients and found that criticism, hostility, and overinvolvement were related to the relapse of positive symptoms, particularly among males. During the nine months after discharge from a psychiatric hospitalization, 58% of the patients from families described as high in expressed emotion relapsed as compared with only 16% in the low expressed emotion group (p < .001). This association was independent of the patients' history of either behavioral or work disturbance. Ratings of expressed emotion among the patients were much less frequent than among relatives and showed no relationship to relapse.

In a replication, Vaughn (1976) used the results of a content analysis to shorten the Camberwell interview to two to three hours and obtained comparable results using only three of the original components of expressed emotion. Based on Brown's findings, she limited the expressed emotion scales to number of critical comments, hostility (again strongly correlated with criticism), and high overinvolvement. She found that two factors, regular medication and reduced familial contact, served to mediate between the measure of expressed emotion and relapse over a nine month period.

She subsequently replicated the study in metropolitan Los Angeles where street drugs complicated the course of treatment and overall outcome of patients suffering from schizophrenia (Vaughn et al., 1984). In spite of this, findings were consistent: relapse of routine symptoms was high among male patients in households characterized by high levels of expressed emotion. Nonetheless it was also clear in these studies that expressed emotion was not the only factor contributing to relapse among the samples since a substantial percent of the patients from the high expressed emotion families did not relapse during the follow-up period.

Cross Cultural Studies

Karno and Jenkins (Karno et al., 1987; Jenkins & Karno, 1992) provided a cross cultural replication of the work on expressed emotion and relapse among low-income Mexican Americans in Los Angeles. They found that high expressed emotion among key family members significantly increased the rate of relapse during a nine month follow-up period among patients suffering from schizophrenia who returned to live at home after an acute hospitalization. However they found a significantly lower rate of high expressed emotion at baseline among the relatives of Mexican descent when compared to their American counterparts. In a separate study conducted in Chandigarh India by Leff and his colleagues (Leff et al., 1987; Wig et al., 1987) among first admission patients, relatively low levels of expressed emotion were reported compared to other studies but high EE, particularly hostility, was still associated with relapse. A reasonable conclusion, in conjunction with general findings that schizophrenia follows a more benign course in developing countries than in developed countries, is that the prevalence of high expressed emotion is determined by cultural, geographic and socioeconomic factors, although it is a major stressor in diverse cultural settings.

The Validity of the Construct

The predictive validity of expressed emotion in relationship to the relapse of the overt psychotic symptoms of schizophrenia over time has been relatively well established in various countries and with various ethnic groups (Brown et al., 1972; Vaughn & Leff, 1976; Vaughn et al., 1984; Moline et al., 1985; Karno et al., 1987; Tarrier et al., 1988; Neuchterlein et al., 1986; Leff et al., 1987). However several studies failed to replicate this finding (Kottgen et al., 1984; Macmillan et al.,

1986; Parker & Johnson, 1987). Kottgen's work has been criticized by Vaughn (1986) for methodological error and because his intervention was an analytically based group treatment (Hogarty et al., 1986). Macmillan (1986) found that expressed emotion and duration of mental illness were both significant predictors of relapse alone, but that duration emerged as the significant predictor in a multivariate analysis, a finding that was not replicated in a study conducted by Nuechterlein and colleagues (1989). In contrast, Parker and Johnston (1987) found that a poor course after hospitalization was best predicted by poor course prior to hospitalization and by living with one parent, rather than by any measure of expressed emotion. In Brown and Vaughn's early work, the predictive power of the construct of expressed emotion remained intact after controlling for symptom patterns, work impairment, severity of behavioral disturbance, duration of illness, age, and premorbid adjustment (Brown & Rutter, 1966; Vaughn & Leff, 1976). Although past impairment and history or disturbed behavior were strongly correlated with relapse, these associations tended to disappear when examined in conjunction with the relative's expressed emotion. Other studies have been less conclusive in terms of control variables. These contradictory findings suggest that 1) sorting out the contributions of various kinds of symptoms to duration of illness, and 2) identifying those characteristics of patients upsetting to family members are key to understanding the relationship between family behavior and patient symptoms.

Findings regarding the relationship between gender and expressed emotion have been more equivocal (Brown et al., 1958, 1962; Hogarty et al., 1986). In his original studies Brown found that the strength of expressed emotions as a predictor variable held only for male patients. In commenting on this finding, Brown speculated that the level of EE in families of male patients probably had to do with the higher expectation placed on male offspring. In a later review of the original studies by Brown, by Vaughn (Vaughn & Leff, 1976; Vaughn et al., 1984) and his own work, Hogarty also found that the expressed emotion variable had only been substantiated as a predictor of relapse for male patients.

Leff and his colleagues evaluated expressed emotion in relationship to psychophysiological studies of the autonomic nervous system (Sturgeon et al., 1984; Tarrier et al., 1988). Using galvanic skin response as a measure both during an acute episode of schizophrenia and during remission, recordings were made with patients alone and then with a relative present. When tested alone patients from high and low expressed emotion homes could not be differentiated. These non-specific responses decreased significantly when a low expressed emotion relative was present but remained high in the presence of a high expressed emotion relative. This was corroborated by the fact that the patients with high expressed emotion relatives described themselves as significantly more tense during the exercise while those with low expressed emotion relatives described a decrease in tension after the relative entered the room. This suggests that low expressed emotion relatives may provide active support as well as non-threatening behavior and a calming presence.

Specificity of the Construct

Other studies have indicated that the phenomenon of expressed emotion is not specific to families in which a patient is suffering from schizophrenia. Research has also been conducted in which the primary diagnosis is depression (Vaughn & Leff, 1976; Hooley et al., 1986), bipolar illness (Miklowitz, 1986; 1988), developmental disability (Greedharry, 1987), and anorexia nervosa (Szmukler et al., 1985). This implies that the expressed emotion scales are valuable in describing certain aspects of family life which are related to both the course and prognosis in a range of psychiatric and related illnesses.

Sources of Expressed Emotion

Patients' symptoms and behavior. In their original work Brown et al (1962) postulated that high expressed emotion was derived from response to disturbed past or current behavior, in part from personality, and in part from the interaction between attitudes toward the patient and the developing illness (especially when there is poor or deteriorating social performance). Given this, it is important to understand how changes in family attitude relate to changes in a patient's ongoing clinical state and outcome. The evidence as to whether expressed emotion is state specific or a stable trait over time is mixed since the rating tends to be lower after the patient's psychotic symptoms improve (Brown et al., 1972; Leff et al., 1982; Dulz & Hand, 1986; Koenigsberg, 1986; Hogarty et al., 1986). In some families expressed emotion may be a situation-specific response while in others it may be a stable trait. Expressed emotion may be simply a response to relapse rather than a cause. There is no study associating relapse with a later expression of expressed emotion so it is unclear as to whether expressed emotion precedes the patient's disturbance and contributes to a florid exacerbation or the behavior triggers high expressed emotion in the household (Falloon, 1988; Bland, 1989). Such a study would add clarity to the much argued question as to whether expressed emotion is derived principally from the relatives' own character structure or induced by particular aspects of a patients premorbid or ill behavior (Koenigsberg, 1986; Mintz, 1987). In the studies conducted by Leff and his colleagues (Leff et al., 1982; 1989), fifty to eighty percent of those rated as high in criticism at baseline were rated as low in criticism nine months after intervention, although in fifteen percent the criticism decreased without intervention. In contrast, overinvolvement scores were generally stable over time, in spite of interventions.

The Components of Expressed Emotion

In addition to the work on relapse and intervention, some attention has also been paid to how expressed emotion and its components (i.e. criticism and overinvolvement) are differentially associated with individual kinds of symptoms as well as with relapse per se. It has been consistently found that patients from high and low expressed emotion households are not significantly different in a clinical sense; that is, they can not be distinguished in terms of premorbid adjustment, severity of psychopathology on admission, or residual symptoms after discharge. As discussed earlier, findings regarding the correlation between high expressed motion and duration of illness are less clear (Miklowitz et al., 1973; Macmillan, 1986; Nuechterlein et al., 1986).

In the early work of Goldstein and others on expressed emotion, no relationship was found between positive symptoms and either low or high expressed emotion (i.e. criticism and overinvolvement combined). Other investigators have supported this finding (Goldstein et al., 1978; Vaughn and Leff, 1976; Miklowitz et al., 1983; Vaughn et al.,1984; Nuechterlein et al., 1986). Brown's early work (Brown et al., 1972) suggested that the level of familial expressed emotion was independent of a patient's clinical condition at baseline but that there was a strong association between expressed emotion and such patient characteristics as work impairment and other disturbed behaviors during the year preceding admission. Hogarty (Hogarty et al., 1986) found a strong relationship between a patient's inappropriate or bizarre behavior (considered a positive symptom) and the level of overall expressed emotion among family members.

These outcomes were more ambiguous when expressed emotion was divided into subcategories of highly overinvolved and highly critical families. The findings on emotional overinvolvement appear to be relatively consistent. For example Goldstein and Miklowitz found that patients from families described as emotionally overinvolved had significantly higher positive symptoms than patients from families described as critical, although not significantly higher than those from low expressed emotion families (Goldstein et al., 1978; Miklowitz et al., 1983; Mujica et al., (1991). They also found that families showed higher levels of overinvolvement if the patient had a history of poor premorbid adjustment and social withdrawal (traditionally considered a negative symptom) and if these symptoms persisted over time. This result was indirectly supported by Mujica et al (1991) who found that a small group of acutely ill patients who showed high levels of anhedonia and asociality at a given point in time tended to have parents with high levels of emotional overinvolvement and low numbers of critical comments.

Attribution by Families

In a study of the relationship between attribution and expressed emotion, Brewin and his colleagues (1991) found that families who attributed the illness to factors external to the patient tended to be overinvolved, while those who viewed the patient as the cause of his or her behavior tended to be critical. In the work by Miklowitz and Goldstein (1983), criticism tended to be associated with higher premorbid functioning and fewer residual symptoms over time. Earlier findings (Brown et al., 1972; Miklowitz et al., 1978; Vaughn et al., 1984; Leff et al., 1987) had also supported this association. In his work, Mujica (Mujica et al., 1991) found that critical comments towards patients were associated with severity of formal thought disorder. The implication here is that criticism may reflect a tendency for parents to react with disappointment to a child of whom more was originally expected and who is less blatantly disabled.

In a recent study Glynn and her colleagues (Glynn et al., 1990) reported that 26 male patients from critical households had higher ratings for positive symptoms, anxious depression, and general psychopathology when compared to a control group of 14 male patients in low expressed emotion families. The number of critical comments was associated with patient's level of thought disorder (in particular, delusions), anxious depression, and anhedonia/asociality. There was no support for a relationship between criticism and other negative symptoms.

In contrast, a relationship between criticism and longstanding interpersonal deficits has also been observed, particularly when these deficits are not attributed to the illness process. In two separate content analyses of the Camberwell Family Interview (Vaughn, 1977; Runions & Prudo, 1983), the findings suggested that critical parents tended to focus on negative personality traits rather than on florid psychotic symptoms.

Vaughn and Leff (1981) later observed that critical responses seemed to be related to negative symptoms as well as to the relapse of the positive symptoms. Based on clinical observation, Beels and McFarlane (1982) also described the tendency for families to criticize withdrawal, lack of motivation and poor hygiene among patients (all considered negative symptoms). Mintz (1989) explored the relationship between criticism and increasing dysfunction on the part of the patient as measured by certain negative symptoms, particularly apathy, inertia, and lack of affection. He argued that exposure to these kinds of symptoms might lead to increasing criticism among parents, and in turn, decreased mastery on the part of the patient might exacerbate that criticism. However, Vaughn (1986) observed that when family members expressed little emotion of any kind (to the point that they appear to have no expectations for the patient), there seemed to be an increase in negative symptoms and in social impairment in particular.

In recent work, Vaughn (1989) described members of families characterized as low in expressed emotion as believing that the patient suffers from a genuine illness, allowing them to combine objective empathy with tolerance of disturbed behavior and an increased ability to remain calm during a crisis. Koenigsberg's (1986) description of low expressed emotion included respect for the patient's desire for privacy and distance, and tolerance of odd or unusual behaviors. But he also noted that although the low expressed emotion family may have a calming influence on a patient's positive symptoms, the price might be an increased tendency toward withdrawal and apathy on the part of the patient for lack of stimulation.

More Complex Models of the Roots of Expressed Emotion

Other interpretations of the relationship between patient and family behavior are also possible. For example, in an interesting reinterpretation of the expressed emotion literature, Greenley (1986) described expressed emotion as a coping behavior and form of social control, i.e. as a means of attempting to influence the patient's behavior in a particular way. He presented two hypotheses: 1) that families who express fear and anxiety regarding the patient would be more likely to express high levels of criticism and overinvolvement; and 2) that such relationship would be modified depending on whether the family attributes the patient's behavior to a "real" illness. In a sample of 101 patients and families from Brown's original data set, Greenley found that the relationship between expressed emotion and relapse was statistically significant and that this particular relationship was strong regardless of how the family perceived the patient's problem. However, when he addressed his own hypotheses, he found that both were supported: first, that family fears and anxiety were positively and significantly associated with expressed emotion in the total sample; and second, that when patients were viewed as not ill, the relationship between fear and anxiety and with expressed emotion was significant, but when viewed as ill, there was little or no relationship with either set of variables.

As Greenley concluded, understanding expressed emotion as a form of social control has important theoretical implications for better understanding the concept of expressed emotion. First, people with schizophrenia may be unusually sensitive to particular types of social control such as criticism and overinvolvement. Further, since social control is viewed as a form of coping, it should be sensitive to changes in the patient's symptoms, and not necessarily a stable attribute of the family. Such social control behaviors could also interact with family characteristics such as family structure or other demographic variables. Moreover, the families' perception of the patient as truly ill should increase as the patient receives psychiatric care, and certainly, by implication, if the family is exposed to even minimal education about the illness over time.

A team of researchers at UCLA has refined our understanding further by attempting to determine if EE represents a transactional process in which parental and offspring/patient behaviors influence each other reciprocally. Cook and colleagues (1989) found that disturbed adolescents had a more oppositional style and their mothers higher ratings of EE than in low-EE, less oppositional parent-child pairs. In the low-EE families, the adolescents had more temporal stability of affect than in the high-EE families. The mothers' EE ratings reflected their tendency to reciprocate the behaviors shown them by their adolescent offspring. The authors concluded that there was a bi-directional process, which is one logical possibility when cross-sectional factors are found to correlate (Cousins and Power, 1986). A similar conclusion arose from another study, in which externalizing or internalizing behavior manifested by schizophrenic patients was associated with high-EE scores in parents, while autonomous or neutral behaviors were associated with low-EE (Strachan et al., 1989). This pattern held over time, even when parental EE scores changed spontaneously from high to low. Data suggested that some patient behavior reflected *former* EE ratings and might be slower to change in response to "improvements" made by relatives. Unfortunately, no study completed to date allows us to clearly identify a transactional process; the data only implies that this is one highly plausible alternative among a narrowing set of possibilities.

CONCLUSION

It is premature to draw final conclusions from the body of research reviewed here. It is clearly in an intermediate stage of development. However, some lessons can be drawn. The first is that proposed in the introduction: it seems highly unlikely that [1] family dysfunction is widespread among those with schizophrenia, [2] that more circum-scribed aspects of family interaction, expressed emotion and communi-cation deviance are unique and ubiquitous, and that [3] these factors cause schizophrenia. However, it is also clear that EE does predict poorer outcome across, and CD is associated with, several psychiatric disorders. What we propose is that the influence of these factors on course and outcome must be examined within a comprehensive systems paradigm in which biological and societal or social network factors are seen as determinants of family responses, at least as much as family interaction is seen as a determinant of patient response. Thus, CD may arise from a common and heritable disorder of attention and information-process-ing, which sets offspring up for being at risk from both biological and social influences during development and on a day-to-day basis after the onset of the manifest disorder. Similarly, the burdens, stigma and isolation may influence the expressed emotion and coping capacities of family members as may patient behavior in itself.

These kinds of hypotheses are possible within a full systems perspec-tive, which also will imply that intervention at any level—via medication or social skills training, to control symptoms and ameliorate disturbing behavior; family psychoeducation, to reduce confusion and misattribu-tion; multiple family groups, to alleviate isolation and stigma and to develop coping strategies collectively; and community education, to reduce stigma and open more rehabilitation possibilities—is likely to enhance outcome. In these interventions, improvements in family com-munication and coping skills serve as intervening variables, although those improvements could be derivative of other interventions at other system levels. One example of an application of this type of paradigm is a clozapine-oriented multiple family group format recently developed at the first author's hospital. In that model family education is linked to treating patients with a more effective antipsychotic medication which for some patients leads to dramatic improvements in social skills and motivation. The family groups then focus on both countering the some-what destabilizing effects on families of such rapid change, and then helping families develop coping strategies to capitalize on those improvements in service of more rapid and more successful rehabilitation. Rather than "finding the nodal interactional sequence", we are simply intervening at every available level and opportunity, with the intention of achieving at least an additive effect, if not some degree of synergy.

Unlike in family systems interventions, it has been our experience that families not only understand the basis for this kind of work, but appear to appreciate the improvements that occur for them in affective and communicational aspects of interactions with their ill relative. We propose that early family theories failed simply because they were not systemic enough to incorporate the actual complexity of the family with a mentally ill person and to then go on and design acceptable and effective strategies for providing assistance. It seems to us that, happily, that era is now behind us.

REFERENCES

Asarnow, J. , Goldstein, M., & Ben-Meir, S. (1988). Parental communication deviance in childhood onset schizophrenia spectrum and depressive disorders. *J. Child. Psychol. Psychiatry.*, 29 (6), 825-38.

Beels, C., McFarlane W. (1983). Thoughts on family therapy and schizophrenia, in W.R. McFarlane (ed): *Family Therapy in Schizophrenia.* New York, Guilford Press, pp 17-40.

Bland, R. (1989). Understanding family variables in outcome research in schizophrenia. *Aust. New Zeal. J. Psychiatr.*, 23, 396-402.

Brewin, C. MacCarthy, B. Duda, K., & Vaughn, C. (1991). Attribution and expressed emotion in the relative of patients with schizophrenia. *J. Abn. Psych.*, 100, 546-554.

Brown, G.W., Rutter M. (1966). The measurement of family activities and relationships. *Human Rel.* 19, 241-263.

Brown, G., Birley J, Wing J. (1972). Influence of family life on the course of schizophrenic disorders: A replication. *Br J Psychiatr*, 121, 241-258.

Brown, G.W., Monck, E.M., Carstairs, G.M. & Wing, J.K. (1958). Influence of family life on the course of schizophrenic illness. *Br. J. Soc. Med.*, 16, 55-68.

Cook, W.L., Strachan, A., Goldstein, M., & Miklowitz, D. (1989). Expressed emotion and reciprocal affective relationships in families of disturbed adolescents. *Fam. Proc.*, 28, 337-348.

Cousins, P., & Power, T. (1986). Quantifying family process: issues in the analysis of interaction sequences. *Fam. Proc.*, 25, 89-105.

Ditton, P. , & Green, R. M. (1987). Communication deviances: A comparison between parents of learning-disabled and normally achieving students. *Fam. Proc.*, *26*, 75-87.

Doane, J. , Jones, J., Fisher, L., Ritzler, B., Singer, M., & Wynne, L. (1982). Parental communication deviance as a predictor of competence in children at risk for adult psychiatric disorder. *Fam. Process.*, *21* (2), 211-23.

Doane, J., & Mintz, J. (1987). Communication deviance in adolescence and adulthood: A longitudinal study. *Psychiatry.*, *50*(1), 5-13.

Dulz, B. & Hand, I. (1986). Short-term relapse in young schizophrenics: can it be predicted and affected by family (CFI), patient and treatment variables? In M. Goldstein, K. Hand, & K. Hahlweg (Eds.), *Treatment of Schizophrenia: Family Assessment and Intervention.* (pp. 85-96). Berlin, Springer Press.

Falloon, I. (1988). Expressed emotion: Current status (Editorial). *Psychol. Med. , 18*, 269-274.

Fisher, L. , & Jones, J. (1980). Child competence and psychiatric risk. II. Areas of relationship between child and family functioning. *J. Nerv. Ment. Dis.*, *168*(6), 332-7.

Glynn, S., Randolph, E., Eth, S., Paz, G., Leona, G., Shaner, A., & Strachan, A. (1990). Patient psychopathology and expressed emotion in schizophrenia. *Br. J. Psychiatr.*, *157*, 887-890.

Goldstein, M. , Rodnick, E., Evans, J., May, P., & Steinberg, M. (1978). Drug and family therapy in the aftercare treatment of acute schizophrenia. *Arch. Gen. Psychiatr.*, *35*, 1169-1177.

Goldstein, M. (1985). Family factors that antedate the onset of schizophrenia and related disorders: The results of a fifteen year prospective longitudinal study. *Acta. Psychiatr. Scand. Suppl.*, *319*, 7-18.

Goldstein, M. (1987). The UCLA highrisk project. *Schizophr Bull.*, *13*(3), 505-14.

Greedharry, R. (1987). Expressed emotion in the families of the mentally handicapped: a pilot study. *Br. J. Psychiatr.*, *150*, 400-402.

Greenley, J. (1986). Social control and expressed emotion. *J. Nerv. Ment. Dis.*, *174*(1), 24-30.

Greenwald, D. (1989). Family interaction and outcome IQ in highrisk boys. *PsycholRep.*, *65*(1), 95-103.

Hatfield, A.B., Lefley, H. 1987. *Families of the Mentally Ill: Coping and Adaptation.* New York, Guilford Press.

Hatfield, A. (1983). What families want of family therapists, in W.R. McFarlane (ed): *Family Therapy in Schizophrenia.* New York, Guilford Press, pp 41-68.

Hogarty, G., Anderson, C., Reiss, D., Kornblith, S., Greenwald, D., Javna, C., & Madonia, M. (1986). Family psychoeducation, social skills training, and maintenance chemotherapy in the aftercare treatment of schizophrenia. *Arch. Gen. Psychiatr.*, *43*, 633-642.

Hooley, J. & Hahlweg, K. (1986). The marriages and interaction patterns of depressed patients and their spouse: Comparison of high and low EE dyads. In M. Goldstein, K. Hand, & K. Hahlweg (Eds.), *Treatment of Schizophrenia: Family Assessment and Intervention.* (pp. 85-96). Berlin, Springer Press.

Johnson, D. (1990). The family's experience of living with mental illness, in H.P. Lefley, D.J. Johnson (ed): *Families as Allies in Treatment of the Mentally Ill.* Washington, D.C., American Psychiatric Press, pp 31-64.

Karno, M., Jenkins, J.H., de la Selva, A., Santana, F., Telles, C., Lopez, S., & Mintz, J. (1987). Expressed emotion and schizophrenic outcome among Mexican-American families. *J. Nerv. Ment. Dis.*, *175*(3), 143-151.

Jenkins, J.H. and Karno, M. (1992). The meaning of expressed emotion: Theoretical issues raised by cross-culture research. *Am. J. Psychiatr.*, *149*(1), 9-21.

Koenigsberg, H., & Handley, R. (1986). Expressed emotion: From predicative index to clinical constrict. *Am. J. Psychiatr.*, *43*, 1361-1373.

Kottgen, C., Sonnichsen, I., Mollenhauer, K., & Jurth, R. (1984). Group therapy with families of schizophrenic patients: Results of the Hamburg Camberwell Family Interview Study III. *Int. J. Fam. Psychiatr.*, *5*, 83-94.

Leff, J., Kuipers L, Berkowitz R, et al (1982). A controlled trial of social intervention in the families of schizophrenic patients: Two year follow-up. *Br J Psychiatr, 146*, 594-600.

Leff, J., Wig, N.N. Ghosh, A., Bedi, H, Menon, D.K., Kuipers, L., Korten, A., Ernberg, G., Day, R., Sartorius, N., & Jablensky, A. (1987). Expressed emotion and schizophrenia in North India, III: Influence of relatives' expressed emotion on the course of schizophrenia in Chandigarh. *Br. J. Psychiatr.*, *151*, 166-173.

Leff, J., Berkowitz, R., Shavit, N., Strachan, A., Glass, I., & Vaughn, C. (1989). A trial of family therapy v. a relatives group for schizophrenia. *Br. J. Psychiatr.*, *154*, 58-66.

MacMillan, J., Gold, A., Crow, T., Johnson, A., & Johnstone, E. (1986). Expressed emotion and relapse. *Br. J. Psychiatr.*, *148*, 133-143.

Madanes, C. Strategic therapy of schizophrenia. In McFarlane, W., (ed.), *Family Therapy in Schizophrenia.* New York, Guilford Press, 1983, pp. 209-226.

Miklowitz, D., Goldstein, M., & Falloon, I. (1983). Premorbid and symptomatic characteristics of schizophrenics from families with high and low levels of expressed emotion. *J. Abn. Psychol.*, 92 (3), 359-367.

Miklowitz, D., Goldstein, M., Nuechterlein, K., Snyder, K. & Doane, J. (1986). Expressed emotion, affective style, lithium compliance, and relapse in recent-onset mania. *Psychopharm. Bull.*, 22, 628-632.

Miklowitz, D., Strachan, A., Goldstein, M., Doane, J., Snyder, K., Hogarty, G., & Falloon, I. (1986). Expressed emotion and communication deviance in the families of schizophrenics. *J. Abnorm. Psychol.*, 95(1), 60-6.

Miklowitz, D., Velligan, D., Goldstein, M., Nuechterlein, K. M., Ranlett, G., & Doane, J. (1991). Communication deviance in families of schizophrenic and manic patients. *J. Abnorm Psychol.*, 100(2), 163-73.

Miklowitz, D., Goldstein M, et al. (1988). Family factors and the course of bipolar affective disorder. *Arch Gen Psychiatr.*, 45, 225-231.

Mintz, L., Nuechterlein, K., Goldstein, M., Mintz, J., & Snyder, K. (1989). The initial onset of schizophrenia and family expressed emotion: Some methodological considerations. *Br. J. Psychiatr.*, 154, 212-217.

Mintz, J., Mintz, L., & Goldstein, M. (1987). Expressed emotion and relapse in first episodes of schizophrenia. A rejoinder to Macmillan et al. (1986). *Br. J. Psychiatr.*, 151, 314-320.

Moline, R., Singh, S., Morris, A., & Meltzer, H. (1985). Family expressed emotion and relapse in 24 urban American patients. *Am. J. Psychiatr.*, 142(9), 1078-1081.

Mujica, E., Haas G., Hien D., et al. (1991). Expressed emotion and positive/negative symptoms in schizophrenia. *American Psychiatric Association* (New Orleans, LA.).

Nuechterlein, K., Goldstein, M., Ventura, J., Dawson, M., & Doane, J. (1989). Patient-environment relationships in schizophrenia. *Br. J. Psychiatry Suppl.*, 5, 84-9.

Nuechterlein, K., & Dawson, M. (1984). A heuristic vulnerability-stress model of schizophrenic episodes. *Schiz. Bull.*, 10, 300-312.

Overall, J., Gorham D. (1962). The brief psychiatric rating scale. *Psychol Reports*, 10, 799-812.

Parker, G. & Johnston, P. (1987). Parenting and schizophrenia: An Australian study of expressed emotion. *Aust. N.Z. J. Psychiatr.*, 21, 60-66.

Rund, B.R., & Blakar, R. (1986). Schizophrenic patients and their parents. A multi-method design and the findings from an illustrative empirical study of cognitive disorders and communication deviances. *Acta. Psychiatr. Scand.*, 74(4), 396-408.

Rutter, M., Brown G. (1966). The reliability and validity of measures of family life and relationships in families containing a psychiatric patient. *Soc Psychiatr 1(1)*, 38-53.

Sass, L., Gunderson, J., Singer, M., & Wynne, L. (1984). Parental communication deviance and forms of thinking in male schizophrenic offspring. *J. Nerv. Ment. Dis.*, 172(9), 513-20.

Scheflen, A. (1981). *Levels of schizophrenia*. New York: Brunner/Mazel,

Singer, M., & Wynne, L. (1985). Schizophrenics, families and communication disorders. R. Cancro, & S.R. Dean (Ed.), *The Stanley R. Dean award lectures. Vol. 1: Research in the schizophrenic disorders* (pp. 231-247). New York: Spectrum Publications.

Strachan, A., Feingold, D., Goldstein, M., Miklowitz, D., & Neuchterlein, K. (1989). Is expressed emotion an index of a transactional process? II. Patient's coping style. *Family Proc.*, 28, 169-181.

Sturgeon, D., Kuipers, L., Berkowitz, R., Turpin, G., & Leff, J. (1981). Psychophysiological responses of schizophrenic patients to high and low expressed emotion relatives. *Brit. J. Psychiatr.*, 138, 40-45.

Szmukler, G., Eisler, I., Russell, G. & Dare, C. (1985). Anorexia nervosa, parental 'expressed emotion' and dropping out of treatment. *Brit. J. Psychiatr.*, 147, 265-271.

Szmukler, G., Berkowitz, R., Eisler, I., Leff, J. & Dare, C. (1987). Expressed emotion in individual and family settings: a comparative study. *Brit. J. Psychiatr.*, 151, 174-178.

Tarrier, N., Barrowclough, C., Porceddu, K., & Watts, S. (1988). The assessment of psychological reactivity to the expressed emotion of the relatives of schizophrenic patients. *Br. J. Psychiatr.*, 152, 618-624.

Vaughn, C. (1986). Patterns of emotional response in the families of schizophrenic patients. In Goldstein, M., Hand, I., Hahlweg, K., (Eds.), *Treatment of Schizophrenia*. New York: Springer-Verlag.

Vaughn, C. (1977). Patterns of interactions in families of schizophrenics. In Katschnig, H. (Ed.), *Schizophrenia: the other side*. Vienna: Urban & Schwarzenberg.

Vaughn, C. (1989). Annotation: Expressed emotion in family relationships. *J. Child Psychol. Psychiatr.*, *30*(1), 13-22.

Vaughn, C.E., Snyder K, Jones S, et al. (1984). Family factors in schizophrenic relapse. *Arch Gen Psychiatr 41*, 1169-1177.

Vaughn, C., Leff, J. (1976). The influence of family and social factors on the course of psychiatric illness: A comparison of schizophrenic and depressed neurotic patients. *Br J Psychiatr.*, *129*, 125-137.

Wagener, D., Hogarty, G., Goldstein, M., Asarnow, R., & Browne, A. (1986). Information processing and communication deviance in schizophrenic patients and their mothers. *Psychiatry Res.*, *18*(4), 365-77.

Wig, N.N., Menon, D.K., Bedi, H., Leff, J., Kuipers, L., Ghosh, A., Day, R., Korten, A., Sartorius, N., Ernberg, G., & Jablensky, A. (1987). Expressed emotion and schizophrenia in North India, II: Distribution of expressed emotion components among relatives of schizophrenic patients in Aarhus and Chandigarh. *Br. J. Psychiatr.*, *151*, 160-165.

Wynne, L.C., Singer M., Bartko J., et al., (1977). Schizophrenics and their families: Research on parental communication, in J.M. Tanner (ed): *Developments in Psychiatric Research*. London, Hodder & Stoughton.

Chapter 6

THE PSYCHODYNAMIC MODEL AND SERVICES FOR FAMILIES: ISSUES AND STRATEGIES

Diane T. Marsh

Given the diversity among family members, a wide range of services offer potential benefits, including such nonclinical services as educational programs and support groups, and such clinical services as individual, marital, family, and group therapy. Indeed, family members may benefit from both nonclinical and clinical intervention, which may meet complementary needs. This chapter focuses on the psychodynamic approach to clinical intervention. As with other services for families, psychodynamic psychotherapy should be recommended when it provides the optimal match for the needs, desires, and resources of particular family members. In that regard, the following topics will be explored: (a) general considerations underlying a recommendation of psychodynamic psychotherapy; (b) an overview of the psychodynamic model; (c) short-term versus long-term psychodynamic psychotherapy; (d) professional practice with family members; and (e) therapeutic foci.

GENERAL CONSIDERATIONS

There are a number of general considerations. First, reflecting the new modes and models of professional practice that were discussed in Chapter 3, effective service delivery is dependent upon a respectful and empathic attitude toward family members, an understanding of their

Appreciation is expressed to Martin S. Willick, M.D., Training and Supervising Analyst, New York Psychoanalytic Institute, for his insightful comments and constructive suggestions.

phenomenological reality, an effort to meet their expressed needs, and a goal of family empowerment.

Second, family consultants can assist families in making an informed choice regarding their use of available services. Consistent with the ethical principle of informed consent, family members should receive information regarding the nature and purpose of specific nonclinical and clinical services; the potential benefits, risks, and costs of these services; and the available alternatives. As Wenning (1993) points out, many long-term psychotherapies begin without sufficient attention to the informed-consent process. He offers a model for informed consent that has applicability to psychoanalysis and other forms of long-term psychodynamic psychotherapy. He suggests that the following topics be discussed: (a) the diagnostic model used and the recommendation for treatment; (b) potential risks and benefits of treatment; (c) availability of less expensive short-term intervention; (d) clarification of the necessity for psychotherapy; (e) limits of insurance coverage; and (f) plans for measuring the patient's response to treatment (patient is the preferred term among most psychodynamic therapists).

Third, from the perspective of differential therapeutics (Clarkin et al., 1992; also see Chapter 3), the objective is to provide the most beneficial type of intervention for particular family members. Accordingly, a recommendation of psychodynamic psychotherapy should follow a careful assessment of indications and contraindications for such treatment, as will be discussed. At the meta level of treatment planning, this recommendation should be based on general knowledge concerned with families of people with serious mental illness, including their experience of a subjective and objective burden (Lefley, 1989). The following account conveys the anguish that an adult child may experience in response to the serious mental illness of a parent.

> *Fearfulness in childhood. Anger at unfairness and apathy of the world to the sufferings of the mentally ill. Grief of seeing Mother when she became ill. Anger at the family members who did not realize that I really lost my mother even though she wasn't dead and [who] never allowed me to express my grief. Guilt because no matter how much I did, it never seemed enough. Relief that she died and no longer had to suffer—and I could finally live life on my own terms.* (Marsh & Dickens, in preparation)

Fourth, at the micro level of treatment planning, the unique circumstances and attributes of individual family members should also receive consideration, including the special needs of parents, spouses, siblings, and children. For example, young family members who are growing up with the mental illness of a parent or sibling are profoundly affected by this family catastrophe, which transforms their lives from the moment of onset. Psychodynamic therapy offers patients a unique opportunity to explore their present circumstances within the context of their life history. Such a developmental model has particular applicability to the experiences of adult siblings and children. Here, for example, are the accounts of two adults who grew up with mental illness in their families.

> *It wasn't until I sought therapy for anxiety upon my divorce that I began to understand some of the dynamics of my family and myself. Therapy opened doors to my self and answered many puzzling questions. The mental illness profoundly changed my life. I have missed much, have just begun to recognize what has been lost or even never realized. It has taken me a long time to finally face the original problem.*
>
> * * *
>
> *I withdrew emotionally from my family. I became an overachiever at school and in extracurricular activities outside the home. I grew increasingly dependent on scholastic and then business achievements at the expense of a rich personal life. I have problems in establishing and maintaining intimate relationships. Through the help of therapy, I am now learning how much of it has to do with my family upbringing.* (Marsh & Dickens, in preparation)

Fifth, since psychodynamic psychotherapy is most likely to assist family members in resolving the subjective burden associated with their relative's illness, they might also benefit from nonclinical services designed to offer information, to improve skills, and to provide opportunities for advocacy. Thus, family consultants who are recommending a course of psychodynamic therapy may also wish to make a referral to a support group in the community, such as those affiliated with the National Alliance for the Mentally Ill (NAMI).

Finally, the risk of negative treatment effects should be kept to a minimum. It was noted in Chapter 3 that there are risks of adverse effects when therapists inappropriately assume that families are pathogenic or dysfunctional. In the past, a general assumption of family pathogenesis was often incorporated into the psychodynamic model, although such an assumption is not supported by a satisfactory empirical database (e.g., Howells & Guirguis, 1985). When an assumption of family pathogenesis underlies the treatment process or is espoused by individual clinicians, there are inherent risks for family members, as the following mother attests.

> My son's therapist told me that his early relationship with me was the central problem—at the same time I was told that his prognosis was poor and he might need institutional care. At the time, I felt as if I were being told my son was dying and I was responsible for his death. It was absolutely devastating. I needed support during the most difficult period of my life. Instead, my pain was intensified by someone who passed judgment without taking the time to understand our family. (Marsh, unpublished interviews)

It is not only parents who are harmed by such negative assumptions about families, as the following adult sibling indicates.

> I was part of a twins and siblings study. I recall no help for my pain. The viewpoint at that time was that the illness was caused by faulty parenting. I am angry at the the doctors for blaming my parents, which hurt them as much as the tragedy of losing a daughter to mental illness. God knows, it pretty much destroyed my parents. (Marsh & Dickens, in preparation)

In light of these negative treatment effects, family members who are interested in psychodynamic psychotherapy should seek a practitioner who does not share these disparaging views of families and who employs an appropriate conceptual framework. Fortunately, the current zeitgeist reflects more favorable attitudes toward families that have been incorporated into present psychodynamic thinking and practice. Writing from a psychoanalytic perspective, for example, Willick (1990) maintains that there is insufficient evidence to conclude that the etiology of the two major adult psychoses can be attributed to failures in development or fixations during the earliest years of life or to deficiencies in the early maternal environment. As McGlashan (1986) has observed, too often the descriptive data that are gathered from psychoanalytic treatment are assumed to be a recreation (via the repetition compulsion) of key past experiences or fantasies, which are then postulated not only to have occurred but also to have been etiologic.

In addition to this new generation of psychodynamic therapists, there are many eclectic therapists who employ a wide range of strategies and techniques, including those based on the psychodynamic model, without necessarily subscribing to the theories that spawned them. Thus, family members who are appropriate candidates for psychodynamic therapy can seek clinical services from a psychodynamic practitioner who does not hold an assumption of family pathogenesis or from an eclectic therapist who is guided primarily by therapeutic efficacy.

THE PSYCHODYNAMIC MODEL

The psychodynamic model is clearly pluralistic, with increasing theoretical and clinical diversity (see Wallerstein's, 1992, discussion of the common ground of psychoanalytic theory). In spite of this diversity, there are some essential elements in a psychodynamic approach to clinical intervention (see Chessick, 1993; Strupp, 1992). Conceptually, these include the notions of the dynamic unconscious, intrapsychic conflict, and psychic determinism, as well as an emphasis on the importance of infantile and childhood experiences, especially preoedipal and oedipal factors. Clinically, essential elements include an emphasis on transference and countertransference, free association, repetition, resistance, the therapist as participant observer, interpretation, and the subjective experience of the patient. These conceptual and clinical elements form the foundation for psychodynamic psychotherapy.

There are also certain strategies and techniques employed in psychodynamic psychotherapy (see Frosch, 1990). In their explication of exploratory psychotherapy (which includes psychoanalysis and psychodynamic psychotherapy), Frances and his colleagues (1984) have examined the following: (a) primary aim; (b) sources of data; (c) therapist's stance; and (d) techniques, strategies, and maneuvers. The primary aim of this form of therapy is to increase understanding of intrapsychic conflicts. Sources of data include developmental history; unconscious derivatives (dreams, fantasies, parapraxes, free associations); transference; and resistances. The therapist's stance is that of a transference figure who functions with relative neutrality, abstinence, and anonymity (see Chessick, 1993). The authors cite four therapeutic techniques: (a) observations; (b) clarifications, in which various associations are organized and made explicit; (c) interpretations designed to help the patient become consciously aware of the meaning of psychic content; and (d) reconstructions of infantile and childhood experiences.

Beginning with psychoanalysis, the psychodynamic model has undergone many changes over its long history. Strupp (1992) has discussed the future of psychodynamic psychotherapy, citing 10 trends of increasing interest that reflect both traditional features and new directions. These include: (a) developmental arrests in infancy and early childhood; (b) focus on treatment of personality disorders and "difficult" patients; (c) the dyadic character of the therapeutic relationship; (d) the therapeutic alliance; (e) developments in neuroscience and pharmacotherapy; (f) group, marital, and family therapies; (g) brief and time-limited therapies; (h) attempts to devise specific treatments for specific disorders; (i) treatment manuals; and (j) continued search for the mechanisms of change in personality and behavior.

Several of these trends are important from the perspective of professional practice with family members. First, as is the case for psychotherapy in general, there is agreement that the quality and nature of the therapeutic alliance is the overarching consideration in psychodynamic psychotherapy. Strupp notes that the therapist has emerged more clearly as a "real" person who manifests commitment, caring, interest, respect, and human concern for the patient. Within the context of the dyadic patient-therapist relationship, the cornerstones of psychodynamic therapy are transference and its complement, countertransference.

During therapy, both patient and therapist continually contribute to the therapeutic process, which always contains both real and transference elements. Consistent with the historical emphasis of the psychodynamic model, Strupp asserts that the troublesome patterns of thinking, feeling, and action that are enacted in psychotherapy typically have a long history; such patterns are assumed to play a central role in the illness being treated. As these patterns of transference are analyzed, they offer the potential for understanding and changing the patient's subjective world. Namely, the patient's experience of the therapist as a significant other whose feelings, attitudes, and values are introjected offers a corrective emotional experience that can modify earlier maladaptive patterns. In the following account, an adult family member who grew up with the mental illness of a close relative describes maladaptive patterns that developed earlier in her life.

> I adapted my behavior at home totally in the interest of keeping the equilibrium in the family. I felt responsible for making everyone happy. I took on emotions of others as something I had to fix. I developed a pattern of putting others before myself, lost my identity in relationships. I have only just begun to identify what I want and who I really am. I am just learning, at age 49, that I can be me. (Marsh & Dickens, in preparation)

Second, following Ackerman's (1959) psychoanalytic approach to the family, there has been more interest in marital, family, and group psychotherapy. For example, Bradley (1987) has formulated a biopsychosocial model that is based on developmental ego psychology and object relations theory. In describing her practice with families, she underscores the adverse consequences of earlier models that stigmatized and emotionally abused families, the importance of an empathic understanding of the dynamic interactions among family members, the potential of families to function as valuable allies for professionals and as sources of strength for patients, and the value of a more balanced view of families that incorporates family strengths as well as limitations. As Strupp (1992) points out, however, individual therapy has remained the mainstay of psychodynamic psychotherapy. Accordingly, in the present chapter, I will focus on the applicability of a psychodynamic model to the treatment of individual family members.

Third, there has been increasing acknowledgement of important advances in neuroscience and pharmacotherapy, particularly in the case of serious mental illness (see Willick, 1990). As a result, the psychodynamic model is less likely to incorporate an assumption of family pathogenesis. On the other hand, as Strupp (1992) remarks, a narrow biological model cannot deal with interpersonal conflicts and other aspects of maladaptive behaviors. Thus, a biopsychosocial model is needed that can integrate important developments in the biological, behavioral, and social sciences (see Levy & Nemeroff, 1993).

Finally, Strupp (1992) notes the renewed emphasis on brief forms of psychotherapy, a development he ascribes to social pressures for accountability, to cost-effectiveness, to the steadily increasing demand for mental health services, and to the desire of various mental health professionals to meet these needs. As he points out, an open-ended approach to dynamic psychotherapy, such as psychoanalysis, will clearly remain a luxury that relatively few members of our society can afford, although an emphasis on personality growth rather than clinical management will undoubtedly survive, at least as an ideal. There is empirical support for the current emphasis on brief psychotherapy. For example, in a longitudinal study of 42 patients who participated in the Menninger Psychotherapy Research Project, Wallerstein (1986) found that brief (supportive) psychotherapy compared favorably with longer-term (exploratory) psychotherapy.

More generally, Howard and his colleagues (1986) examined the "dose-effect" relationship in psychotherapy, based on a meta-analytic pooling of research findings that provided estimates of the expected benefits of specific doses of psychotherapy. They reported that by eight sessions, approximately 50% of patients are measurably improved, and approximately 75% are improved by 26 sessions. The researchers estimate that maximum improvement would be reached in approximately 52 once-weekly sessions, although there is variability among individuals. As Rockland (1989) has discussed, it is difficult to demonstrate empirically that long-term exploratory treatment leads to better outcomes than either brief or supportive treatments.

SHORT-TERM VERSUS LONG-TERM DYNAMIC PSYCHOTHERAPY

For both economic and clinical reasons, then, there is increasing interest in short-term dynamic psychotherapy. In their discussion of the process of differential therapeutics, Clarkin and his colleagues (1992) cite the following as general indications for brief therapy: (a) a definite focus, precipitating event, or intervention target; (b) sufficient (if limited) motivation and goals for brief treatment; (c) capacity for separation from treatment; (d) adequate level of functioning; (e) limited financial and/or time resources; and (f) a desire to avoid secondary gain, negative therapeutic reactions, unmanageable therapeutic attachments, or other iatrogenic effects. The distinction between short-term and long-term dynamic psychotherapy is sometimes discussed in terms of supportive and exploratory (expressive) modalities, respectively. As Rockland (1989) observes, however, all psychotherapies are mixtures of supportive and exploratory interventions, the balance between them determined by the level of psychic organization, motivation, capacity for introspection, and ego strengths and weaknesses, as well as present degrees of anxiety, regression, and disorganization.

Bemporad and Vasile (1990) state that suitability for all forms of psychodynamic psychotherapy rests on the capacity to maintain a therapeutic alliance, to constructively use the transference neurosis to develop insight, and to build on this insight to develop a corrective emotional experience. Patients must have the ability to explore current relationships, including the real patient-therapist relationship in psychotherapy, the transference relationship, and past relationships, all of which exist in dynamic equilibrium. In long-term psychodynamic psychotherapy, the aim is to increase conscious knowledge of crucial aspects of psychological makeup and functioning.

Bemporad and Vasile list two major goals of such psychotherapy: first, to make the here-and-now experience between patient and therapist reveal those unconscious processes that still influence and direct the individual's current life; and second, to help the patient understand how the present is different, in terms of autonomy and control, from those times in the distant past when the unconscious aspects were learned and subsequently repressed. In contrast, the authors state that supportive psychotherapy focuses on abreaction in the present, is time limited, and does not rely on the activation of transference or an exploration of unconscious determinants of illness. Namely, as Frosch (1990) states, in a supportive approach, the therapist accepts the existing basic psychic structure and tries to work within this framework.

In their treatment manual for time-limited dynamic psychotherapy (TLDP), Strupp and Binder (1984) describe a representative approach to short-term dynamic psychotherapy. They hypothesize that earlier difficulties with significant others have given rise to patterns of inter-personal relatedness that originally served a self-protective function but are now self-defeating and maladaptive. To the extent that these patterns reflect basic aspects of personality structure and the interpersonal repertoire, they tend to come into play whenever the patient forms a relationship with a significant other, including the therapist, which offers an opportunity for correction. Here, for example, are the accounts of two adult children of parents with mental illness whose early experiences resulted in distorted roles and relationships.

> As the eldest daughter I had a unique relationship with my father. I became his confidant and fellow decision maker in the family. This relationship was comforting, and I clung to it emotionally. Little did I realize how unhealthy it was, until as an adult, I have had great difficulty in my relationships with men as a result.
>
>   * * *
>
> I feel a great sadness for the loss of the very close and special (sick, as it turns out) relationship with my mother. And some-times I still hurt for her, as I still can feel her pain at the loneliness and rejection that accompany her illness. [When I was younger], I thought she was a prophet who was just being misunderstood by the rest of the world. I had no yardstick to measure by. (Marsh & Dickens, in preparation)

Strupp and Binder specify the principle tools of TLDP as empathic listening, understanding of the psychodynamics of current problems in terms of life history, and clarification of their self-defeating character. The authors view TLDP as appropriate for patients whose problems include anxiety, depression, and conflicts in interpersonal relationships, such as inability to achieve intimacy. The goal is to offer a constructive experience in living that results in improvements in self-concept and quality of interpersonal relationships. The following adult child of a parent with mental illness might benefit from this approach.

> *I have spent the last 25 years trying to find confidence, love, acceptance. I am extremely sensitive and weep easily. I avoid intimacy but crave it desperately. I want more friends but fear to trust. I took on a role of peacemaker at a young age and developed some exceptional coping skills: problem solving, soothing, getting along with difficult people, and intellectual searching. I am a doer and a fixer, but paid a price.* (Marsh & Dickens, in preparation)

In general, a course of short-term psychodynamic psychotherapy should be considered initially for family members who have chosen to pursue this form of therapy. For example, a course of brief therapy would be suggested by satisfactory prior functioning, the presence of precipitating stress, the relatively poor match between the expressed needs of families and ambitious treatment goals, and the likelihood of poor motivation for extended therapy among families who are coping with a catastrophic event.

Although the recent literature reflects increasing interest in short-term psychodynamic psychotherapy (e.g., Groves, 1992), there are circumstances when long-term psychotherapy is appropriate. As Clarkin and his associates (1992) point out, the latter should be considered for problems that are ingrained, complex, and extensive. Indications for long-term therapy include multiple problems areas, few enabling factors for treatment, relatively poor premorbid functioning, and an unsatisfactory response to brief treatment. Accordingly, a recommendation of long-term psychotherapy is appropriate for family members who are experiencing severe problems in several areas of their lives. It is also necessary for those who have chosen to pursue psychoanalysis, which typically requires multiple sessions per week over a period of several years.

Here, for example, is the account of an adult child whose mother has mental illness. Her description points to the kinds of ingrained, complex, and extensive problems that are indications for long-term psychotherapy.

As a child, I tried desperately never to have a problem because our family had so many. So I became perfectionistic and hid my fears, concerns, and needs from everyone. On the outside, I always appeared strong, self-assured, and able to handle anything. But I developed a lot of self-depreciation and shame, felt that I was going crazy too. I always had tremendous anxiety that someday, somebody would find out that I was a fraud. I've probably always had a certain degree of depression as a result of my mother's illness. When my father died, I suffered a major depression and went into therapy. (Marsh & Dickens, in preparation)

PROFESSIONAL PRACTICE WITH FAMILY MEMBERS

As this discussion demonstrates, a psychodynamic approach to therapy may be beneficial for some family members. Before making a referral for psychodynamic therapy, however, family consultants should weigh a number of factors. These include: (a) the relative value of nonclinical and clinical intervention; (b) differential therapeutics; and (c) selection criteria for psychodynamic therapy.

Nonclinical Versus Clinical Intervention

Initially, family consultants should consider the relative value of nonclinical and clinical services, since there is empirical evidence that nonclinical intervention can meet the needs of many family members. For example, researchers have consistently found that nonclinical services, such as educational programs and support groups, are rated as more helpful than various forms of psychotherapy by adult relatives (primarily parents) of people with mental illness (Hatfield, 1979; Lefley, 1987). These family members have pressing needs for the information, skills, and support that will enhance their coping effectiveness under conditions of severe stress. Emphasis on the historical roots of intrapsychic conflict is incongruent with these needs, and parents may find psychodynamic therapy irrelevant and intrusive under these circumstances.

Here, for example, is the account of a mother who responded negatively to psychodynamic therapy, although she found a support group very helpful.

I went to see the therapist specifically to see how I was going to live through my pain and how to deal with my son's mental illness. He wanted me to deal with my childhood, something I had already dealt with. My son's illness wasn't caused by my

*childhood. I didn't feel he was willing to help me with my goals,
so I quit after three sessions.* (Marsh, 1992, p. 207)

In contrast, in two national surveys of adult siblings and children of
people with mental illness (Marsh et al., 1993), respondents affirmed
the value of both nonclinical and clinical intervention. Over three-
fourths (77%) of all respondents had received personal psychotherapy.
A majority (63%) reported therapy was very or extremely helpful; only
one respondent rated it not helpful. Moreover, 90% of those who were
age 10 or younger at the onset of their relative's illness or who had both
a parent and a sibling with mental illness had sought personal therapy.
The following respondents convey the feelings of anguish and demoralization that may prompt these family members to seek therapy.

> *I am certainly not the person in any way that I might have been
> had my family not been struck with such tragedy. I suffered the
> dual "taboos" of mental illness and divorce. My parents di-
> vorced as a result of my father's mental illness. Losing the family
> that I was born into and loved, and losing my father to a living
> death. I have a driving need to "re-create" the family that I lost.*
>
> * * *
>
> *I have become an angry person. A person who is afraid to not
> be liked by others. A person who fears close relationships but
> longs for them daily. A person who is afraid of change but who
> longs for adventure and loves to travel. I believe it has hardened
> me. I can't seem to love myself. I take care of and please others,
> but when I try to take care of me, I fail.* (Marsh & Dickens, in
> preparation)

Thus, based on the available research, nonclinical services appear to
be the intervention of choice for most parents. In contrast, siblings and
children appear to be good candidates for psychotherapy, both as young
family members and as adults.

Differential Therapeutics

Once family members have made an informed choice regarding their
use of clinical services, family consultants can employ a process of
differential therapeutics to assist them in recommending the most efficacious form of therapy. Relevant considerations include the presence
of psychodynamic issues, differences associated with particular roles

within the family, personal mental health status, individual characteristics, and selection criteria for psychodynamic therapy.

Psychodynamic issues. There are a number of indications for psychodynamic therapy among family members. These include the presence of an unresolved or pathological grieving process, of an entrenched pattern of denial, of intrapsychic conflict, of inappropriate anger that is directed inward or at other family members, of earlier feelings of loss that may have been resurrected in the present, or of family-of-origin issues. For example, the following adult child describes unresolved issues pertaining to her family of origin.

> *My mother still has a major impact on my life as an adult. Feelings of becoming mentally ill myself. Relationships with people, especially men. Self-esteem. Guilt about almost everything—never good enough, not worthy. Feelings of rejection or abandonment. I always try to make everyone feel good. Finally, [I went] to a counselor for my depression and low self-esteem.* (Marsh & Dickens, in preparation)

Family roles. Based on the research findings with different family members (e.g., Lefley, 1987; Marsh et al., 1993), family roles should be given consideration. For example, some parents may prefer to meet their own needs through a confidential therapeutic relationship rather than a support group. For most of these parents, relatively limited treatment goals are appropriate, including the provision of support, the strengthening of relevant competencies and coping effectiveness, the reframing of personal and familial experience, and the expression and working through of painful affects. Bernheim's (1982) supportive family counseling offers a therapeutic approach that is likely to be beneficial for these family members.

The following mother had no history of mental health problems and was functioning well in spite of her feelings of grief and loss. She spent two years in psychodynamic psychotherapy. Her evaluation of therapy suggests that a more supportive and less exploratory approach to therapy would have been more appropriate.

> *I was both helped and hurt by therapy. I needed an opportunity to unburden my soul, and my therapist was a caring and empathic listener. But that is all that I needed. When my own goals were met, and I was ready to terminate, I was talked into remaining in therapy. . . . As a result, I spent another year in*

therapy that didn't benefit me in any way that I can see and that added significantly to my problems. It seemed as if everything I said was treated as an irrational symptom to be analyzed. My desire to terminate was labeled resistance, and my genuine feelings and legitimate concerns about other matters were repeatedly labeled transference. The overall process distorted my very real feelings and problems, and undermined my ability to deal with them. (Marsh, 1992, p. 209)

In contrast, research with adult siblings and children suggests that they may be good candidates for therapy in general and for psychodynamic therapy in particular. In the following accounts, two family members who grew up with mental illness in their families discuss the legacy for their own lives.

To validate your own sense of worth or value, you must grow up with affection and approval as a child. If you don't have those things, you don't know if you're a valuable person or not. When I was a child, my mother never said, "I love you." I was so very, very sensitive. I wanted to be liked and loved by everyone. I was insecure because I didn't have validation of the quality of the person that I really was.

* * *

It was like a large cloud moved over our heads and everyone was paralyzed for years. This mental illness business affected all aspects of my life—self-esteem, trust, intimacy, hope, and emotional development. I lost my ability to feel for many years. Loss of hope, helplessness, confusion, powerlessness. We needed professional understanding and validation of our experience. (Marsh & Dickens, in preparation)

Personal mental health status. In addition to problems that are largely reactive to their relative's illness, family members may have personal mental health problems or serious mental illness themselves, which should obviously be considered in making treatment recommendations. In our survey of adult siblings and children of people with mental illness, for example, two-thirds (66%) of respondents indicated they experienced feelings of depression at least sometimes; almost one-fifth (19%) experienced depression often or always. In the following accounts, two family members describe the personal mental health problems that motivated them to seek treatment.

I was in Mental Health myself for attempting suicide after my husband left me and a combination of a lot of things. I have had a great deal of counseling, which has helped me very much. I have been mentally abused by my husband, and so have my children. Counseling has made us all stronger. (Marsh, 1992a, p. 197)

* * *

I am so full of problems. [In] early childhood, I had anxiety disorder (panic attack), depression, hypochondriasis. Later depersonalization disorder, which persists to this day. I have difficulty expressing my own opinions, have poor relationships with men, no sex drive. Therapy since 16, on and off. Good therapists and medication ultimately gave me hope. (Marsh & Dickens, in preparation)

Personal characteristics. In addition to these general considerations, the overarching objective is to recommend the most appropriate form of therapy for particular family members. Although many adult siblings and children appear to be good candidates for psychodynamic therapy, almost one-fourth (23%) did not seek personal therapy. These family members were members of support groups sponsored by the Siblings and Adult Children (SAC)Council of NAMI, which met many of their essential needs. Similarly, although the needs of many parents can be met through nonclinical intervention or supportive therapy, some parents may benefit from psychodynamic therapy. Reflecting the central importance of goodness-of-fit, for example, the following family members offer different evaluations of their experiences in therapy. In the first case, a mother comments on the relatively poor match between her needs and the psychodynamic therapy she received.

I feel now that it was a mistake to get into therapy, that the costs outweighed the benefits. In many respects, there was a poor match between what I wanted and needed and what psychotherapy offered. I was not mentally ill and did not need treatment or analysis. The usual interpretations were largely irrelevant to my concerns, and I had no need to deal with my mother at that point in my life. Nor was it constructive for me to become a patient or to become involved in a process that seemed to emphasize my vulnerability and to drain my energy. . . .The last thing I needed was to be treated as if I were the problem instead of my daughter. (Marsh, 1992, p. 204)

In contrast, the following family member, an adult child, found long-term psychotherapy a good match for her needs.

> *My mother's illness completely interrupted my life. Her illness progressed, and I found myself isolated and powerless in dealing with it. My mother would not agree to see a doctor. The establishment repeatedly told me that there was nothing they could do unless my mother wished help. She didn't. I sank into an eight-year depression. I've been in therapy for 11 years now. That helped me develop more healthily. That's the only good result I can see coming out of this tragedy.* (Marsh & Dickens, in preparation).

Selection criteria for psychodynamic therapy. The selection criteria for psychodynamic therapy should also influence recommendations for this form of therapy. In their discussion of differential therapeutics, Frances and his colleagues (1984) discuss the relative indications for psychodynamic therapy, which include the presence of intrapsychic conflict and a goal of character change (as opposed to symptom reduction). They list the following enabling factors: (a) motivation for psychodynamic psychotherapy; (b) willingness to make sacrifices; (c) honesty; (d) psychological mindedness; (e) ability to experience, tolerate, and discuss painful affects; (f) relatively high ego strength; and (g) intelligence and verbal facility.

Relative contraindications include poor response to prior psychodynamic psychotherapy and the presence of specific symptoms that demand immediate attention (although such therapy may become an option once those initial problems have been addressed). In addition, as Frances and his associates discuss (1984), the lack of structure in psychoanalysis may be harmful for patients who do not have the capacity to form a trusting relationship with the analyst, to tolerate the frustration inherent in this form of treatment, or to analyze constructively the distortions that develop within the transference relationship. Such individuals should be referred for other services.

THERAPEUTIC FOCI

A number of therapeutic foci are likely to emerge in psychodynamic therapy with family members. Some of these are universal foci, including the subjective burden that is experienced by family members in response to the mental illness their relative. Other foci have more limited applicability to clinical practice with this population, including those related to an unresolved grieving process or to the reactivation of earlier losses. Still other foci are associated with particular roles in the family, such as adult siblings and children.

Subjective Burden

In response to the mental illness of their relative, family members often experience a subjective burden that includes intense feelings of grief and loss, of demoralization, of guilt and responsibility, of hopelessness and helplessness, and of chronic sorrow. A psychodynamic approach to therapy is likely to promote the expression and working through of this emotional burden. From the perspective of a bereavement model, it is assumed that family members undergo a grieving process as they mourn the loss of the healthy family member they knew and loved prior to the onset of mental illness. The grieving process also encompasses symbolic losses, including the loss of hopes and dreams, and perhaps of the potential for a meaningful and productive life. The bereavement model makes intuitive sense to many family members, who often refer spontaneously to the experience of loss and grieving.

> *The problems with my daughter were like a black hole inside of me into which everything else had been drawn. My grief and pain were so intense sometimes that I barely got through the day. It felt like a mourning process, as if I were dealing with the loss of the daughter I had loved for 18 years, for whom there was so much potential. That daughter was now lost to me, and I had to adjust to another one who was mentally ill, who might need a lifetime of care, and who was not going to survive in any meaningful sense.* (Marsh, 1992, p. 10)

It is also important to note the limitations of the bereavement model for family members, who are likely to experience a pattern of chronic sorrow, which is characterized by continuing distress that varies in intensity, rather than a time-bound, progressive mourning process (see Marsh, 1992). Furthermore, the bereavement model is largely predicated on the experience of biological death, an actual loss that is tangible and permanent, and that receives social validation. In contrast, people with mental illness are very much alive, and some have the potential for recovery.

In spite of these limitations, the profound feelings of anguish and loss experienced by family members offer fertile ground for psychodynamic therapy. There is an extensive psychodynamic literature concerned with normal and pathological mourning, which provides the context for such psychotherapy. Piper and his associates (1992) have described a program of psychodynamic group psychotherapy that incorporates the unique psychoanalytic vision and understanding of loss, and that has potential applicability to professional practice with family members.

Unresolved Grieving Process

A subjective burden is experienced in some form by all family members, who may resolve their emotional burden with the assistance of family and friends, a family support group, or supportive counseling. Family members who have difficulty resolving their emotional burden are at risk for an unresolved grieving process. As Rando (1984) has discussed, the risk of unresolved grief is increased by the presence of guilt, loss of an extension of the self, reawakening of an old loss, multiple losses, social negation of the loss, socially unspeakable loss, and social isolation. All of these factors may be present in the case of serious mental illness. As a result, normal grief may be absent, inhibited, delayed, conflicted, chronic, unanticipated, or abbreviated. The following family member refers to his own experience of unresolved grief.

> *A big part of my problem was unresolved feelings of grief and loss. Our family has lost so much as the result of Mom's illness, but it has happened a little at a time, so there hasn't really been an opportunity to grieve. Eventually I realized I had been deprived of the opportunity to mourn my losses—my loss of a healthy mother, a normal childhood, and a stable home. I wanted to give the scared little boy inside me every opportunity to mourn.* (Marsh & Dickens, in preparation)

Resurrection of Earlier Losses

The powerful emotional impact of a relative's mental illness is likely to have a pervasive impact on the subjective world of family members. In response to the intense emotions experienced in the present, earlier conflicts may be reactivated and earlier losses resurrected. For instance, the following mother found that the anguish she experienced in response to her son's involuntary commitment evoked similar feelings she endured at the time of her father's premature death

> *The court order is hell for any parent to go through. My son kept saying, "I'm not a criminal, what are they taking me for?"*

They put handcuffs and leg chains on him. . . .That was the worst ordeal. Even after all these years, it hurts, it hurts inside. . . . just [as it did] when my father died. My father died when he was very young. It hurt very bad. . . .And this, too, every time I bring it back, it hurts. (Marsh, 1992, p. 215).

Issues of Adult Siblings and Children

Because siblings and children of people with mental illness are exposed to this catastrophic family event as they are growing up, the event has a pervasive impact on all aspects of their personal and interpersonal lives. There are a number of issues and concerns that are likely to emerge in psychodynamic therapy with this population, including problems with basic trust and security, with reality testing, with self-concept and self-esteem, with guilt and responsibility, with emotional anesthesia and anhedonia, with perfectionism and control, with separation, with social isolation and isolation, with unfulfilled potential, with intimacy, and with caregiving. The following vignettes (from Marsh & Dickens, in preparation) highlight some of these issues, which may emerge as therapeutic foci.

Family members who are confronted with the mental illness of a close relative very early in life are at risk for a number of problems, including the failure to develop a sense of basic trust and security.

Mother's illness had a profound effect. Safety, security, trust were shattered. I was very scared and very confused. I changed from a "good girl" into someone who was always in trouble. I was screaming for help but didn't know how or what for. A strong need to protect myself from any hurt. A lot of anger.

Young family members may also become involved in the psychotic system, which may place them at risk for problems in reality testing themselves.

Before I entered therapy, I had one foot in reality and one foot in the legacy of psychosis. I'd been going around like that for years, and finally the discomfort of the contradiction grew too great. New I feel like I have moved my right foot from psychosis into reality, so both feet are planted in reality.

In their effort to protect themselves from the anguish associated with mental illness, young siblings and children may repress disturbing experiences or strip them of painful affect through dissociation, banishing these events to an unconscious territory that continues to have amorphous jurisdiction over their lives.

> *I shut down emotionally sometime in my youth, and this carried over into my adulthood. I didn't know how to relate to other people, especially women, beyond the superficial. I have become less human, less trusting, less vulnerable, more of a mechanical man [who] is hollow inside. It has put my life on emotional hold for 15 years.*

Siblings and children often report feelings of poor self-esteem, self-efficacy, and self-confidence in response to the pervasive stigmatization that enshrouds the family, as well as their continuing feelings of loss and helplessness.

> *I constantly battle low self-esteem and shame. Our family has lost a great deal to this illness. My father committed suicide. My sister went into the state hospital and is still there. I [visit] the hospital with dread, anxiety, and great sadness. I carry pain about my sister every day. I sometimes expect life to be one bad thing after another.*

Feelings of guilt and responsibility appear to be universal components of the legacy of these family members, who may engage in magical thinking regarding their ability to rescue their ill relative, if not in the present, then in some indefinite future.

> *I survived childhood largely on the belief that if I could hurry and grow up, I could fix my mother. I also believed that adulthood would bring wonderful things for me, since I was having all my hard times as a child. The shattering of these beliefs, which hit me in my thirties, created an extreme crisis for me. In therapy I have resolved my feelings about my mother, but it was still very difficult to face the fact that I failed to fix my mother when she died.*

The feelings of helplessness and insecurity experienced by young family members may leave them with an inordinate need for perfection and control later in their lives, and perhaps with a "survivor's guilt" that renders them incapable of deriving satisfaction from their own lives and accomplishments.

*I became the perfect child to spare my parents any more grief. I
was forced to become responsible. In many ways it forced me to
accomplish things in my life I might not have otherwise done. But
I have spent my life trying to run away from this problem. Feeling
guilty and helpless, the unending sorrow for not being able to help.
I have not felt entitled to be happy most of my adult life.*

As a result of the mental illness in their families, siblings and children
may experience difficulties in separation and individuation, including
problems separating from beleaguered family members who have come
to depend upon them.

*I continued to work toward my own self-preservation. I felt
that my family would drag me down and that I had to do
whatever I could to salvage my own life. I constantly worried
about my mother. I found a good therapist who convinced me
that I really needed to separate from my mother, who worked
with me on knowing what behavior is a function of the illness
and what isn't.*

Adult siblings and children often report feelings of social isolation
and alienation, fear of abandonment and rejection, and difficulty establishing and sustaining intimate relationships, as the following family
member attests.

*I have not had a relationship with a woman longer than one
year. I withdrew socially, became very introverted, had low
self-esteem. I was still introverted in my early twenties. Seeing
my brother homeless. I was trying to achieve, but it felt like I
was working on only one or two cylinders out of four.*

A recurrent theme among adult siblings and children is their sense of
depleted energy as a result of the mental illness in their families. The
chronic family stress may deflect them from their own educational and
career goals, which may be moved to the periphery as they attempt to
meet the needs of their distressed family.

*My potential can't be tapped because of the pain. I feel bitter
resentment because of the devastation I've been through. Unable to have parenting because parents were both ill and in and
out of the hospital. Fear, rage. Isolated, desperate, confused.*

> *Lack of trust, lack of money, lack of support. Little sense of self, low self-esteem. Unable to address my needs or wants.*

Our research underscored the central importance of caregiving concerns among adult siblings and children, who often struggle to balance their commitments to their families and to themselves.

> *The most difficult thing I've encountered is knowing that my father is still alive, but I have lost him to a dreadful and torturing mental illness. Four years ago, I [became] my father's caretaker. Anything he needed, I was there with it. [I was] told something I had been needing to hear for a very long time—that I have a life of my own to live. Since then I've learned to take better care of my life.*

In addition to delineating the legacy of mental illness for adult siblings and children, our research provided impressive evidence of their capacity for resilience. As a result of their experience with mental illness, these family members reported many positive changes in self-concept and self-efficacy, in compassion and tolerance toward others, in contributions to society, in family relationships and social life, and in attitudes and priorities. Accordingly, it is important to avoid pathologizing family members who may already have concerns about personal mental health. The following family member affirms this potential for a resilient response to a catastrophic family event.

> *My adolescent years were filled with a hollow dread. I felt somehow that I was responsible. I felt incredibly angry, resentful toward my mother, unable to escape, and very guilty. Gradually, I have come to see my mother's mental illness as just one part of my life. I have my own life, dreams, and goals. Her illness has caused me to develop tremendous strength, discipline, and personal stability.*

Finally, there are many potential benefits for family members who are considering a course of psychotherapy. In particular, psychodynamic psychotherapy offers family members an opportunity to resolve long-standing problems and to understand present circumstances within the context of their life history. For family members who are experiencing the anguish and demoralization associated with a relative's mental illness, these are meaningful goals indeed.

I did not explore therapy until age 35. Professionals can be a wonderful vehicle to bring out repressed pain and guilt. Don't be afraid to admit to yourself you cannot handle certain situations. It's hard to move forward without opening up blocked tears. Once I allowed myself to really cry, I unburdened more than I ever thought I could carry. Besides making me feel relieved, I felt human—a healthy human for the first time.

* * *

I was so depressed and lonely. I even thought of suicide. For many years, I looked for answers for my brother's problems, never realizing I had to find myself first. I had to leave home to survive. I have—being in therapy, learning I'm okay. I'm now married and successful in my job as an elementary guidance counselor. I am what I wanted to be—a caring, nurturing person.

REFERENCES

Ackerman, N. W. (1959). The psychoanalytic approach to the family. In J. H. Masserman (Ed.), *Individual and family dynamics* (pp. 105-121). New York: Grune & Stratton.

Bemporad, J. R., & Vasile, R. G. (1990). Psychotherapy. In A. S. Bellack & M. Hersen (Eds.), *Handbook of comparative treatments for adult disorders* (pp. 51-63). New York: Wiley.

Bernheim, K. F. (1982). Supportive family counseling. *Schizophrenia Bulletin, 8*, 634-641.

Bradley, S. S. (1987). Family treatment within a psychodynamic treatment milieu. *Psychiatric Clinics of North American, 10*, 289-308.

Chessick, R. D. (1993). *A dictionary for psychotherapists: Dynamic concepts in psychotherapy.* Northvale, NJ: Aronson.

Clarkin, J. F. et al. (1992). Differential therapeutics: Macro and micro levels of treatment planning. In J. C. Norcross & M. R. Goldfried (Eds.), *Handbook of psychotherapy integration* (pp. 463-502). New York: Basic Books.

Frances, A. et al. (1984). *Differential therapeutics in psychiatry: The art and science of treatment selection.* New York: Brunner/Mazel.

Frosch, J. (1990). *Psychodynamic psychiatry: Theory and practice. Vols. I & II.* Madison, CT: International Universities Press.

Groves, J. E. (1992). The short-term dynamic psychotherapies: An overview. In J. S. Rutan (Ed.), *Psychotherapy for the 1990s* (pp. 35-59). New York: Guilford.

Hatfield, A. B. (1979). Help-seeking behavior in families of schizophrenics. *American Journal of Community Psychology, 7*, 563-569.

Howard, K. I. et al. (1986). The dose-effect relationship in psychotherapy. *American Psychologist, 41*, 159-164.

Howells, J. G., & Guirguis, W. R. (1985). *The family and schizophrenia.* New York: International Universities Press.

Lefley, H. P. (1987). Impact of mental illness in families of mental health professionals. *Journal of Nervous and Mental Disease, 175*, 613-619.

Lefley, H. P. (1989). Family burden and family stigma in major mental illness. *American Psychologist, 44*, 556-560.

Levy, S. T., & Nemeroff, C. B. (1993). From psychoanalysis to neurobiology. *National Forum, 73*(1), 18-21.

Marsh, D. T. (1992) *Families and mental illness: New directions in professional practice.* New York: Praeger.

Marsh, D. T., & Dickens, R. M. (in preparation). *Troubled journey: Siblings and children of people with mental illness.*

Marsh, D. T. et al. (1993). Troubled journey: Siblings and children of people with mental illness. *Innovations & Research, 2*(2), 17-28.

McGlashan, T. H. (1986). Dr. Pao on diagnosis. In D. Feinsilver (Ed.), *Towards a comprehensive model for schizophrenic disorders* (pp. 3-14). Hillsdale, NJ: Analytic Press.

Piper, W. E. et al. (1992). *Adaptation to loss through short-term group psychotherapy.* New York: Guilford.

Rando, T. A. (1984). *Grief, dying, and death.* Champaign, IL: Research Press.

Rockland, L. H. (1989). Psychoanalytically oriented supportive therapy: Literature review and techniques. *Journal of the American Academy of Psychoanalysis, 17*, 451-462.

Strupp, H. H. (1992). The future of psychodynamic psychotherapy. *Psychotherapy, 29*, 21-27.

Strupp, H. H., & Binder, J. L. (1984). *Psychotherapy in a new key: A guide to time-limited dynamic psychotherapy.* New York: Basic Books.

Wallerstein, R. S. (1986). *Forty-two lives in treatment.* New York: Guilford.

Wallerstein, R. S. (Ed.). (1992). *The common ground of psychoanalysis.* Northvale, NJ: Aronson.

Wenning, K. (1993). Long-term psychotherapy and informed consent. *Hospital and Community Psychiatry, 44*, 364-367.

Willick, M. S. (1990). Psychoanalytic concepts of the etiology of mental illness. *Journal of the American Psychoanalytic Association, 38*, 1049-1081.

PART III

SERVICE-RELATED ISSUES

Chapter 7

COPING STRATEGIES FOR FAMILIES OF PEOPLE WHO HAVE A MENTAL ILLNESS

LeRoy Spaniol and Anthony M. Zipple

INTRODUCTION

Families of people who have a mental illness are frequently confronted with the need to deal with problems requiring practical coping skills. Yet many families report not knowing how to deal effectively with commonly recurring problems. For the purposes of this chapter the authors will be focusing on coping concerns related to the family member with a mental illness. Problems including social withdrawal, poor hygiene, bizarre behavior, self-destructive behavior, assaultiveness and lack of cooperation with treatment are common sources of concern for families. These behaviors can be distressing and generate profound feelings of anxiety, anger, guilt and worry. Families often feel frightened and quite helpless. Certain behaviors such as suicidal threats are especially distressing. Unfortunately, professionals often lack the information and skills required to assist families with their practical coping needs (Spaniol, 1987).

Lazarus and Folkman (1984) have stated that how we react to potential stressors in our lives is a function of our conscious and unconscious appraisal of how threatening or non-threatening the particular stressor is to us. Our appraisal is closely linked to the information, skills and supports we feel are available to us to deal with the stressor. If we perceive the stressor to exceed our resources we will begin to experience physical and emotional stress reactions. The intensity of these reactions will depend on how serious we perceive the threat to be. By increasing the range of options for dealing with potentially stressful situations, professionals can be more helpful to families, and families can increase their confidence in their ability to cope more adequately.

131

The onset of a serious mental illness may leave the family member with the illness profoundly disconnected from him/herself, from others, from their living, learning and working environments, and from the larger meanings or purposes in life. The purpose of the coping strategies discussed in this chapter is not simply to reduce conflict or stress, to manage the illness, or to "keep the peace." The purpose of these strategies is to help the family and the family member with the mental illness to repair and further build these important connections. What families often find most stressful is the loss of the person they once knew. The loss of the "person they once knew" is also what is most distressing to the person with the mental illness. The authors hope these strategies help family members to reconnect more meaningfully with one another.

This chapter will provide families and professionals with practical information on how to deal with a wide variety of situations that often require coping. We generated these strategies from families themselves, from our experience in training professionals to work collaboratively with families, from our work with people with mental illness and from the stress and coping literature.

THE FAMILY RECOVERY PROCESS

The onset of mental illness can be a traumatic experience for the family. While the mental illness in their family member may be life-long, we have found that families can experience their own recovery from the trauma, just as their family member with a mental illness can experience recovery (Power, Dell'Orto & Gibbons, 1988; Spaniol & Koehler, 1993a; Van der Kolk, 1987). Recovery is a process of readjusting our attitudes, feelings, perceptions, and beliefs about ourselves, others, and life in general. It is a process of self-discovery, self-renewal, and transformation. All people experience recovery at various times in their lives. The more threatening the precipitating event, the more it shakes the roots of who we are and how we experience our lives, the more it breaks connections we took for granted, the more it shatters the dreams and fantasies we hoped for, the deeper and more profound the required recovery process will be. Recovery is painful and difficult. Yet its outcome can be the emergence of a new sense of self, more vital, more connected to who we really are, more connected to others, and to a greater sense of meaning and purpose in life.

While there is not a great deal of information on the recovery process in families, there are a number of aspects of family recovery that can be identified (Tessler, Killian & Gubman, 1987). Understanding the recovery process can provide a welcome long-term perspective to families. It can bring some relief when they are caught up in the many difficult daily events of caring for a family member with a mental illness. Professionals also need to understand how families react to the trauma of mental illness in a family member. This knowledge can help professionals understand the family's experience and respond to it in a helpful way.

There are some general characteristics of family recovery that should be noted. (1) Recovery is a growth process—a transforming process. While it may not feel transformative at the time, and can be very painful, it is still a growth process. (2) Each individual in the family recovers at his or her own rate. Family members may be in different phases of recovery at any given time. (3) The particular impact of the illness differs in family members. A mother's experience is different from a father's experience (Thurer, 1983). A parent's experience differs from a sibling's experience. A younger sibling's experience is not the same as a sibling who is older than the family member with the illness (Marsh, 1993a,b.). (4) Families need to be aware of each other's phase of recovery. Each phase of the recovery process has its own reactions and its own developmental tasks. As family members acquire the knowledge, skills and support to complete these tasks they grow personally. (5) Recovery is not linear, so family members will recycle themselves through the phases as they gradually complete tasks that will facilitate moving ahead. (6) Emotional reactions of family members during the recovery process, even intense ones, are natural reactions and do not imply there is something wrong with the family members.

Discovery/denial

As family members begin to become aware of what is happening they may try to explain it away. The family may believe that it is not really so serious. They may have negative or exaggerated images of people with mental illness from the media and their family member does not conform to those images. Or they may feel the family member's behavior is caused by alcohol, drugs, laziness or bad friends. As the relationship with the family member begins to change, family tensions and frustrations increase. The family often attempts to find answers through any possible source, such as friends, other families, clergy and professionals. Denial can be persistent and can linger throughout other aspects of the recovery process. Each individual must deal with his/her own recovery. Other members of the family cannot do it for them.

Recognition/acceptance

The family gradually becomes aware that their family member has a major mental illness. Initially this awareness increases their faith and hope in professionals because professionals are expected to know the answers. As awareness of the seriousness of the illness increases, so may feelings of guilt, embarrassment, and self-blame. Families are part of the general culture which has supported these feelings. If families encounter professionals who maintain that families are responsible for the illness, then families have a double burden (Terkelsen, 1983), because their worst fears seem to be confirmed by an "expert."

As families begin to accept the illness, they experience a deep sense of loss. The loss includes the vision of the life they had envisioned for their family member. This feeling of loss is also experienced by the family member with the illness. All family members share this deep sense of loss in common. Acceptance of the loss is often made more difficult by the cyclical nature of the illness. Improvement of the family member raises hope that their family member will return to normal previous functioning. This on-again, off-again experience becomes an emotional roller coaster ride for the family. Gradually the persistence of the illness becomes obvious to the family. Then the grieving process can begin more fully as families let go of old hopes and expectations and begin to create new ones. Awareness also creates a crisis in meaning. Questions about oneself, one's relationships to others, to one's work, and to larger meanings or purpose in life become important. As these meanings change, families change.

Coping

Coping implies struggling with a problem with inadequate knowledge, skills or support. This is how families begin to cope. Coping begins to take the place of grieving. Families cope with the disruption in normal family life. They cope with recurrent crises, the persistence of the illness, the loss of faith in some professionals and the mental health system. Professionals may feel families are intrusive at this stage because families may become more angry and assertive. They may question professional competency. Their anger at professionals and the mental health system derives from their frustrations when seeking adequate care. Sometimes it derives from poorly trained professionals. The anger families feel is augmented by the hopelessness they often feel. They cope with pessimism and despair. Belief in family expertise grows. Families value the support of other families and learn to accept the limits of what they can do about the illness. They focus increasingly on the management of symptoms and improving the functioning of their family member. They become more interested in improved inpatient care, community services, housing and rehabilitation. They gradually identify professionals on whom they can rely, and work more closely with them. Families come to see valued professionals as necessary, but not sufficient.

Personal and political advocacy

Families gradually come to a new awareness of themselves in the recovery process. This awareness includes a greater level of personal advocacy and increased assertiveness. Families say they feel differently about themselves. Even though the illness of their family member continues, they have changed. They blame themselves less. They let go of what they can't change or don't want to change and become more focused on efforts to bring about the changes they see as necessary. They work out new roles and relationships with professionals which are more collaborative and based on equality. Their interest in the training of professionals may increase. They become more persistent over the long run. For many, political advocacy becomes more important. United action to change the system becomes more valued. Families experience their power, often for the first time in their life. They experience their ability to influence the systems that are supposed to support their family member. At this point, they have integrated and/or deepened new meanings and values about themselves, others, their work, and larger concerns in life.

PRACTICAL COPING STRATEGIES

During the last decade we conducted research in the area of family needs and we have trained professionals to respond to family needs with practical strategies (Zipple & Spaniol, 1987a,b; Zipple, Spaniol & Rogers, 1990). In our work with families, they themselves have identified many areas of concern and strategies for dealing with families. In addition to our work with families and professionals, we also worked extensively with people with mental illness who identified their own coping needs (Spaniol & Koehler, 1993a,b,c). They made many suggestions about how they would like family members to respond when they are confused or in crisis. The following sections identify the most common problem areas facing families and the strategies which they and their family members with a mental illness have suggested for coping effectively.

Bizarre or unusual behavior

Families often have difficulty coping with the symptoms that accompany schizophrenia and other serious mental illnesses. Families suggested a number of strategies for managing such behavior in the home. They stress the importance of becoming more tolerant of symptom-related behavior. Some behavior may be benign although eccentric. Learning to identify harmful or unacceptable behaviors is an important skill.

It is important to take the time to sit down and talk calmly with the family member about their concerns and the family's concerns about behavior before behavior becomes harmful or unacceptable. It is important to be clear with the family member about the behaviors which the rest of the family expects and those it dislikes. However, families have noted that relying on threats is counter-productive. It is better to remind the family member clearly, firmly and repeatedly about behavior which is and is not acceptable. It is useful to ask the family member what is helpful to them, what they would like done, and who they would like to do it. Early negotiating can create responses that are more effective in helping family members and their family member with a mental illness through difficult times.

Sometimes families find it necessary to gently confront hallucinations or delusions by reminding the family member that what he or she is experiencing is a part of their illness. For example, they might refuse to discuss paranoia because it is a distortion of reality. Or, they may identify behavior suggesting that a manic episode may be building. This kind of feedback can be very reassuring to the family member with the illness because they are often as frightened by their behavior as other family members are. Many families suggest that gentle physical contact, humor and consistent reassurance are essential in connecting with the family member and reducing their fears. Other families suggest that distraction can be a useful strategy, such as involving the family member in family activities and in the day-to-day rhythm of the household.

Families know that their family member can become skilled at challenging his or her own symptoms with adequate skills and support. Discuss with your family member the possibility of receiving training in symptom management strategies. Self-management is ultimately the most effective. Manuals and workbooks on symptom management strategies have become available over the past five years (Wallace, Liberman MacKain, Blackwell & Eckman, 1992; Spaniol & Koehler, 1993).

Families have also suggested the importance of coordinating in-home efforts with the efforts of mental health practitioners. Regular contact with the treatment practitioners for the purposes of soliciting information, advice and support in helping the family member with the illness to manage his/her symptoms can be useful. Coping with overt symptoms can be a challenge and an active partnership between the family, the family member with the mental illness and mental health practitioners can increase the chances of finding successful solutions.

Aggressive behavior

Aggressive behavior on the part of the family member with the illness towards other family members is a particularly difficult problem. Assaults and the threat of assault, while not common, are crises of major importance when they occur. Families have suggested the importance of remaining calm in these situations and speaking to the family member in a firm but normal voice. They emphasize the need to be clear about what behavior is acceptable and unacceptable in the family and to explain the reasons. Other families have indicated that it is helpful to let the family member know about the effect that their assaultive and aggressive behavior has on other family members. This is not done to induce guilt. Rather, it is done to help the family member stay connected with the other family members and to understand how distressing the aggressive behavior can be to others.

If the family member with the illness is angry it is important to listen to their concerns while they are still at a low level. Expressing feelings before they build up to a crisis helps build connectedness and intimacy. It is a way to let each other know that each person counts and has value within the family. Listening is a way of acknowledging a family member's value. It is particularly important because mental illness and the consequent stigma often challenge a person's sense of value.

Families also report that they must rely on outside help to manage severely aggressive behavior. They quickly learn that others can also make a difference. In areas where crisis outreach services are available, early contact with the crisis team may provide helpful suggestions and support for managing aggressive behavior and insure more effective responses if these strategies do not work. Many families report that they call the police when they believe that their family member's behavior has become dangerous. Calling the police is often traumatic for the family and the family member with the mental illness. Yet, it is a coping option that families sometimes feel they must use.

Families also mention the importance of working on problems with the family member while they are calm. Everyone has limits and it is important not to wait until a person is pushed over the edge. During calm periods the family member with the illness and other family members can work together to outline a successive set of interventions of gradually increasing intensity. Discussion can help the family member with the illness identify early interventions that would help eliminate aggressive behavior before a major crisis erupts. Family decisions arouse many strong emotions in all family members. Living with upset caused by limits can be difficult, even when these limits are mutually agreed upon. It is important for families to get support as they hold to these limits.

Self-destructive and suicidal behavior

Self-destructive and suicidal behavior seem to generate the most intense feeling of anger, guilt and helplessness in family members. It is important to note that many families support their family member with the illness through many difficult years of suicidal feelings and self-destructive behavior. These families indicate that it is important to listen to their family member and to their concerns sympathetically. It is important to allow them to talk about their depressed or self-destructive feelings and what is happening to bring on these feelings.

Sometimes gentle confrontation by family members about the value of life and the importance of the family member with the illness to the rest of the family is helpful. Everyone needs to know that he/she is valued, especially when distressed. Sometimes simply sitting quietly with the family member and keeping him/her company is sufficient.

Active collaboration with treatment professionals is reported by families as essential to avoiding suicidal behavior. Medication, regular outpatient therapy and support from peers can help many people. Making use of mental health practitioners can also relieve families from the stress of being the only active support for the family member with the mental illness.

Like aggressive behavior, it is helpful to discuss these situations with the family member when they are not actively suicidal. For example, ask them what they want you to do or say when they are feeling suicidal? What would be helpful to them? During these discussions, develop a set of mutually agreed upon interventions for coping with the suicidal behavior. Mutual identification of early warning signs and strategies allows the family and the family member with the mental illness to intervene before suicidal behavior begins.

Families also emphasize the importance of recognizing what they can realistically manage in the home and what is beyond their ability to manage. When self-destructive or suicidal behavior or thoughts do not subside or increase to where the family and/or the person with the mental illness can no longer manage it, it becomes necessary to call the local crisis team or police. They have the skills required to get the family member to an emergency room for evaluation and possible hospitalization. If the family member is actively engaged in self-destructive behavior, it may be necessary for the family to interrupt the behavior physically. Again, calling for assistance from peers, the local crisis team, emergency room, or police may be necessary. Families emphasize that they must deal with the immediate crisis in these situations and wait to discuss the situation with the family and the family member with the illness once the immediate crisis has been resolved.

Social withdrawal

Many individuals with serious mental illnesses withdraw from family members and friends. This can happen even when the family member with the illness is living in the family household with active and supportive loved ones. Many families experience this withdrawl as a painful rejection. Others worry that the isolation will lead to an exacerbation of the illness. Still other families find that they grieve the loss of the full participation of the family member in the life of the family.

Families suggested a two-prong approach to coping with withdrawal and isolation. First, they advised against forcing the family member to be unreasonably social and active. The family member may need significantly more "down time" than most people to integrate and sort out his/her experiences. It is important to acknowledge that the family member may need to be alone at times and to create physical and emotional space for him/her. For some people with mental illness, this need for emotional space can be a lifelong condition. This may be expecially true for individuals with persistent symptoms.

Second, it is helpful to gently and consistently encourage additional social activities. This may mean increased involvement in family social activities and the day-to-day rhythms of the household. For example, grocery shopping and other necessary household activities provide many opportunities for social engagement. Involvement also reassures the family member that he/she is a valued person in the family. It may also be helpful to encourage the family member to participate in a social/vocational rehabilitation, a clubhouse program or a peer support group. Families may need to advocate for these services in the community because families consistently report that one of their greatest concerns is the lack of social and vocational rehabilitation services (Skinner et al, 1992; Spaniol et al., 1987). It is important to advocate with the family member's practitioners for more support in helping the family member access and utilize these resources. However, families need to continue to recognize the limits that their family member with an illness may have and not push them beyond their tolerance for social activity. It may be helpful to work with therapists, case managers and their family member to develop meaningful schedules of social activity which are appropriately demanding.

Hygiene and appearance

At times the physical appearance and hygiene of the family member with the illness differs from the rest of the family. Their appearance may be a source of worry, irritation and embarrassment to themselves and other family members. Families have encouraged acknowledging the range of styles that may be acceptable among the family member's peers and suggest that family members increase their tolerance for a broader acceptance of appearance and hygiene.

Other families indicated that frequent and gentle reminders about cleanliness in terms of clothes and bathing can be useful, as well as sharing their feelings directly with their family member in a supportive manner. It is helpful to find out what the family member's concerns are about clothing and hygiene. Ask them how would they like to dress and care for themselves and what would be helpful. How would they like people to let them know that hygiene or appearance is not acceptable? Becoming a source of support rather than a source of criticism and additional demands can be liberating for the whole family.

Families indicate that sometimes the family member may not be aware that their appearance and hygiene have worsened. Arranging for special instruction on hair care, makeup and wardrobe may give the family member the information, skills and encouragement necessary to improve his/her appearance. Actively involving the family member in selecting new clothes and consistently praising him/her for improvement in appearance and hygiene is also helpful. Supporting the family member for positive achievements helps to build self-esteem and self-respect.

Cooperation with treatment

Families are usually very concerned about their family member's participation in recommended treatment. This is especially true in the area of medication. Family members indicated willingness to take medication is the single most important variable in predicting whether the family member with the illness will function well in the home. They indicate that supportive reminders to take medication and helping the family member understand and manage the medication and its side effects are essential.

Medication raises strong feelings in families and in people with mental illness. It is important that everyone in the family understands the family member's medication and its side effects. If families have a clear understanding of the family member's concerns about the medication, they are more likely to help their family member manage the medication and its side effects. Families understand the reluctance of their family member to take medication because they are also very concerned about potential side effects. All members of the family struggle with the balancing of benefits and costs. Discussing medications and mutual concerns together can help relieve some of the fears and anxieties everyone in the family feels.

Families also report discussing how willingness to take medication can reduce symptoms and prevent hospitalization. Some families have taken a very firm stance on medication, requiring that the family member take medication as prescribed in order to remain at home or to visit the home. This decision is very painful for everyone, but some families have indicated that it was important and helpful.

Reminders and support for the family member (including transportation) to attend psychiatrist and therapist appointments may be helpful. Also, consumer/survivor support groups can often be of assistance in understanding the importance of medication. Families also emphasize the importance of working collaboratively with practitioners to support the ongoing cooperation with the treatment. Finally, some families have encouraged their family member to assume responsibility for his/her own life and live with the consequences of taking or not taking his/her medications. This "school of hard knocks" or "logical consequences" approach seems most feasible in situations where the family member does not reside in the family home.

Stress management

There are times when the preceding suggestions are adequate to help families cope with the demands of caring for their family member with the mental illness. Yet families must also work hard to manage their own personal levels of stress and cope with the feelings and changes in their lives generated by the stress. The most useful source of support for families is other families. Sharing experiences and feelings in a family support group with other families can help reduce personal and familial tension and can identify practical solutions that other families have found useful. Sharing also helps families experience part of the recovery process as they feel their pain, move through it, and move on to other feelings.

In addition to sharing feelings and experiences, group sharing can facilitate exploration and deepening of the family's beliefs and values. Beliefs and values are important advocacy tools. They indicate personal and political initiatives families can take. As families move beyond the telling of their stories they need support for initiatives that increase the effectiveness of the service delivery system for their family member with the mental illness. Family support groups can help families deal more effectively with the service system. The family support group can help families to finally accept the need to change the mental health system.

Families realize that the stress of dealing with the mental illness of one family member places a great burden on relationships with other family members. Siblings are especially vulnerable to the onset of a mental illness in a member of their family. Research on the impact on siblings is just beginning to become available (Marsh, 1993a,b). We know, for example, that younger siblings of a family member with a mental illness have a more difficult time coping than older siblings who have already left the home when the illness occurs. Families need to take the time to pay attention to how other family members are experiencing this family trauma. Active listening, setting aside time for special activities, and providing information are important resources for siblings. Encouraging siblings to join their own sibling support group can also be helpful.

Because the mental illness of a family member can be so demanding of time and energy, many families recognize the importance of balance in their lives. When families are under stress they often eliminate the very things that have comforted and soothed them in the past, just when they need them most. Familiar activities that had been enjoyed should be reintroduced into the life of the family. Family members need their own lives, and they must secure them for themselves. No one else can do this for them.

The onset of severe mental illness in a family challenges how family members see themselves, their relationships with others (especially relatives), their living, learning and working environment, and their larger meaning or purpose in life. Similar challenges are also being faced by the family member with the illness. Families need validation for themselves. The family support group can give this to them. A mutual discussion of challenges with their family member with the mental illness can deepen their relationship. Each share the same challenge. What one person experiences is not that different from what others experience.

Families experience it together. Together they can confront their feelings and the challenges that provoke them.

Families take different approaches to building a life for themselves. Some find it helpful to be involved in activities that are not related to mental illness. Some find meaningful work away from the home. Some use regular exercise and proper nutrition to break the cycle of their stress. Some find that scheduling time with friends is helpful. Whatever options they choose, they are effective because they break the cycle of stress. In addition, they promote self-care, ground themselves in important ways, and offset the debilitating effects of stress.

Maintaining a realistic hope is important for families. They know there are no miracles, yet they are also aware that much remains to be discovered by neurobiology, rehabilitation and service system design. Some people with severe mental illness do very well with adequate information, skills, and support. Others do not. The hope is that we will find a way to reach even those who appear to be unreachable. The vision most useful for families is the vision of recovery. That is, that the family and the person with the mental illness will find a way to rebuild the personal, social, environmental, and spiritual connections that have been so severely broken by the illness.

SUMMARY

Major mental illnesses affect families as well as individuals. Families struggle to cope with the changes and often difficult behavior of their family member with a mental illness. There are no simple answers for families as they struggle to cope. Rather, every day is a process of trial and error. Families look towards professionals and each other for support and assistance in identifying effective methods of coping. It is important that practitioners are available to family members to support their efforts to manage the challenges at home.

It is also important for practitioners to listen to families and to learn from them. Families often have significantly more experience than practitioners in struggling and responding to the difficulties of their family member with the illness. If practitioners are willing to listen to and learn from families they will gradually increase their own repertoire of strategies that are effective for coping and become more helpful to subsequent families.

REFERENCES

Lazarus, R.S. and Folkman, S. (1984) *Stress, appraisal, and coping.* New York: Springer Publishing Company.

Marsh, D. (1993a). *Innovations and Research*, 2(2).

Marsh, D. (1993b). *Innovations and Research*, 2(2).

Power, P.W., Dell'Orto, A.E. & Gibbons, M.B. (Eds.) (1988). *Family interventions throughout chronic illness and disability.* New York: Springer Publishing Co.

Skinner, E.A., Steinwachs, D.M. & Kasper, J.A. (1992). Family perspectives on the service needs of people with serious and persistent mental illness: Part I: Characteristics of families and consumers. *Innovations and Research*, 1(3), 23-30.

Spaniol, L. (1992). *Beyond stress management: A holistic approach.* Human Services Associates, 218 Newtonville Avenue, Newton, MA 02158.

Spaniol, L. Coping strategies of family caregivers. In A.B. Hatfield & H. Lefley (Eds.). *Families of the mentally ill: Coping and adaptation.* New York: Guilford Press, 1987.

Spaniol, L. & Koehler, M. (1993a). *The recovery workbook: Practical strategies for facilitating the recovery of people with mental illness.* The Center for Psychiatric Rehabilitation, Boston University.

Spaniol, L. & Koehler, M. (1993b). *Recovery: Self-reports by people with mental illness.* The Center for Psychiatric Rehabilitation, Boston University.

Spaniol, L., Koehler, M. & Gagne, C. (1993c). *Psychological and social aspects of mental illness.* The Center for Psychiatric Rehabilitation, Boston University (draft).

Spaniol, L., Jung. H., Zipple, A.M. & Fitzgerald, S. (1987). Families as a resource in the rehabilitation of the severely psychiatrically disabled. In A. Hatfield and H. Lefley (Eds.), *Families of the mentally ill: Coping and adaptation.* New York: Guilford Press.

Terkelsen, K.G. (1983). Schizophrenia and the family: II, Adverse effects of family therapy. *Family Process*, 22, 191-200.

Tessler, R.C., Killian, L.M. & Gubman, G. (1987). Stages in family response to mental illness: An ideal type. *Psychosocial Rehabilitation Journal*, 10(4), 3-17.

Thurer, S. (1983) Deinstitutionalization and women: Where the buck stops. *Hospital and Community Psychiatry*, 34(12), 1162-1163.

Van der Kolk, B. (1987). *Psychological trauma.* Washington, DC: American Psychiatric Press.

Wallace, C.J., Liberman, R.P., MacKain, S.J., Blackwell, G. & Eckman, T.A. (1992).

Effectiveness and replicability of modules for teaching social and instrumental skills to the severely mentally ill. *American Journal of Psychiatry*, 149(5), 654-658.

Zipple, A.M. & Spaniol, L. (1987a). *Families that include a person with a mental illness: What they need and how to provide it.* (A Trainer's manual). The Center for Psychiatric Rehabilitation, 730 Commonwealth Ave., Boston, MA 02215.

Zipple, A.M. & Spaniol, L. (1987b). *Families that include a person with a mental illness: What they need and how to provide it.* (A Student's manual). The Center for Psychiatric Rehabilitation.

Zipple, A.M., Spaniol, L. & Rogers, S. (1990). Training mental health professionals to assist families of persons who are mentally ill. *Rehabilitation Psychology*, 35(2), 121-129.

Chapter 8

DETERMINING AND IMPLEMENTING
THE FAMILY SERVICE PLAN

Kayla F. Bernheim

It is now widely recognized that state-of-the-art treatment planning for any psychiatrically disabled person necessarily includes attention to the role the family will play in rehabilitation efforts, and to the type and intensity of professional activities that will be necessary to support their competently filling that role. In short, the family service plan should be an integral part of the patient's treatment plan. This chapter will i) offer a frame of reference for conceptualizing the clinician's role in working with families. 2) review the skills and knowledge base which are necessary for the family clinician, 3) discuss the goals and procedures for the initial phase of family contact, 4) consider the steps necessary to arrive at a family service plan, and 5) explore some of the implementation issues involved in working with families.

FAMILY CONSULTATION

Developing a cooperative alliance with families is a relatively new goal of professional practice. Until recently, families (when they were seen at all) were seen as the recipients of treatment, the "unidentified patients" as it were. Just as the patient role is not conducive to the development of assertive interactions, nor to feelings of competence and mastery, the therapist role is not conducive to sharing knowledge and power, nor to acknowledging the expertise and autonomy of the non-therapist participants. 'Thus, it has been argued that a therapeutic orientation to work with families of persons with serious marital illness may be ineffective if not iatrogenically harmful. (Drake and Sederer, 1986; Terkelsen. 1983; Spaniol et al., 1984). Therefore, an alternative model for professional practice with families, currently characterized as "family consultation" has recently gained acceptance (Bernheim, 1989; Wynne et al., 1986; Kanter, 1985).

While family therapy is based on a model of family pathogenesis, family consultation is based on a notion about family functioning that Pinsof (1983) has described as the "assumption of least pathology," Hatfield and Lefley (1987) have called a "coping/adaptation" model, and Marsh (1992a) has characterized as a "family competence" paradigm. Through these lenses, mental illness is seen as a catastrophe that befalls a family, much like flood, death, or loss of livelihood might befall a family. As such, it challenges the adaptive capacities of individual family members and of the family system as a whole. Families of the mentally ill are presumed to be much like other families in their pre-existing capacities to manage the various stressors and to solve the various problems connected with the illness. Therefore, intervention is not oriented to reducing dysfunction, since none is presumed, a priori, to exist. Rather it is aimed towards increasing both emotional and practical mastery skills of family members.

The word "consultation" is defined as "deliberating together" (C. and G. Merriam Co., 1963). This implies a structural equality between the deliberating parties—in this case, the mental health professional and the family member. In family consultation, the agenda is mutually set, unlike family therapy in which the therapist may have the a priori (and generally unstated) goal of emancipating the patient from the family of origin or of reducing the level of "expressed emotion" in relatives. Note that consultation is different from family education in the same way: course goals and syllabus are set by the instructor (with, perhaps, some input from students). Family consultation implies a "doing with" rather than a "doing to" or even a "doing for." Relatives are acknowledged to bring to the process information and expertise which will be useful in rehabilitation efforts. Consultation implies a mutual sharing rather than a withholding of information and does not admit the use of paradoxical, mystifying, or authoritarian techniques.

Having said what consultation is not, what can we say about what it is? Consultation is a process in which most of us have participated at some time or another. We have consulted with financial planners, attorneys, physicians, interior decorators, even hairdressers and butchers. In each case, the consultative aspect of our interaction with these professionals involves goal-setting and strategy-planning.

Perhaps the most analogous consultation is that between the primary care physician and the specialist, in which the ongoing care is provided by one health care professional, with advice and occasional participation provided by the other.

In family consultation interested family members (who often function as primary caregivers for their ill relative) and mental health professionals exchange information to increase the competence of each, and to develop a mutual understanding about how each will participate and contribute to rehabilitation efforts. It contains large doses of listening, supporting, educating, advising, and negotiating by both parties. It is a dialogue which should begin early in treatment and which should occur periodically as treatment progresses. There may be times when regular, frequent. and intensive consultation is required, and other times when "as needed," infrequent, or informal consultation may be more appropriate. This will vary with the family's needs and wishes, the level of activity of the illness and rehabilitation efforts, and the agreed upon goals of consultation at any particular time.

Consultation may be viewed as the core service for families out of which other clinical and non-clinical services might evolve. For example, following an initial consultation, a family might participate in a family education or psychoeducation program before returning for additional consultation. They might be encouraged to attend Alliance for the Mentally Ill (AMI) support group meetings as an adjunct to ongoing consultation. One or more family members might decide, as a result of consultation, to enter individual psychotherapy. Whatever happens. the family consultant remains available to interpret and negotiate changes in the patient's rehabilitation plan, to reassess relatives' current needs, and to provide support and information. Consultation should be seen as an ongoing process in the context of a more or less chronic condition.

Not all family members will attend all consultation sessions. It is sometimes most efficient and appropriate to consult with the family as a whole (including, in some instances the ill person). Examples would include sessions in which the goals of the current rehabilitation program are being discussed, or in which the patient and family share their subjective experiences associated with the illness, or in which ground rules for living at home are negotiated. However, there may be times when relatives need to ventilate feelings in private, or when the ill person is too delusional or disruptive to participate in a useful way. Siblings or children of the ill person may need consultation for themselves, as their issues and needs are different from those of their parents. Often. the primary caregiver will elect to consult alone, sharing information with other relatives as needed.

Occasionally the mental health professional and relatives may conflict about who should attend a meeting. In these situations, reviewing the goals each holds for the consultation may reveal the source of the problem and point the way to its resolution.

SKILLS AND KNOWLEDGE BASE

Family consultation requires a wide range at knowledge and skills. Training in family therapy or individual therapy is widely regarded as insufficient (Wynne et al., 1988). The family consultant should be a senior clinician with specialized expertise in serious mental illness. He or she may be called upon to answer questions about etiology. symptoms, treatment options, course, and prognosis. Questions about what behaviors the patient can control are common as are those about whether and when the patient can be expected to continue with school or work.

The consultant should be familiar with the family burden literature (Johnson, 1990; Lefley, 1987a) and should be able to demonstrate understanding of the ways in which culture, phase of adaptation, and other variables can affect family members' experience of mental illness in their own families (Marsh, 1992b; Lefley, 1987b; Terkelsen, 1987; Bernheim and Lehman, 1985).

The clinician will need good pedagogical skills—the ability to simplify and synthesize, to organize material and communicate clearly, to tailor teaching pace and techniques to the learner's needs, and to cheek frequently that what is being taught is what is being learned. The ability to train relatives in certain behavioral skill areas. including communication, conflict resolution, problem-solving. and stress management, is an additional asset. Further, the family consultant will need skills similar to those of a good clinical supervisor—the ability to modify the amount of direction offered based on the needs of the consultee, and the ability to blend task orientation with attention to the emotional processes of the consultee.

Finally, the family consultant will need negotiating and conflict-resolution skills in order to assist the patient's treatment team to consider the needs. wishes, and opinions of relatives in treatment plan development. While the perspectives of team, patient and family often overlap, divergent views are also common. Without an ombudsman or advocate, relatives' opinions may neither be sought nor seriously considered.

In general, a warm, engaging, active style is preferable to a distant, formal, reserved posture. Invariably, relatives have suffered an assault on their self confidence, self-esteem, and ability to cope. It is likely that they have had experiences with professionals that have exacerbated these problems. They are prone to demoralization and guilt and can easily misinterpret ambiguous professional behavior as blaming or demeaning in intent. Therefore, the ability to demonstrate warmth, empathy, and support is fairly critical to gaining their trust and repairing their damaged sense of personal competence.

GOALS AND STRATEGIES FOR THE INITIAL SESSIONS

Ideally, the first family consultation occurs soon after the patient's illness is identified and treatment has begun. However, in reality, relatives may have gone months or even years before being provided adequate consultation. Therefore, the goals of the initial sessions will vary somewhat depending on the unique circumstances, the setting (inpatient, outpatient, residential), and the length of time the consultant predicts being available to the family. In general, four goals can be identified:

1. establishing an empathic/supportive connection
2. evaluating current needs, including informational needs
3. orienting relatives to the current situation
4. developing an initial plan for family services/involvement.

Establishing an Empathic/Supportive Connection

This goal has many names. Anderson et al. (1986) call it "joining." Others have identified the "therapeutic alliance" or the "working relationship." Typically, relatives will enter the treatment system after a period of turmoil or crisis. They can be expected to be demoralized, exhausted, and fearful. Often, they are also angry, guilt-ridden and despairing. Occasionally, they are relieved and even hopeful. At the beginning, it is important to allow relatives to ventilate, communicating to them that their feelings are both expectable and acceptable. The clinician should set enough time aside to allow relatives to tell their story in their own way if they seem to wish to do so. Often. an open-ended question ("what would you most like to tell me about your experiences with John's illness?") or empathic comment ("you folks have really had a rough couple of months, haven't you?") will put the first session on the right footing.

The experienced clinician who is familiar with the family burden literature will have multiple opportunities to demonstrate empathy. For example, one might encourage the family to talk about sadness and loss, or the sense of isolation and stigma that they may have experienced, or about the frustrations attendant upon attempts to secure help. In any case, the focus should be on the family's *experience* of the illness rather than on collecting a more formal, "objective" history.

In addition to demonstrating empathy and support, the clinician should look for opportunities to demonstrate trustworthiness. Admitting uncertainty or ignorance, clarifying expectations, taking care to be respectful of relatives' experiences and attempts to cope, and asking for feedback about one's own behavior (e.g. , "do you feel that this conversation has been useful to you? is there anything else I could do that would be helpful to you right now?") are examples of behaviors which can enhance trust.

It is often particularly useful to explore the family's previous experiences with mental health providers as their expectations will be colored by this history. If they have felt disrespected, held responsible for the illness, neglected, or abused, they will be understandably wary. If, on the other hand, they have had positive experiences, they may be able to develop a working alliance more rapidly (unless, or course, they are mourning the loss of the previous clinician). This is the context in which to explore how confidentiality issues have been handled in the past and to develop mutual understandings about how they will be handled in the future. Successful management of boundary issues is one of the keys to establishing a supportive trusting relationship with family members.

As the family's story unfolds, the clinician will choose some areas to highlight and others to downplay. It is generally advisable to focus on areas of strength and competence rather than on deficits or mistakes, at least early in the developing relationship. Not only will this boost relatives' self-esteem, but it will create a sense of safety for family members who have been highly self-critical or who have felt criticized or belittled by family, friends, or other mental health workers.

Finally, achieving an empathic/supportive connection is dependent upon allowing the family to set (or at the very least to participate in setting) the agenda. The clinician's agenda—taking a history, giving certain information, promoting a certain kind of behavior change—should take a back seat to the family's agenda if at all possible. The questions of "who is in charge here" and "whose needs are to be met here" are paramount and will be answered, in the family's mind, quite early, for better or for worse.

Evaluating the Family's Current Needs

Clearly, relatives will have different needs at different points in their experience with mental illness. They may be actively seeking information at point A, needing to learn certain skills at point B, grieving their loss at point C, and dealing with non-illness related concerns at point D. Therefore, it is inappropriate to provide a group format psychoeducational experience for all relatives. Over the course of the first few family meetings, the clinician will be developing a picture of the unique strengths, resources, and problems that each family member brings at that particular moment to the challenge of coping with mental illness. An individualized plan should take into account as many of these variables as possible.

The family's phase of adaptation to the illness will be relevant to relatives' needs (Terkelsen. 1987; Marsh, 1992b). For the family whose ill relative has just suffered an acute, traumatic, first psychotic episode, crisis intervention, respite and very basic information about the initial phase of treatment may be all that is needed. At this point, extended educational interventions would likely be inappropriate. Referral to AMI groups might also be premature for many relatives at this point, since the issue of chronicity has not yet been faced. Some skills-building interventions are most useful prior to discharge from inpatient services or at other times when family-patient interaction is anticipated to be high. Emotional support (including, possibly, supportive psychotherapy) should be extended to relatives when emotional issues, like grieving, surface. The clinician will want to take a developmental approach to needs assessment, building in opportunities to change the service plan as relatives' experiences and expertise evolve.

Of course, it is important to assess relatives' knowledge and sophistication about behavioral disorders. Do they subscribe to an illness model. or do they frame the problem as laziness, moral failure, or possession by the devil? What assumptions do they make about the ill person's level of responsibility for symptoms, or about their own? What information has been provided by previous mental health professionals about the illness. its causes, prognosis, and treatment? Do relatives have faith in this account? Are there gaps or distortions in their knowledge? One of the goals of family consultation will be to develop, if possible, an explanatory construct that is held mutually by the patient, the family. and the clinical team. However, in the beginning it will be enough to respectfully explore participants' ideas about what has happened and why.

Relatives' expectations for the patient should be explored. Both short and long term goals can be discussed with a view towards assessing how realistic the goals are, in light of current understanding. Frequently, relatives need help in walking the fine line between hopelessness (and its attendant demoralizing effects on the patient as well as others) and unrealistic hopes of complete cure which can raise the level of stress experienced by all members of the family.

The clinician will also want to assess the family's skills as well as knowledge. How successful are they at managing symptoms? Have they been able to contain or minimize the disruptive effects of the illness on their own lives? Do they know how to effectively interact with the mental health system and access appropriate responses? If some skills are inadequate to the task, what services might help relatives becomes more proficient? Generally, family members' stress management, problem-solving, conflict-resolution, and communication skills (at a minimum) should be evaluated since behavioral training may be useful to those with weaker skills.

In order to plan for the future, the clinician will need to assess relatives' wishes for involvement in rehabilitation efforts. How "burnt out" are family caregivers? What responsibilities have they assumed? What input have they had so far? What modifications in their role do they wish to make? How consonant are their expectations and wishes with the perspective and goals of the treatment team? What are the potential areas of conflict? How might these be ameliorated? Again, needs may differ over time: family members may need respite and a low level of involvement immediately following a crisis but they may want substantial participation later in the process.

Finally, initial assessment should include attention to relatives' access to outside supports, as well as the nature and extent of non-illness related stressors. For examples a single parent with no car and few friends will have different needs from a married sister with children of her own. Aging parents with health problems or a fixed income will have yet another set of concerns, needs, and resources, as will a large, extended family with many intrafamilial and community ties. To the extent that caregivers are isolated, support may need to be provided by the mental health system; to the extent that care givers are burdened by additional life problems, the system may need to address those before the full adaptive capacities of the family can be brought to bear on the problem of mental illness.

Orienting Relatives to the Current Situation

Confusion is a major block on the road to mastery. Inadequate orientation is common. It undermines relatives' sense of efficacy and gets the family-professional relationship off to a rocky start. For example, many community residence programs are meant to be transitional, but families may perceive them as permanent asylum. When, later, discharge is attempted, the family's anxiety and resistance may have a negative impact. Equally commonly, relatives often expect more of acute inpatient treatment than it is able to provide As one father said "when the doctor said he had to stay four or five days, I thought that was a long time, but I thought he'd be all healed up—you know, that he'd be a new man or something, a new kid." (Bernheim et al., 1982). Letting families know what reasonably can be expected is a great help.

As with other aspects of working with families, orientation should be geared to the particular needs of specific families. Some will need a painstaking and comprehensive orientation to the mental health system as a whole. This may include describing stages and levels of care (for examples what is day treatment, how is it different from outpatient treatment, and when is it appropriate?), discussing the range of outcomes that might be expected, and explaining the various financial resources that may be available and how these would be accessed. Providing written material to augment the discussion is generally advisable as memory is short when stress is great.

Other families may require only a more specific orientation to the particular treatment setting in which the professional works. What is its role in the larger system? What is the time frame with which it works? Does it have a utilization review mechanism? If so, what are the criteria for retention? What are the goals? Who are the players and what are their roles? How do they relate to professionals from other involved agencies and to each other? What input and responsibilities should relatives expect to have? Who should they contact if there is a problems? Are there formal mechanisms to address grievances? If so, how do they work?

This kind of orientation may be done in a group setting. In addition to the cost and time advantage, such a setting gives relatives the chance to hear answers to questions they hadn't thought to ask. They may be stimulated by the conversation to address their own concerns.

Developing an Initial Plan for Family Service/Involvement

The initial phase of family consultation moves towards conclusion when relatives have established rapport with and trust in the professional, when they understand the current situation, and where the professional understands their feelings, strengths, wishes, and needs. This may take one session or it may take several. The end product is a plan that specifies 1) how and for what purpose relatives will continue to be involved with both the patient and the mental health system, 2) what clinical or non-clinical services will be provided to the family, and 3) when and how the plan will be reviewed. For some families, the plan may consist of nothing more than an occasional phone call. Some may read about mental illness. Others will attend case conferences, family support meetings, psychoeducational or skills-training sessions. Others may request ongoing consultation or psychotherapy of some kind for themselves. In some families the primary caregiver will liaison with the treatment team, while in others, more or other members at the family may be involved in some way.

Ideally, the plan should consider the needs of all family members, even those to whom it is decided that services won't be directly provided. For example, siblings of a young adult patient may have concerns that their parents can address. Consultation can help the parents become sensitive to, anticipate, and respond to those concerns more adequately. In addition, the person with the illness should be included in planning for family involvement as his or her wishes for autonomy and privacy may conflict with the family's desire for involvement and need for information. These conflicts can be negotiated at the beginning of treatment and agreements can be modified as needed. In all cases, flexibility is the watchword—there is no one right way to interact with all families, or even with one family over time.

IMPLEMENTATION ISSUES

As in any complex situation with multiple actors, each with a unique agenda, conflicts may arise. Of paramount concern to clinicians interested in family consultation has been the issue of confidentiality in particular, and boundary issues in general.

Confidentiality mandates, both ethical and legal, only occasionally present an insurmountable barrier to collaboration with family members (Zipple et al., 1990; Pepper and Ryglewicz, 1984). Rather, misunderstandings about and misuse of the confidentiality issue abound. First, clinicians should keep in mind the distinction between confidential and non-confidential information. For example, while telling relatives a patient's diagnosis may invoke confidentiality guidelines, educating them about the implications of that diagnosis does not, as this information is in the public domain. Second, listening to family members is never barred. Confidentiality refers to disclosure, not receipt of information. Third, individuals must be competent to give informed consent (or refusal). A patient who believes family members are really space aliens in disguise probably is not competent to give or withhold consent for information exchange. Fourth, confidentiality is not an all-or-none issue.

It is a rare patient who, for non-psychotic reasons, refuses to allow the clinician any contact with relatives. More commonly, even in cases where distance and distrust impair cooperation, permission for limited release of information can be obtained. Strategies for doing so include: 1) presenting the need for information exchange in a matter-of-fact manner, 2) taking time to explore patients' hesitancies rather than terminating the process if consent is initially withheld, 3) clarifying what information will and will not be exchanged, and 4) treating the consent issue as a process over time rather than as a single event.

Nonetheless, there are some situations in which it will not be feasible or advisable for the clinician who is working most directly with the patient to consult with the family. in these rare instances, referral of the family to a colleague or program that does not have a confidential relationship with the ill person can be helpful. In fact, many of the goals of family consultation can be met by a clinician who does not have personal knowledge of this patient, and many of the support and educational functions can be achieved through AMI group participation. Referral may also be in order when the clinician feels that the patient and the family have genuinely conflicting goals. In these instances, the clinician may feel unable to provide adequate advocacy for either. However, more often, these conflicts become more grist for the consultative mill, as conflict-resolution skills can be taught and practiced.

The question of who should provide consultation and who should participate in the development of the family service plan is complicated by more than confidentiality problems. The issues run the gamut from clinical to administrative, from individual to systemic. For example, in inpatient units social workers often are assigned the task of working with families, but relatives are often frustrated if they don't have access to the physician on the team. This problem can be solved in a number of ways, including occasional joint consultations with the physician and social worker, or by demonstrating the social worker's expertise in answering relatives' questions and addressing their concerns.

On the other hand, team members become frustrated when they're faced with calls from several members of the same family who appear to be unable to coordinate or cooperate among themselves. Working with the family to organize itself and to delegate one or two members to communicate with the team may be one of the first consultative tasks.

If multiple agencies are involved, who should consult to the family? While the case manager would, in some ways be the ideal person, only clinical case managers with advanced degrees are likely to have the necessary skills and expertise. When the case manager is not sufficiently skilled, team consultations which include representatives of each of the agencies may be necessary.

Other implementation questions may arise. When is it appropriate to include the ill person in family sessions? When are group sessions more beneficial than individual ones? When are home-based services preferable to agency-based services? How will family services be funded when the patient is not present (and, presumably insurance won't cover the session)? The answers to these questions will depend upon the unique circumstances of the patient, family, and agency.

How will we train, supervise, and support clinicians who are struggling to disengage from a family pathogenesis model, embrace a family competence model, and develop cooperative alliances with relatives of their patients? It is clear that a commitment to both preservice and inservice training will be required. There must also be administrative and supervisory support for the notion that successful engagement of the family is often as critical to rehabilitation as is a successful medication strategy. A system of care must be created in which it is unacceptable for a clinical team to decide it hasn't the time to work with families.

While the implementation issues are significant, the problems are not insurmountable. The development of a family service component to treatment should be considered an evolutionary process which begins by providing staff with opportunities to interact with relatives in new ways and to develop some comfort in doing so. Agencies might wish to form a family advisory group to begin a dialogue about needs and to break down family-agency barriers. At the same time, efforts might be made to train supervisory staff in a family competence paradigm. Or, one might ask staff to facilitate family support meetings or to provide family education lectures. Or records audits by quality assurance staff might attend to inclusion of a family service component (based on comprehensive assessment of the individual family) in the treatment plan. Or, several interactive agencies might come together to discuss how family services might be incorporated at a systemic level.

What is important is for clinicians to learn to listen, not just to their patients, but to relatives whose lives have also been disrupted, often catastrophically, by mental illness. As we get to know them, we will often find that they have developed expertise and resources that can help us as we endeavor to help them. In the end, to the extent that we can support the family's competence and reduce the distress of its members, we will be increasing the probability of successful community reintegration for the person with the illness.

REFERENCES

Anderson, C.M., Reiss, D.J., and Hogarty, G.E. (1986). *Schizophrenia and the family: A practitioner's guide to psychoeducation and management.* New York: Guilford.

Bernheim, K.F. (1989). Psychologists and families of the severely mentally ill: The role of family consultation. *American Psychologist. 44,* 561-564.

Bernheim, K.F. and Lehman, A.T. (1985). *Working with families of the mentally ill..* New York: Norton.

Bernheim, K.F., Lewine, R.R.J., and Beale, C.T. (1982). *The caring family: Living with chronic mental illness.* p. 12. New York: Random House.

Drake, R.E. and Sederer, L.I. (1986). The adverse effectsof intensive treatment of chronic schizophrenia. *Comprehensive Psychiatry, 27,* 313-326.

G. and C. Merriam Co. (1963). *Webster's Seventh New Collegiate Dictionary*, p. 179. Springfield, MA: G. and C. Merriam Co.

Hatfield, A.B. and Lefley, H.P. (Eds.) (1987). *Families of the mentally ill: Coping and adaptation.* New York: Guilford.

Johnson, D.L. (1990). The family's experience of living with mental illness. In HP Lefley and DL Johnson (eds) *Families as allies in treatment of the mentally ill: New directions for mental health professionals* (pp. 31-64). Washington, D.C.: American Psychiatric Association Press.

Kanter, J.S. (1985). Consulting with families of the chronic mentally ill. In J.S. Kanter (Ed) *Clinical issues in treating the chronic mentally ill* (pp. 21-32). San Francisco, CA: Jossey-Bass.

Lefley, H.P. (1987a). The family's response to mental illness in a relative. In A.B. Hatfield (ed.), *Families of the mentally ill: Meeting the challenges* (pp. 3-21). San Francisco, CA: Jossey-Bass

Lefley, H.P. (1987b). Culture and mental illness: The family role in AB Hatfield and HP Lefley (eds.) *Families of the mentally ill: Coping and adaptation* (pp. 30-59). New York: Guilford.

Lefley, H.P. and Johnson, D.L. (1990). *Families as allies in treatment of the mentally ill: New directions for mental health professionals.* Washington, D.C.: American Psychiatric Association Press.

Marsh, D.T. (1992a). *Families and mental illness: New directions in professional practice.* New York: Praeger.

Marsh, D.T. (1992b). Life-span perspectives in D.T. Marsh *Families and Mental Illness: New directions in professional practice* (pp. 61-78). New York: Praeger.

Pepper, B. and Ryglewicz, B (1984, November). Families and clinicians of young adult chronic patients: How can we bridge the gap? *TIE-Lines*, pp. 1-3, 6-7.

Pinsof, W. (1983). Integrative problem-solving therapy: toward the synthesis of family and individual psychotherapies. *Journal of Marital and Family Therapy, 9*, 19-36.

Spaniol, L. Jung, H. Zipple, A.M., and Fitzgerald, S. (1984). *Families as a central resource in the rehabilitation of the severely psychiatrically disabled: Report of a national survey.* Unpublished Manuscript, Boston Center for Psychiatric Rehabilitation, Boston, MA.

Terkelsen, K.G. (1987). The evolution of family responses to mental illness through time in A.B. Hatfield and H.P. Lefley (eds.) *Families of the mentally ill: Coping and adaptation* (pp. 151-166). New York: Guilford.

Terkelsen, K.G. (1983). Schizophrenia and the family. II. Adverse effects of family therapy. *Family Process, 22*, 191-200.

Wynne, L.C., Bernheim, K.F., and Wynne, A.R. (1988). Key issues for training in family therapy with the long-term, seriously mentally ill patients and their families, in *Clinical training in serious mental illness: Proceedings of the national forum for educating mental health professionals to work with the seriously mentally ill and their families.* National Institute of Mental Health, Chevy Chase, Maryland.

Wynne, L.C., McDaniel, S.H., and Weber, T.T. (1986). *Systems consultation: A new perspective for family therapy.* New York: Guilford.

Zipple, A.M., Langle, S., Spaniol, L., and Fisher, H. (1990). *Client confidentiality and the family's need to know: Strategies for resolving the conflict.* Unpublished manuscript, Boston University Center for Psychiatric Rehabilitation, Boston, MA.

Chapter 9

SERVING CHILDREN, SIBLINGS, AND SPOUSES: UNDERSTANDING THE NEEDS OF OTHER FAMILY MEMBERS

Katherine A. Judge

I. INTRODUCTION

Theories on family stress have been challenged for their failure to incorporate the notion that a stressful event will have unique meaning for each member of the family (Walker, 1985; Montgomery, 1985). Similar criticisms apply to research and services pertaining to families of persons with serious mental illness. Thus far, service providers primarily target parental caregivers for psychoeducational training. Likewise, the burgeoning research on families of the mentally ill most often relies on the report of a parent, i.e. the mother. While it is essential to address the needs of parental caregivers, this limited scope omits the experience of siblings within these uniquely stressed families, and overlooks the serious needs of children and spouse-caregivers of people with mental illness. To omit the divergent perceptions of individual family members is to underestimate the complex task families face as they work toward crisis resolution and reorganization (Walker, 1985; Montgomery, 1985).

This chapter focuses on the experience of children, siblings, and spouses of persons with major mental illness[1]. Because research and practice can and should inform each other, the chapter begins with a brief historical overview of the research on these three groups. The subsequent sections each concentrate on one of the three groups, begin-

---

1. Throughout this chapter "mental illness" refers primarily to severe and persistent forms of schizophrenia, bipolar disorder, and unipolar depression.

ning with children and ending with spouses of persons with serious mental illness. The relevance or significance of the particular relationship is discussed within a life-span development perspective. A review of the available literature is provided in hopes of illuminating the family experience from the unique perspective of each group. Similarly, each section attempts to explore the personal consequences for the individual whose parent, sibling, or spouse has a serious mental illness.

Finally, each section closes with a discussion of implications for services and service providers. Using Hatfield's (1988) distinctions between support, consultation, and education, the implications for service providers are discussed within a primarily psychoeducational framework. It is apparent throughout the chapter, however, that some family members have direct service needs which go beyond the objectives of psychoeducation. The discussion of service needs is not intended to be exhaustive. Instead, the reader is encouraged to derive methods for addressing the varied needs of family members which are congruent with their practical training, the needs of the families they serve, and the service setting.

II. BRIEF OVERVIEW OF RESEARCH IN THESE THREE AREAS

Historically, the *children* of people with mental illness have been studied more than any other family members. Originally termed "high-risk" studies, the early research focused on the genesis of mental illness and centered primarily on the mother-child dyad (Mednick, 1967). Within this research paradigm, the psychiatrically ill parents provide a genetic and environmental legacy for their children which puts them at high-risk for the development of severe mental illness. The avowed goal of such work was to discover the prevalence and predictors of psychopathology in the children studied. Eventually, researchers recognized that a significant proportion of these children never developed a mental illness and some, in fact, seemed to thrive. This led to the description and study of the "invulnerable" or "resilient" child and the factors that predict such successful outcomes (See Anthony & Cohler, 1987). Lander, Anthony, Cass et al. (1987) describe resilient children as competent in their thinking, their reality testing, their coping skills, their capacity to relate, their sense of identity, and their self-control. Unfortunately, this literature seldom speaks in the voice of the children studied, and fosters little understanding of how children perceive their families and their lives.

The experience of *siblings* of persons with serious mental illness has, for the most part, been overlooked by family researchers. The few early research efforts specific to well siblings sought to understand the pathology of the "schizophrenic family" through examination of well siblings (Lidz, Fleck, Alanen, & Cornelison, 1963; Day & Kwitkowska, 1962). More recently, however, the experience of siblings has been described in terms of their subjective burden (Riebschleger, 1991; Miller, Dworkin, Ward, & Barone, 1990) and the resources they offer their brother or sister with mental illness (Horwitz, Tessler, Fisher & Gamache, 1992). In addition, the voices of siblings have emerged powerfully through their own writing and research (Johnson, 1988; Riebschleger, 1991; Aranowitz, 1988; Moorman, 1988; Moorman, 1992).

Investigations of *spouses* of persons with serious mental illness were instrumental in generating the concept of "burden" as it relates to families of persons with mental illness. As the movement toward deinstitutionalization began in the late 1950s, researchers began to investigate the consequences of this transition for the patient's relatives. Spouses were among the first to be studied, as Clausen & Yarrow (1955) investigated the experience of women for six months to one year following their husbands' first admission to a psychiatric hospital. Except for studies which examine the effects of depression in marriage (Merikangas, Prusoff, Kupfer, & Frank, 1985; Biglen, Hops, Sherman, Friedman, Arthur, & Osteen, 1985), spouses are rarely the focus of contemporary research on families of persons with mental illness.

This overview reveals the serious limitations in the present state of knowledge regarding the experience and needs of these three groups. While the children's literature is vast, it is also full of inconsistent findings and rarely addresses practice implications. The sibling and spouse literature is so small as to be virtually non-existent. This chapter, though not exhaustive in its review, will draw upon the existing literature as well as related literatures to construct a provisional picture of the unique experience and needs of these family members.

III. CHILDREN OF PERSONS WITH SERIOUS MENTAL ILLNESS

For *children*, the parent-child relationship has a profound influence throughout life but commands primacy during infancy and the early childhood years. Object-relations (Winnicott, 1972) and attachment theorists (Bowlby, 1988) consider infancy the crucial period for the development of a core faith in self and other persons. Winnicott (1972) asserts that the "good-enough" parent not only meets the child's basic human needs, but also allows the infant a full range of experience without allowing need, emotion, or stimulation to be too overwhelming. The parent-child relationship is the most fundamental relational context; it is within this context that psychological growth unfolds (Jossel-son, 1992).

Kaplan and Sadock (1988) report that the number of children born to people with schizophrenia doubled from 1935 to 1955. The current rate of births to persons with schizophrenia and affective disorders is believed to resemble that of the general population (Kaplan & Sadock, 1988; Fadden, 1989). Studies suggest that many women with severe mental illness, whether institutionalized or not, wish to experience motherhood and do in fact give birth (McEvoy, Hatcher, Applebaum & Abernethy, 1983; Rudolph, Larson, Sweeny, Hough & Arorian, 1990). There is some evidence that persons with serious mental illness lose custody of their children and/or parental rights at disproportion-ately high rates (Fialkov, 1988; Knitzer, 1982), despite the purportedly low rates of child abuse among this population (Friedrich & Wheeler, 1982; Spinetta & Rigler, 1972).

Children of persons with serious mental illness have a higher risk of developing a major mental illness than the general population[2]. The fact remains, however, that an overwhelming majority of these children never develop the psychiatric disorder of their parent(s). While research reveals that some children thrive despite parental mental illness (An-thony & Cohler, 1987), there is much evidence to indicate that the stress and crises surrounding the mental illness of a parent lead to problems in adjustment and development (Radke-Yarrow, Nottelmann, Martinez, 1992; Silverman, 1989). In a study of children of persons hospitalized for psychiatric illness, Schacnow (1987) discovered that all the children displayed stress symptoms in reaction to the parent's decompensation and psychotic behavior. For children under 12 years of age, stress symp-toms included sleep disturbance, diminished appetite, more dependent and attention-seeking behavior, crying at night, social withdrawal, and problems with attention and learning at school. Children 12 years of age or older "verbalized a painful awareness of their parent's bizarre, deteriorated or self-destructive state" (p. 71). While the majority of the adolescents concurrently experienced a decline in school performance, 14% excelled academically. Adolescents, like their younger counter-parts, reported sleep disturbance and social withdrawal due to feeling different from peers and having increased responsibilities at home.

---

2. See Appendix 1 for the lifetime risk of developing bipolar disorder, unipolar depression, and schizophrenia for relatives of persons with these disorders.

The plight of some adolescent children is made alarmingly clear by Drake, Raucsin, and Murphy (1990) as they alert service providers to the risk of suicide among adolescent children of people with severe and persistent mental illness. The adolescents who committed suicide differed in terms of parental diagnosis, academic performance, and social competence. Each of them, however, had recently experienced the departure of a family member from the parental home, which consequently left the child to live alone with a seriously ill parent.

The experience of children of persons with serious mental illness will vary dramatically depending upon whether a well parent is in the home. When both parents have a serious mental illness, children are at increased risk for behavior problems and mental illness (Stiffman, Jung, & Feldman, 1988). But the presence of a well parent in the home consistently reveals beneficial outcomes (Rutter, 1987; Anthony, 1974; Kellamm, Ensminger, & Turner, 1977). A well parent has the potential to provide support, consistency, and a model for coping (Rutter, 1987; Castleberry, 1988). The well parent is also, however, a spouse who is grappling with the many stresses and demands of having a husband or wife with a mental illness[3], which may result in a decreased ability to meet the needs of the children (Grunebaum, 1984; Schacnow, 1987).

While boys may be more vulnerable to stress than their female counterparts (Rutter, 1970), boys appear to have better outcomes when their well father is in the household (Fisher, Kokes, Cole, Perkins, & Wynne, 1987). Furthermore, a cohesive sibling group plays an important role in mediating the stress associated with parental mental illness (Werner & Smith, 1982).

Well parents may underestimate the hardships experienced by children, and provide little explanation of the ill parent's behavior (Schacnow, 1987; Grunebaum, 1984). Reid and Morrison (1983) emphasize the importance of acknowledging the mental illness, and assert that the child's ability to cope effectively depends upon a realistic appraisal of the situation. Numerous studies indicate that a child's ability to achieve a psychological distance from the ill parent's behavior is essential for resilience (Anthony, 1987; Fisher et al., 1987; Schacnow, 1987; Worland, Janes, Anthony, McGinnis, & Cass, 1984). This objective stance may be especially difficult for the child who is incorporated into the delusional system of the parent (Anthony, 1987). With information

---

3. See section in this chapter on well spouses of persons with mental illness.

regarding the parent's mental illness and assistance with "reality testing," the child is better able to cope with the confusing and frightening symptoms of the parent's illness (Fisher et al., 1987; Anthony, 1987; Schacnow, 1987). The child must learn how to identify behaviors which are illness-related and avoid involvement in the affective state or psychosis of the ill parent.

The stress, and hence the risk, for children is compounded when the parent's illness is severe and chronic (Garmezy, 1984; Grunebaum, 1984), the family lives in poverty (Sameroff & Seifer, 1981), and there are repeated moves and separations (Rolf & Garmezy, 1974). The diagnosis of the afflicted parent may affect child outcome less than the severity and chronicity of the illness (Fisher et al., 1987), the general stress and chaos at home (Weintraub, Winters, & Neale, 1982), and the parent's level of social functioning (Kauffman, et al., 1979). Similarly, Musick et al. (1987) assert that the capacity to be an adequate parent is not related to diagnosis per se, but rather to a "constellation of maternal factors that seem related to the children's capacity to seek and use growth-fostering influences beyond the mother's orbit" (p. 240). According to Musick et al. (1987) young children fare better if: (1) the parent has attained a psychological distance from the child which facilitates decision-making that is in the child's best interest, (2) the parent is able to provide tasks for the child which are appropriate to the child's developmental needs, and (3) the parent is able to empathize with the feelings and needs of the child.

The child's age at the onset of the parent's mental illness is an important factor in determining resilience. Several studies indicate that a good parent-child relationship during the first year of life is key to healthy development (Anthony, 1987; Fisher et al., 1987; Werner & Smith, 1982). This notion is consistent with a range of psychological theories which view infant bonding with a parental figure (traditionally the maternal figure) as essential to the development of self (Winnicott, 1972; Bowlby, 1988). Anthony (1987) suggests that a sense of self lays the seeds of resilience and can only develop through parental availability, warmth, and responsiveness in the first year of life. Musick et al. (1987) point out that some mothers are able to provide their children with such contact despite their psychiatric disorder. Studies reveal inconsistent findings regarding the relationship between diagnosis and parental characteristics of withdrawal and emotional unavailability (Kauffman et al., 1979; Goodman & Brumley, 1990).

Social support including interaction with extrafamilial adults and the presence of many caretakers may protect children from stress and enhance their coping efforts (Werner & Smith, 1982; Kauffman et al., 1979). All of the children identified as good copers in Schacnow's study (1987) had an "empathic" adult available to them. An empathic adult is someone who discusses the parental illness openly with the child and whose report about the child's experience/feelings very closely matches the child's own report (Schacnow, 1987).

Finally, a child's coping skills can promote mastery of the stressful environment, modify its meaning, and alleviate stress symptoms (Feldman, Stiffman, & Jung, 1987). Intelligence, social skills, problem-solving ability, self-esteem and self-efficacy all contribute to a child's ability to cope with a stressful environment (Garmezy, 1981; Rutter, 1987). These factors have strong implications for service providers.

Adult Children

Investigators caution that, in their attempt to master their stressful family life, some children may become parental surrogates. Anthony (1974) describes some children as exhibiting a self-reliance and autonomy which is beyond their developmental years. Such self-reliance may lead to difficulty relying on others and asking for help in adulthood. Similarly, Anthony (1987) suggests that some resilient children pay a price for their competence and may find that the coping strategies of childhood and adolescence make intimacy difficult to achieve in adulthood. Coping through the construction of rigid personal boundaries, suppression of feelings and needs, and intellectualization may significantly interfere with both friendships and love relationships.

Anthony (1987) states that despite success and achievement, resilient adult children may experience a persistent, amorphous sense of dysphoria in adulthood. Bleuler (1978) suggests that a childhood dominated by the frightening symptoms of a fragile parent leaves painful memories for years to come, in addition to anger at an adult world that offered so little help. Adult children may experience grief over the loss of a normal childhood.

> When you've been through that . . . you can never really be happy; you can never laugh as others do, you always have to be ashamed of yourself and take care not to break down yourself (Bleuler, 1978, p. 410).

One of the few studies of this adult population corroborates Bleuler's findings. Williams and Corrigan (1992) studied college students who were the adult offspring of persons with serious mental illness. These adult children reported subclinical dysphoria, anhedonia, worry, and nervousness which likely diminished their quality of life. Williams & Corrigan report that anxiety and depression were greater for the off-spring of persons with mental illness than for adult children of alcoholics, though satisfaction with one's support network mediated reports of psychological distress. It is important to note that the adult children in this study were college students, hence these were the reports of "resilient" children.

Finally, many adult children eventually face the prospect of caregiving for their aging parent with mental illness (Bleuler, 1978). Painful childhood experiences and the demands of one's own life, may make caregiving in adulthood an emotionally overwhelming task.

Implications for Service Providers

Of course, not nearly all offspring of schizophrenics experience an adverse childhood development. There are vast numbers of examples that show how even schizophrenic parents can be good parents. Some children learn to distinguish what it is about their father or mother that is peculiar or sick, and what is good and lovable about him or her. Sometimes gifted, warm-hearted spouses are able to nullify all the evil influences of the other partner who is schizophrenic (Bleuler, 1978, p. 406).

Despite the expansive literature on children of persons with serious mental illness, there is surprisingly little formal support for these children. Those who treat adults with serious mental illness may not even be aware that their clients have children, let alone address the needs of these children (Silverman, 1989; Drake et al., 1990; Schacnow, 1987). It is incumbent upon mental health service providers to establish whether the adults they treat for major mental illness have children. When children are present, every effort should be made to assess their needs and well-being. Formal evaluations of developmental progress and psychological well-being at various stages of development are advisable (Silverman, 1989; Drake et al., 1990).

The service needs of the children of persons with serious mental illness vary depending upon their the age and developmental stage. Generally, the task of the service provider is to reduce the child's exposure to risk factors, and facilitate the development of protective factors in the child and the social network (Benard, 1987; Rutter, 1987; Silverman, 1989).

The most fundamental way to reduce the child's exposure to risk is to provide assertive treatment to the parent with serious mental illness. The prevention of relapse will reduce the child's risk of exposure to frightening symptoms, inadequate parenting, and disruptive separations. Ideally, such interventions would begin in infancy, when the seeds of resilience are planted (See Cohler & Musick, 1984, for examples of programs for infants and children).

Another strategy to reduce children's exposure to risk is to provide education and consultation to all family members. Both parents will benefit from information regarding the psychiatric disorder, its symptoms, the treatments, and strategies for coping. Education should also include information on the children's developmental needs, how the illness might effect parenting issues, and how to discuss the mental illness with their children[4]. In addition to education, parents may benefit from on-going practical assistance in providing effective parenting. The children must also receive education regarding the parent's illness in a manner which is appropriate to their cognitive capacity (Bernheim & Lehman, 1985). In early childhood the child can be helped to differentiate between reality and the parent's symptoms (reality-testing), e.g. your parent is sad because he/she has a mental illness, not because you make him/her unhappy. Such education should occur in a manner which conveys respect and positive regard for the parent. As the child grows, more sophisticated information about the illness, its symptoms, and coping behaviors is both appropriate and necessary.

Finally, exposure to risk may be reduced by encouraging growth-fostering activities for the child outside of the home. This may consist of a therapeutic nursery for the infant (Musick et al., 1987), day care for the pre-school child (Goodman, 1984), and a range of activities outside the home for the school-age child and adolescent (Benard, 1987). Such opportunities not only reduce exposure to stress, but also have the potential to provide important socialization experiences and opportunities for feelings of success and accomplishment. Furthermore, the parent may also benefit from respite.

Protective factors encompass both the resources within the child and the resources within the larger social system. Benard (1987) recommends a range of skills training interventions to develop the competencies of the child. Children of people with major mental illness may benefit from

---

4. Resources which may assist the service provider and parent in this area can be found in the Resource List at the end of the chapter.

training in social problem solving and critical thinking, assertiveness and communication skills, stress and health management, planning and goal setting, and academic skills. In addition, Rutter (1987) asserts that children can be helped to establish or maintain a sense of self-esteem and efficacy. Self-esteem may develop through secure and harmonious parent-child relationships in childhood and/or good interpersonal relationships with significant others throughout life (Rutter, 1987). Furthermore, both self-esteem and self-efficacy can be built through the accomplishment of tasks that are important to the child. Success in school, with friends, and non-academic pursuits builds the child's sense of self-worth and, hence, facilitates coping (Rutter, 1987).

Service providers can also cultivate protective conditions in the child's social system. The healing potential of significant others is cited consistently throughout the research. Some point to the protective influence of the well parent (Rutter, 1987), others declare the importance of siblings (Werner & Smith, 1982), and still others point to the influence of an "empathic" adult (Schacnow, 1987). Josselson (1992) asserts that human development does not rely solely on the parent-child relationship, rather it is the "whole interpersonal network that ultimately shapes development" (p. 28). Facilitating the formation or maintenance of consistent and empathic relationships with extended family, peers, trusted adults, or "mentors" may do much to provide protection for a child. Finally, community organizations (e.g. school, boy/girl scouts, sports, religious communities) can provide opportunities for children to participate in meaningful tasks and activities which foster social competence, self-esteem, and self-efficacy (Benard, 1987; Rutter, 1987).

Support Groups for Adult Children

The stigma surrounding mental illness may lead adult children to feel embarrassed about their childhood, sharing their unique family experience with no one (Bleuler, 1978). Throughout life, humans have a fundamental need to be known, understood, and accepted (Josselson, 1992). To be alone with a secret, believing that no one else has lived through what you have, is a horrendous form of isolation. In 1984 a support group was established for adult children and siblings of persons with mental illness. Affiliated with the National Alliance for the Mentally Ill, The *Sibling and Adult Children's Network* now has support groups in 35 states and Canada, publishes a newsletter, and serves as a clearinghouse of information for adult children and siblings[5]. Such

---

5. See resource list for contact information.

support groups allow adult children to talk with others who have experienced similar life experiences, thus decreasing their sense of aloneness. In addition, the support group provides a forum for the safe ventilation of feelings and facilitates recovery through validation and support (Moorman, 1988). Coping mechanisms are strengthened by the belief that someone else knows what one is going through (Josselson, 1992); support groups composed of similar others may meet this need.

In addition, adult children may have a range of service needs. They may need support regarding the role they decide to play in the ill parent's life and a range of clinical services to address feelings of dysphoria, loss, and issues surrounding intimacy. Julie Tallard Johnson (1988; 1989) has pioneered clinical interventions and self-help groups for adult children and other family members of persons with serious mental illness. For many family members, supportive counseling or therapy may be necessary as they seek to understand their family experience and its consequence.

IV. SIBLINGS

The life-long sibling relationship is the most enduring of human connections, extending beyond the relationships with one's parents, and preceding the connection with a life-mate and/or offspring (Cicirelli, 1982). The sibling relationship has special significance in human growth and development as siblings look to each other as models, friends, and competitors throughout childhood and adolescence (Goetting, 1986; Dunn, 1984; Bank & Kahn, 1975; Ross & Milgram, 1980). Siblings often serve as primary sources of emotional support in preadolescence and adolescence, a time when friends are capricious and parents less attractive as confidants (Lamb, 1982). Many now recognize that sibling relationships can have a profound influence on child and adolescent development, and often a source of support and connection throughout adulthood (Sandmaier, 1944).

The onset of serious mental illness generally occurs in late adolescent or adult years. One consequence of these relatively late disability onsets is the disruption of a sibling relationship. It is not uncommon for siblings to have had a close relationship with a highly functional brother or sister prior to the onset of mental illness. Consequently, like parents and spouses, the experience of siblings has often been explained in terms of the process of grief and loss (Riebschleger, 1991; Miller et al., 1990; Johnson, 1988; Titelman & Psyk, 1991). Researchers compare the onset of mental illness to a death in the family which is complicated by stigma, the cyclical nature of the illness, and the continuing physical presence of the bereaved. In a preliminary study of unresolved grief, Miller et al. (1990) found considerable grief among family members of persons with serious mental illness, and no difference between parents and siblings in their level of grief. Their research suggests that a prolonged period of time passes before families realize the scope of their loss.

Remarkably similar to the literature on sibling bereavement, the theme of survivor's guilt pervades the literature on siblings of persons with severe mental illness (Titelman & Psyk, 1991; Samuels & Chase, 1979; Bank & Kahn, 1982). Survivor's guilt may be more common among younger siblings of persons with serious mental illness, especially same-gender younger siblings (Samuels & Chase, 1979). "They had lived to tell the story, while the sibling who had often shown early promise had failed. The consequence was a sense of guilt, a feeling that they were not deserving of a good life" (Samuels & Chase, 1979, p. 32). Bank & Kahn support this finding. "Many well siblings ask themselves, 'By what right do I live a relatively normal life when my sibling suffers so much?'" (Bank & Kahn, 1982, p. 264).

Sibling bereavement studies indicate that persons who were adolescents at the time of their sibling's death experience more long-term distress than both older and younger groups (Fanos & Nickerson, 1991; Davies, 1991). Similarly, research on siblings of persons with severe mental illness suggests more disruption in the lives of same-gender and younger siblings than cross-gender, or older siblings (Samuels & Chase, 1979). This is consistent with sibling research which indicates that later born children are importantly influenced by older siblings, whereas first-borns are more influenced by their relationship with their parents (Sutton-Smith & Rosenberg, 1970).

In addition to grief and survivor's guilt, subjective burdens such as fear, shame, and anger are commonly reported by siblings of persons with serious mental illness. Fear is experienced as a consequence of witnessing the peculiar and seemingly erratic behavior of the ill sibling (Harris, 1988; Samuels & Chase, 1979). Siblings report anxiety regarding the unpredictability of home life and fear that someone will be hurt (Johnson, 1988). In addition, siblings report fear that they too might acquire a mental illness (Harris, 1988; Samuels & Chase, 1979; Titelman & Psyk, 1991). This fear regarding heredity extends to concern about the genetic transmission of the illness to one's children (Schulz, Schulz, Dibble, Targum, VanKammen, & Gershon, 1982). Stigma has been described as the most pervasive subjective burden experienced by families of persons with mental illness (Greenberg, Greenley, McKee, Brown, & Francell, 1993). The socially unacceptable behaviors of an ill brother or sister often result in a sense of shame and embarrassment on the part of well siblings (Harris, 1988; Yarrow, Clausen & Robbins, 1955). Families make efforts to minimize the opportunity that they, or their ill relative, will experience stigma (Yarrow, et al., 1955). For example, siblings may stop bringing friends home and may avoid public appearances with their ill brother or sister (Link & Cullen, 1990; Hatfield, 1978). Hence, stigma surrounding mental illness may restrict interactions and relationships with the outside world as well as one's family.

Kates & Hastie (1987) suggest that the perpetual crises experienced by families of persons with mental illness results in a decreased ability to meet the developmental growth needs of its members. One mother attributed this to being "mentally and emotionally exhausted and therefore having little patience to cope" (p. 356). The literature on distressed families similarly indicates that an environment of family crisis may not be conducive to nurturing the healthy growth and development of children and adolescents (McKeever, 1983; McHale & Gamble, 1987). Hatfield's (1978) study of parents reveals that other children in the family suffer hardship and are frequently neglected.

Adolescents may be especially vulnerable to family crises because of the developmental tasks of this age-group. Within Erikson's theory of psychosocial development, adolescents are faced with the task of defining and stabilizing personal identity (1968). Research suggests that the crisis of identity is intensified when one's environment includes both sibling and family distress (Balk, 1990; Hogan & Greenfield, 1991). Bank and Kahn (1982) argue that siblings serve as principal referents for each other in the development of identity. For adolescent siblings of the mentally ill, the task of defining and stabilizing personal identity must now occur in the context of a distressed and deteriorating principal referent, i.e. one's brother or sister with mental illness.

The sibling bereavement literature reveals that, despite trauma, some adolescents experience growth through crisis. Examples of growth include a sensitive outlook on life, feeling good about oneself, increased maturity and seriousness, a belief in one's ability to cope, and increased creativity (Balk, 1990; Davies, 1991; Hogan & Greenfield, 1991). Davies (1991) cautions, however, that while an increase in maturity and seriousness may involve growth, such outcomes have the potential to isolate adolescents from their peers. The task of forming one's identity through relationships with a peer group is made more difficult for those adolescents who withdraw from the social world (Davies, 1991). Davies found that bereft siblings who experienced negative long-term outcomes were those who withdrew from peers because of their altered view of the world. Conversely, factors which contribute to positive outcomes include the emotional availability of parents, social support through peers and significant others, and family environments characterized by both cohesion and an emphasis on the social environment (Hogan & Greenfield, 1991; Davies, 1991; Fanos & Nickerson, 1991). Similarly, research on adolescents experiencing high life stress combined with low family support report high psychological distress symptoms (Tyerman & Humphrey, 1983). However, evidence suggests that some high-risk adolescents maintain their well-being in the face of a stressful family life by developing extrafamily social ties (Hirsch, 1985; Prasinos & Tittler, 1981).

Little is known about the adult sibling relationship when a brother or sister has a serious mental illness. Because the majority of persons with serious mental illness do not have spouses or children, siblings are generally expected to assume caregiving responsibility when parents relinquish or are unable to perform this role (Finch, 1989). This may be a source of considerable concern to adult siblings as they struggle with the competing demands of helping a needy brother or sister and meeting the challenges of one's own life (Bank & Kahn, 1982). Especially in adulthood, time becomes scarce and siblings work to balance their allegiance to their new families with that felt toward their family of origin. Bank and Kahn (1982) assert that "for most people, it is impossible to do a job well and care for a home, spouse, and a sibling [with severe mental illness]" (p. 265).

Most siblings, at one time or another, attempt to provide help to their brother or sister with mental illness (Bank & Kahn, 1982; Titelman & Psyk, 1991). A pilot study conducted by the author indicates that despite their efforts to help, many siblings feel confused and uncertain regarding how to help, how to interact with, and how to alleviate the distress of the ill brother or sister (Judge, 1991). Lacking experience in helping a person with severe mental illness, siblings may overtax themselves in this helping process (Bank & Kahn, 1982). Bank & Kahn (1982) accuse the mental health system of exacerbating the well sibling's sense of impotence by failing to provide information regarding constructive strategies for supporting their brother or sister.

Implications for Service Providers

Service providers too often assume that education and support offered to parents will "trickle down" to other family members. While many parents do a remarkable job of educating their other children, it is a mistake to assume that siblings get their educational needs met through their over-burdened parents. Education regarding etiology, genetic risks, treatments, and symptoms of mental illness may enhance empathy, increase coping skills, and address concerns regarding sibling vulnerability to mental illness. In addition, education can provide siblings with information regarding how best to communicate with a brother or sister who is experiencing the symptoms of psychosis or a mood disorder, and set realistic expectations regarding the process and outcome of their interactions. Such information may decrease feelings of helplessness on the part of well siblings, and enhance the sibling relationship.

In this culture, the sibling relationship is unique among family relationships in that sibling contact may have a negative effect on morale if it undermines one's sense of competence or independence, if it is not equitable or reciprocal, or if the volitional nature of the relationship is violated (Avioli, 1989). In addition, social relationships characterized by approval, integration, and reciprocal relating are perceived as helpful by persons with serious mental illness (Brier & Strauss, 1984). Therefore, sibling relationships have potential to provide important emotional support to the individual with serious mental illness through friendship behavior (approval, integration, and reciprocal relating), as opposed to "caretaking" or "rescuing." So while siblings have a meaningful and positive role to play in their sibling capacity, there is potential for tension and conflict if, and when, this relationship is characterized by caregiving.

Many themes of emotional distress or subjective burden (e.g. loss, survivor's guilt) point to the siblings' need for support. Service providers should be aware that adolescents, especially siblings who are younger and the same-gender as their brother or sister are at special risk (Samuels & Chase, 1979). Survivor's guilt combined with a family consumed by the needs of the brother or sister with mental illness, place siblings in danger of internalizing a sense that their own needs do not matter. Josselson (1992) asserts that human beings have a deep need to matter, to feel that they really "count" to someone. Parents are not the only people who are able to meet this need for siblings, however. A special extended family member, an adult friend, or even a counselor can provide such validation to siblings.

Siblings must be supported as they struggle to balance their own developmental and mental health needs with those of their brother or sister. Service providers and significant others can ensure that siblings understand that neglecting goals and needs does not change the brother's or sister's situation (Johnson, 1988). In childhood and adolescence, significant others can encourage involvement with friends and/or supportive adults as well as separation from the turmoil at home through outside activities. As with children of persons with mental illness, academic, social or creative accomplishments instill a sense of control over one's fate and foster the self-esteem that is necessary for resilience. In adulthood, siblings may require considerable support and consultation services as they confront the possibility that they will inherit caregiving responsibilities for their brother or sister.

Psychoeducation should help families recover from crisis in a manner which addresses the needs of all family members, including siblings. Parents need information regarding the developmental tasks of siblings and the unique issues they face. Siblings may benefit from time spent alone with parents, as well as an occasional family activity which does not include the brother or sister with mental illness. The condition of a brother or sister with mental illness may make it difficult for siblings to speak about the progress of their own lives. They need the space and permission to share their development and life with parents, without guilt or fear of rubbing salt in the wounds of the brother or sister with mental illness.

As with children of persons with serious mental illness, stigma may compel siblings to cope privately with the unique plight of their family, rarely sharing their experience with people outside the family (Harris, 1988). Support groups of similar others may provide a powerful source validation and support (Moorman, 1988).[6]

V. SPOUSES OF PERSONS WITH SERIOUS MENTAL ILLNESS

The later the onset of mental illness, the more likely it is that people will have achieved the developmental task of marriage. Schizophrenia generally strikes males in their late adolescence, while females typically don't experience onset until their late twenties. Thus one would expect more women than men marry prior to the onset of schizophrenia. Similarly, the average age of the onset for unipolar depression is forty years old, for bipolar disorder the mean age of onset is thirty (Kaplan & Sadock, 1988). Accordingly, persons with affective disorders are more

---

6. See resource list for information regarding the Sibling and Adult Children's Network. Refer to the section on service needs for adult children for a discussion of the benefits of support groups and clinical intervention.

likely to be married and living with life-partners than are people with schizophrenia (Fadden, 1989; Fadden, Bebbington, Kiupers, 1987b).

The Spouse Experience

> [My spouse] and I were living two different lives, I skittered along the ground, a fallen kite. I no longer had . . . what the novels called a heart's companion (Strong, 1988, p. 93).[7]

Life-span development theorists assert that development continues throughout life (Wrightsman, 1988). In adulthood, individuals grow with and through their relationship with a spouse or life-mate. Still, the notion of love as a foundation for marriage is a relatively recent social idea (Skolnick, 1992). Josselson (1992) asserts that marriage represents fundamental and universal human needs to feel chosen, to feel cared for, and to feel like a priority in someone else's life. In the spousal relationship, unlike the parental and sibling relationship, our culture permits us to *choose* a partner with whom to face the complex demands of adulthood.

Well spouses of persons with a chronic illness experience many losses. Like siblings and parents, spouses report that mental illness often trans-forms the person they once knew, resulting in grief for the loss of the pre-illness spouse (Fadden, Bebbington, & Kiupers, 1987b; Miller et al., 1992). The symptoms of serious mental illness involve impaired thinking and significant functional limitations, the consequences of which are major changes in lifestyle and altered plans for the future. Hence, many spouses report a sense of loss for their dreams and their future (Fadden et al., 1987b; Strong, 1988). In addition, the symptoms of mental illness cause spouses to mourn the suffering of their partner, and the loss of companionship and intimacy (Strong, 1988). Finally, faced with the overwhelming needs of the ill husband or wife, spouses

---

7. Excerpt from Maggie Strong's (1988) insightful book, *Mainstay: For The Well Spouse of the Chronically Ill*, recalling her own experience with her physically ill husband. While the book concentrates on chronic physical illness, Strong includes well spouses of persons with mental illness in her discussion. Similar issues are faced by spouses of persons with chronic illness and spouses of persons with mental illness. Strong recognizes, however, that "when thinking is impaired, the spouse becomes far more alone in the marriage and the children basically bereaved" (p. 218).

of persons with chronic illness may mourn the loss of self, and the loss of the "luxury" of having one's own needs met (Strong, 1988).

Like parental caregivers, spouses face the extraordinary demands inherent in caring for a person with serious mental illness, except they are without the benefit of an adult partner who offers support and assistance. As with chronic physical illness, the responsibilities for household chores, economic sustenance, and family maintenance multiply for the well spouse while the energy to perform these tasks is depleted (Strong, 1988; Bernheim & Lehman, 1985; Fadden et al., 1987b). There is some indication that females experience more burden than their male counterparts when caring for a companion with mental illness (Fadden, Bebbington, & Kiupers, 1987a). When women are faced with becoming the sole breadwinner, the family may experience a decrease in financial status (Fadden et al., 1987a; Strong, 1988). Husbands may have a broader range of alternatives. It has been reported that husbands of women with chronic *physical* illness are more likely to increase their work hours outside the home and hire help with household and family duties (Strong, 1988). Financial burden may take on a different level of urgency for spouses of persons with bipolar disorder, however, as the spending sprees characteristic of mania may deplete the family's resources.

In addition to the tasks of managing the household, well spouses of persons with mental illness must cope with the unique issues surrounding mental illness. The symptoms of serious mental illness are initially frightening and often confusing. Gubman, Tessler, & Willis (1987) examined the behaviors which elicit family member complaints and found no differences between spouses and parents. The most common problematic behaviors were temper tantrums, bizarre behavior, failure to perform household chores independently, and failure to socialize with friends. Many studies indicate that, while positive symptoms (hallucinations, delusions) are distressing, it is the negative symptoms (social withdrawal, amotivation, anhedonia) which are most difficult for spouses and other family members to cope with (Creer & Wing, 1974; Fadden, 1989). Some hypothesize that negative symptoms are more challenging for family members because they pose questions regarding which behaviors can be attributed to the illness and which are under the control of the individual (Fadden, 1989; Creer & Wing, 1974). When behaviors can be attributed to the illness, family members are less likely to engage in the power struggles inherent in changing another's behavior (Greenley, Greenberg, & McKee, 1993). The concern regarding failure to socialize with friends may have little to do with attributions, however. When the husband or wife with mental illness lacks friends this may represent a lack of respite for spouse caregivers. In addition, well spouses may experience sadness as they perceive the loneliness of their husband or wife.

The burdens faced by the well spouse are compounded when the couple has children in the home (Gibbons, Horn, Powell, & Gibbons, 1984; Noh & Avison, 1988). Noh & Avison (1988) note that the presence of children contributed especially to the burden of women. When a parent is ill, the children have serious needs for information, care, and support. At the same time, the family no longer centers around the children's needs. Rather, the needs of the ill member become the focus. While some parents manage to meet their children's needs for information, comfort, and predictability (Castleberry, 1988), many are confused themselves about the mental illness and are at a loss as to how to explain it to their children. In addition, well spouses often find that their role as a parent conflicts with their role as a spouse. Family matters become difficult to negotiate when the spouse must thwart the parental alliance to meet a child's need, or vice versa.

Considerable conflict may arise within the marital relationship be-cause of the shifts and eventual imbalance in marital roles (Fadden, 1989). The husband or wife with mental illness may resent his/her dependence and declining authority within the family. The well spouse has the difficult task of compensating in the areas where the husband or wife has limitations, while trying not to infantilize him or her (Strong, 1988). A study of the spouses of persons with affective disorders revealed that almost half of the spouses came to view their husband or wife as another child: someone who needs to be supervised (Fadden et al., 1987b).

A range of issues may converge to negatively affect the couple's sexual relationship. For example, medications may cause impotence, and per-sons with bipolar disorder may experience a sex drive which mirrors the extremes of the disorder. Disparate expectations and desires may cause serious problems for the well spouse.

Spouses of persons with serious mental illness may differ significantly from spouses of the chronically physically ill in their level of social isolation. The stigma of mental illness leads some spouses to conceal the illness of their spouse from friends and even family (Yarrow et al., 1955). In addition, they may not share their feelings with their husband or wife for fear of upsetting them (Fadden, 1989), or not being under-stood. In the face of extraordinarily stressful circumstances many spouses may have no one they can confide in. Some hypothesize that such isolation may help explain the increased rate of depression among spouses of persons with serious mental illness (Brown & Harris, 1978; Fadden, 1989). Fadden et al. (1987b) report that spouses of persons with mental illness have very few social and leisure activities, with some couples spending as many as 65 hours a week in face-to-face contact with each other. For some, work was their only respite from the husband or wife with serious mental illness. Strong (1988) makes the point that the love exchanged between the well spouse and the husband or wife with chronic illness is often colored by the demands of the illness. She asserts that well spouses need the intimacy, support and nurturance of outside friendships.

Most parents believe that it is in the best interest of both the family and the consumer for the adult child with mental illness to reside outside the family home (Hatfield, 1988). But unlike the parental relationship, the spousal relationship usually requires physical proximity for its maintenance. Thus the options for spouses are more painful when in-home care exceeds their physical, emotional, or financial resources. To both spouses, separate residences may represent a threat to a highly valued relationship. Fadden et al. (1987b) assert that there are high rates of divorce and separation when a husband or wife has a serious mental illness. The divorce rate for the average population increased dramatically from the late sixties through the mid-eighties (Skolnik, 1992). Still, the divorce and separation rates for one 1966 sample of persons with serious mental illness were 3 to 4 times the rate of the national average (Brown, Bone, Dalison, & Wing, 1966).

While many marriages dissolve under the strain of mental illness, a considerable number of spouses remain despite the hardships (Fadden et al., 1987b). The decision to leave a marriage when a partner is chronically ill may be deeply agonizing. In fact, Strong (1988) suggests that the well spouse who leaves may experience residual heart-ache for years to come. We live in a culture that currently expects intimacy, understanding, companionship, and satisfying sexual relations within marriage (Skolnick, 1992). For the spouse of a person with mental illness these expectations are often not met. The well spouse thus confronts moral and ethical dilemmas concerning a commitment to care for someone you love (or once loved) when they are ill.

Implications for Service Providers
Spouses have been almost uniformly neglected by service providers: many have never received information about the nature of the illness or practical assistance regarding how to cope with it (Deasy & Quinn,

1955; Fadden, 1989; Fadden et al., 1987b). The spousal desire to receive information about etiology, diagnosis, prognosis, and skills for dealing with the illness was documented almost four decades ago (Deasy & Quinn, 1955). Information to spouses must include issues relevant to medications, sexuality, and the legal and practical options for dealing with the spending sprees of the partner with hypomania or mania. Education potentially mediates the infantilization of the husband or wife by helping well spouses discern realistic ways one's partner can contribute to the household. Similarly, tensions may decrease as spouses learn what behaviors are attributable to the illness and which are not. Spouses need education in order to enhance coping skills and their sense of mastery. Consultation alone, or in conjunction with multiple family members, may be useful in dealing with the specific concerns and issues faced by the family as it attempts to adapt.

Well spouses of persons with serious mental illness are in dire need of support. Spouses are grieving many losses and caregiving for a chronically ill family member, while often dealing with the demands of parenthood and the needs of similarly distressed children. Erikson claims that adults (ages 30-49) undergo a process of self-evaluation in mid-life which involves reflection on personal needs and values in conjunction with the needs of significant others (see Wrightsman, 1988). Adults must ask themselves what kind of life they desire. In the context of a marital relationship altered by mental illness, this will be a challenging process requiring the support of a trusted other.

With support as its aim, service providers may help well spouses address their needs for companionship, intimacy and social support. The service provider might encourage the well spouse to take an inventory of extended family members who may provide both tangible aid and friendship. In addition, an important function of supportive relationships is to remind well spouses that they do exist, and that their feelings and needs do matter (Strong, 1988). If spouses are to remain healthy, they must shore up social support and develop their own interests and potentials. Support groups for well spouses of persons with mental illness may provide invaluable support and practical assistance.[8]

Service providers can also assist well spouses by providing information and support surrounding parenting issues and the needs of the children (Castleberry, 1988). Parents can benefit from information about how

---

8. See Resource List for information about support groups for well spouses.

to discuss mental illness with their children, how to support their children, and the developmental issues their children face[9]. The service provider may help parents devise a plan to cultivate social support for their other children: weekly outings with a relative or trusted adult friend, for example.

Finally, in this culture, the institution of marriage is overloaded with so many expectations that it often collapses under the psychological burden (Josselson, 1992). This burden is compounded in marriages where a husband or wife has a serious mental illness. Service providers can help alleviate the hardships well spouses face by providing comprehensive services to the ill family member. The dangers of reducing the spousal relationship to that of nurse-patient may be mitigated if a trusted service provider (in collaboration with the couple) monitors medication issues, provides oversight on money management, coordinates transportation to appointments, negotiates services, deals with hygiene issues, etc.

The spouse's burden likely increases when she/he has sole responsibility for meeting the varied needs of the husband or wife with mental illness. The heavy responsibility placed on spouses can be reduced by ensuring the ill relative has meaningful activity outside the family-home, including vocational activity and social relationships. An innovative program, called "Compeer," is an example of a formal effort to facilitate one-to-one friendships between persons with mental illness and volunteers in the community.[10] In addition, there may be untapped resources in extended family members and old friends who, with guidance and encouragement, would be glad to provide support and assistance.

VI. CONCLUSION

Human relationships are the context within which development takes place: we grow with and through the significant others in our lives (Josselson, 1992). For children, siblings, and spouses, a formative relationship has been disrupted by severe and persistent mental illness. For each of these family members, the developmental significance of this relationship acquires prominence at different stages in the life cycle.

---

9. See Resource List at the conclusion of this chapter for recommendations on books and resources for children. Also see section on children of persons with mental illness.

10. See Resource List for more information on "Compeer."

Generally speaking, the parent-child relationship commands primacy in infancy and childhood, the sibling relationship supports and shapes growth during childhood and adolescence, and the spousal relationship provides a context for adult development. As Josselson (1992) contends, however, a dyadic relationship with a significant other does not determine one's fate:

> It is not how things go with a particular person but the whole interpersonal network that ultimately shapes development. We must extend our view to observe the healing effects of later nutrients on early deprivation. Although people harm each other, they also offer solace and sustenance to assuage prior hurt. And as individuals grow, more people become available to meet their developmental needs (p. 28).

Whether family members thrive or languish when confronted with mental illness may largely depend on the supports available outside of the dyadic relationship.

The task of the service provider is to decrease exposure to crippling stress through assertive treatment for the family member with mental illness; to empower coping through the provision of education, support, and consultation to family members; and to enhance opportunities for growth through natural and formal support systems. In order to adequately address the needs of particular family members, service providers must understand the significance of the relationship, the unique burdens experienced by the well family member, and the personal consequences of both for the individual whose parent, sibling, or spouse has a serious mental illness.

APPENDIX 1

Lifetime Risk for the Development of Schizophrenia or Affective Disorders based on relationship to the patient

BIPOLAR DISORDER
Table modified from S. Targum, 1988, p. 202

RELATIONSHIP TO THE PATIENT	LIFETIME RISK OF DEVELOPING A MAJOR AFFECTIVE DISORDER
Offspring: One ill person	15-20%
Offspring: Two ill parents	50-75%
Sibling/DZ twin	15-25%
Monozygotic twin	75%
General population	1%

UNIPOLAR DEPRESSION
Table modified from S. Targum, 1988, p. 202

RELATIONSHIP TO THE PATIENT	LIFETIME RISK OF DEVELOPING A MAJOR AFFECTIVE DISORDER
Offspring:	15-20%
Sibling	10-15%
Monozygotic twin	40-50%
General population	2-3%

SCHIZOPHRENIA
Table modified from I. Gottesman, 1991, p. 96.

RELATIONSHIP TO THE PATIENT	LIFETIME RISK OF DEVELOPING A MAJOR AFFECTIVE DISORDER
Offspring: 1 parent has schizophrenia:	13%
Offspring: 2 parents have schizo-phrenia	46%
Sibling	9%
Monozygotic twin	48%
General population	1%

RESOURCE LIST FOR FAMILIES AND SERVICE PROVIDERS

YOUNG FAMILY MEMBERS

Castleberry, K.S. (1987). *Helping Children Adapt*. Radford, VA: Commonwealth Press. Provides practical suggestions to help children whose family members have been hospitalized for the treatment of mental illness. To order contact: Dr. Karma Castleberry, School of Nursing, Radford University, Radford, VA 24142. Phone: (703) 831-5415.

Dinner, S. (1989). *Nothing to be Ashamed of: Growing up with Mental Illness in your family*. New York: Lothrop, Lee & Shepard

Johnson, J.T. (1989). *Understanding Mental Illness: For Teens Who Care about Someone with Mental Illness*. Minneapolis: Lerner

United Mental Health, Inc. (1989). *After the Tears: Teens Talk About Mental Illness in their Families*. Pittsburgh: United Mental Health, Inc. 20 minute VHS and 3/4" cassette. Excellent orientation for service providers, parents, and spouses in addition to its intended audience (siblings and children). To order, write: UMH, Inc., 1945 Fifth Avenue, Pittsburgh, PA 15219. Phone: (412) 391-3820.

SERVICE PROVIDERS

Bernheim, K.F., & Lehman, A.F. (1985). *Working with Families of the Mentally Ill*. New York: Norton.

Brown, E.M. (1989). *My Parent's Keeper: Adult Children of the Emotionally Disturbed*. Oakland: New Harbinger Publications, Inc.

Johnson, J.T. (1989). *The Eight Stage Healing Process for Families of the Mentally Ill: A Training Manual for Therapists*. To order write: Eight Stage Healing Process, P.O. Box 19067, Minneapolis, MN 55419. Phone: (612) 872-1565.

ADULT FAMILY MEMBERS

Bernheim, Lewine, & Beale (1982). *The Caring Family: Living with Chronic Mental Illness*. Chicago: Contemporary Books.

Brown, E.M. (1989). *My Parent's Keeper: Adult Children of the Emotionally Disturbed*. Oakland: New Harbinger Publications, Inc.

Copeland, M.E. (1992). *The Depression Workbook: A Guide for Living with Depression and Manic Depression*. New Harbinger Publications.

Hatfield, A.B. (1990). *Family Education in Mental Illness*. New York: Guilford.

Johnson, J.T. (1988). *Hidden Victims: An Eight-stage Healing Process for Families and Friends of the Mentally Ill*. New York: Doubleday.

Torrey, E.F. (1988) *Surviving Schizophrenia*. New York: Harper & Row.
Woolis, R. (1992). *When Someone You Love Has a Mental Illness: A Handbook for Family, Friends, and Caregivers*. New York: Perigee Books.

SUPPORT GROUPS

Sibling and Adult Children's Network. National Alliance for the Mentally Ill, 2101 Wilson Blvd., Suite 302, Arlington, VA 22201. Phone: (703) 524-7600.

Spouse Support Group. National Alliance for the Mentally Ill, 2101 Wilson Blvd., Suite 302, Arlington, VA 22201. Phone: (703) 524-7600.

OTHER

Compeer, Inc., Monroe Square—Suite B-1, 259 Monroe Avenue, Rochester New York, 14607. Phone: (716) 546-8280. Compeer is a formal program which matches volunteers from the community and individuals with mental illness who desire a one-on-one friendship. The Compeer Network provides training information and resources to persons who wish to start a Compeer program.

BIBLIOGRAPHY

Anthony, E. J. (1974). The syndrome of the psychologically invulnerable child. In E. Anthony & C. Koupernik (Eds.) *The Child in his Family: Children at Psychiatric Risk*. New York: Wiley and Sons.

Anthony, E.J. (1987). Children at high risk for psychosis growing up successfully. In E.J. Anthony & B.J. Cohler (Eds.) *The Invulnerable Child* (pp. 147-184). New York: Guilford Press.

Anthony, E.J., & Cohler, B.J. (1987). *The Invulnerable Child*. New York: The Guilford Press.

Aranowitz, P. (1988). A brother's dreams. *New York Times Magazine*, 1/24/88, p. 35.

Avioli, P. (1989). The social support functions of siblings in later life: A theoretical model. *American Behavioral Scientist, 33*, 45-57.

Balk, D. (1990). The self-concepts of bereaved adolescents: sibling death and its aftermath. *Journal of Adolescent Research, 5*(1), 112-132.

Bank, S. P., & Kahn, M. D. (1975). Sisterhood-brotherhood is powerful: Sibling subsystems and family therapy. *Family Process, 14*, 311-337.

Bank, S., & Kahn, M. (1982a). *The Sibling Bond*. New York: Basic Books.

Bank, S. P., & Kahn, M. D. (1982b). The embroiled family: "Well" and "disturbed" siblings. In S. P. Bank & M. D. Kahn (Eds.). *The Sibling Bond* (pp. 232-270). New York: Basic Books.

Benard, B. (1987). *Protective Factor Research: What we Can Learn from Resilient Children.* Springfield, Ill: AHTDS Prevention Resource Center.

Bernheim, K.F., & Lehman, A.F. (1985). *Working with Families of the Mentally Ill.* New York: Norton.

Biglen, A., Hops, H., Sherman, L., Friedman, L.S., Arthur, J., & Osteen, V. (1985). Problem-solving interactions of depressed women and their husbands. *Behavior Therapy, 16,* 431-451.

Bleuler, M. (1978). *The Schizophrenic Mental Disorders in the Light of Long-Term Patients and Family Histories.* New Haven: Yale University Press.

Bowlby, J. (1988). *A Secure Base.* New York: Basic Books.

Brier, A. & Strauss, J. (1984). The role of social relationships in recovery from psychotic disorders. *American Journal of Psychiatry, 141*(8), 949-955.

Brown, G.W., Bone, M., Dalison, B., & Wing, J.K. (1966). Schizophrenia and social care: A comparative follow-up study of 339 schizophrenic patients. *Institute of Psychiatry Maudsley Monographs: Number 17.* New York: Oxford University Press.

Brown, G.W., & Harris, T. (1978). *Social Origins of Depression: A Study of Psychiatric Disorder in Women.* London: Tavistock Publications.

Castleberry, K.S. (1987). *Helping Children Adapt.* Radford, VA: Commonwealth Press.

Castleberry, K. (1988). Helping children adapt to the psychiatric hospitalization of a parent. *The Psychiatric Hospital, 19*(4), 155-160.

Cicirelli, V. (1982). In M. E. Lamb & B. Sutton-Smith (Eds.) *Sibling Relationships: Their Nature and Significance Across the Lifespan* (pp. 267-284). Hillsdale, NJ: Erlbaum.

Clausen, J.A. & Yarrow, M.R. (1955). The impact of mental illness on the family. *Journal of Social Issues, 11,* 3-64.

Cohler, B.J., & Musick, J.S. (1984). Intervention among psychiatrically impaired parents and their young children. *New Directions for Mental Health Services, Volume 24.* San Francisco: Jossey-Bass.

Creer, C., & Wing, J. (1974). *Schizophrenia at Home.* London: Institute of Psychiatry.

Davies, B. (1991). Long-term outcomes of adolescent sibling bereavement. *Journal of Adolescent Research, 6*(1), 83-96.

Day, J., & Kwitkowska, H. (1962). The psychiatric patient and his "well" sibling: A comparison through their art productions. *Bulletin of Art Therapy*, 1, 51-66.

Deasy, L.C. & Quinn, O.W. (1955). The wife of the mental patient and the hospital psychiatrist. *Journal of Social Issues*, 11, 49-60.

Downey, G., & Coyne, J. (1990). Children of depressed parents: An integrative review. *Psychological Bulletin*, 108(1), 50-76.

Drake, R.E., Racusin, R.J., Murphy, T.A. (1990). Suicide among adolescents with mentally ill parents. *Hospital and Community Psychiatry*, 41(8), 921-922.

Dunn, J. (1984). Sibling studies and the developmental impact of critical incidents. *Life-Span Development and Behavior*, 6, 335-353.

Erikson, E. (1959). Identity and the life cycle: Selected papers. *Psychological Issues*, 1(1), 5-165.

Erikson, E. (1968). *Identity: Youth and Crisis*. New York: Norton.

Fadden, G. (1989). Pity the spouse! Depression within marriage. *Stress Medicine*, 5, 99-107.

Fadden, G., Bebbington, P., & Kuipers, L. (1987a). The burden of care: The impact of functional psychiatric illness on the patient's family. *British Journal of Psychiatry*, 150, 285-292.

Fadden, G., Bebbington, P., Kuipers, L. (1987b). Caring and its burdens: A study of the spouses of depressed patients. *British Journal of Psychiatry*, 151, 660-667.

Fanos, J., & Nickerson, B. (1991). Long-term effects of sibling death during adolescence. *Journal of Adolescent Research*, 6(1), 70-82.

Feldman, R.A., Stiffman, A.R., & Jung, K.(1987) *Children at Risk: In the Web of Parental Mental Illness*. New Brunswick: Rutgers University Press.

Fialkov, M.J. (1988). Fostering permanency of children in out-of-home care: Psycho-legal aspects. *Bulletin of the American Academy of Psychiatry and Law*, 16(40, 3434-357.

Finch, J. (1989). *Family Obligations and Social Change*. Cambridge: Polity Press.

Fisher, L., Kokes, R. F., Cole, R. E., Perkins, P. M, & Wynne, L. C. (1987) Competent children at risk: A study of well-functioning offspring of disturbed parents. In E.J. Anthony & B.J. Cohler (Eds.) *The Invulnerable Child* (pp. 211- 228). New York: Guilford Press.

Friedrich, W., & Wheeler, K. (1982). The abusing parent revisited: A decade of psychological research. *Journal of Nervous and Mental Disease*, 170, 577-587.

Garmezy, N. (1981). Children under stress: Perspectives on antecedents and correlates of vulnerability and resistance to psychopathology. In A. I. Rabin, J. Aranoff, A.M. Barclay, & R. Zucker (Eds.), *Further Explorations in Personality.* New York: Wiley-Interscience.

Garmezy, N. (1984). Children vulnerable to major mental disorders: risk and protective factors. In L. Grinspoon (Ed.) *Psychiatry Update, Vol. III.* Washington, D.C.: American Psychiatric Press.

Gibbons, J.S., Horn, S.H., Powell, J.M., & Gibbons, J.L. (1984). Schizophrenic patients and their families: A survey in a psychiatric service based on a DGH unit. *British Journal of Psychiatry, 144,* 70-77.

Goetting, A. (1986). The developmental tasks of siblingship over the life cycle. *Journal of Marriage and the Family, 48,* 703-714.

Goodman, S.H. (1984). Children of disturbed parents: A research-based model for intervention. In B.J. Cohler & J.S. Musick (Eds.) *New Directions for Mental Health Services, Volume 24* (pp. 33-51). San Francisco: Jossey-Bass.

Goodman, S.H. & Brumley, H.E. (1990). Schizophrenic and depressed mothers: Relational deficits in parenting. *Developmental Psychology,* 26(1), 31-39.

Goodman, S.H., & Isaacs, L.D. (1984). Primary prevention with children of severely disturbed mothers. *Journal of Preventive Psychiatry,* 2, 387-402.

Gottesman, I. (1991). *Schizophrenia Genesis: The Origins of Madness.* New York: Freeman & Co.

Greenberg, J., Greenley, J., McKee, D., Brown, R., & Francell, C. (1993). Mothers caring for an adult child with schizophrenia: The effects of subjective burden on maternal health. *Family Relations,* 42(2), 205-211.

Greenley, J.R., Greenberg, J., & McKee, D. (1993). Family Stress and Coping with Chronic Mental Illness: A Theoretical Model. Unpublished manuscript, University of Wisconsin-Madison, School of Social Work (J. Greenberg).

Grunebaum, H. (1984). Parenting and children at risk. In L. Grinspoon (Ed.) *Psychiatry Update, Vol. III.* Washington, D.C.: American Psychiatric Press.

Gubman, G.D., Tessler, C., & Wilis, G. (1987). Living with the mentally ill: Factors affecting household complaints. *Schizophrenia Bulletin,* 13(4), 727-736.

Harris, E.B. (1988). My brother's keeper: Siblings of chronic patients as allies in family treatment. *Siblings in Therapy.* New York: W.W. Norton & Co.

Hatfield, A. (1978). Psychological costs of schizophrenia to the family. *Social Work*, September, 355-359.

Hatfield, A. (1988). Issues in psychoeducation for families of the mentally ill. *International Journal of Mental Health*, 17(1), 48-64.

Hirsch, B. (1985). Adolescent coping and support across multiple social environments. *American Journal of Community Psychology*, 13, 381-392.

Hogan, N., & Greenfield, D. (1991). Adolescent sibling bereavement symptomatology in a large community sample. *Journal of Adolescent Research*, 6(1), 97-112.

Hooley, J.M., & Hahlweg, K. (1986). The marriages and interaction patterns of depressed patients and their spouses: Comparison of high and low EE dyads. In M. Goldstein et al. (Eds.) *Treatment of Schizophrenia* (pp. 85-95). Berlin: Springer-Verlag.

Horwitz, A.V., Tessler, R.C., Fisher, G., & Gamache, G.M. (1992). The role of adult siblings in providing social support to the severely mentally ill. *Journal of Marriage and the Family*, 54, 233-241.

Johnson, J.T. (1988). *Hidden victims: An eight-stage healing process for families and friends of the mentally ill*. New York: Doubleday.

Johnson, J.T. (1989). *The Eight Stage Healing Process for Families of the Mentally Ill: A Training Manual for Therapists*. P.O. Box 19067, Minneapolis, MN 55419.

Josselson, R. (1992). *The Space Between Us: Exploring the Dimensions of Human Relationships*. San Francisco: Jossey-Bass.

Judge, K. (1991). One family's experience: Siblings of persons with schizophrenia. Unpublished manuscript.

Kaplan, H., & Sadock, B. (1988). *Synopsis of Psychiatry: Behavioral Sciences, Clinical Psychiatry*. Baltimore: William & Wilkins.

Kates, N., & Hastie, J. (1987). The family and schizophrenia: Recovery and adaptation. *International Journal of Mental Health*, 15(4), 70-79.

Kauffman, C. et al. (1979). Superkids: competent children of psychotic mothers. *American Journal of Psychiatry*, 136, 1398-1402.

Kellam, S.G., Ensminger, M.A., & Turner, J. (1977). Family structure and the mental health of children. *Archives of General Psychiatry*, 34, 1012-1022.

Knitzer, J. (1982). *Unclaimed Children*. Washington D.C.: The Children's Defense Fund.

Lamb, M. (1982). Sibling relationships across the life span: An overview and introduction. In M. E. Lamb & B. Sutton-Smith (Eds.), *Sibling Relationships: Their Nature and Significance Across the Lifespan*. (pp. 1-11) Hillsdale, NJ: Erlbaum.

Lander, H., Anthony, E.J., Cass, L., Franklin, L., & Bass, L. (1978). A measure of vulnerability to risk of parental psychosis. In E. J. Anthony, C. Koupernik & C. Chiland (Eds.), *The Child in His Family: Vulnerable Children* (International yearbook, Vol. 4). New York: Wiley.

Lidz, T., Fleck, S., Alanen, Y. O., & Cornelison, A. (1963). Schizophrenic patients and their siblings. *Psychiatry, 26*, 1-18.

Link, B., & Cullen, F. (1990). The labelling theory of mental disorder: A review of the evidence. In J. Greenley (Ed.) *Research in Community and Mental Health: Mental Disorder in Social Context* (pp. 75-105). Greenwich, CT: JAI Press.

McEvoy, J., Hatcher, A., Appelbaum, P. & Abernethy, V. (1983). Chronic schizophrenic women's attitudes toward sex, pregnancy, birth control, and childrearing. *Hospital and Community Psychiatry, 34*(6), 536-539.

McHale, S., & Gamble, W. (1989). Sibling relationships of children with disabled and nondisabled brother and sisters. *Developmental Psychology, 25*, 421-429.

McKeever, P. (1983). Siblings of chronically ill children: A literature review and implications for research and practice. *American Journal of Orthopsychiatry, 53*(2), 209-218.

Mednick, S. (1967). The children of schizophrenics: serious difficulties in current research methodologies which suggest the use of the "high-risk group" method. In J. Romano (Ed.) *Exerpta Medica Foundation,* Amsterdam.

Merikangas, K.R., Prusoff, B.A., Kupfer, D.J. & Frank. E. (1985). Marital adjustment in major depression. *Journal of Affective Disorders, 9*, 5-11.

Miller, F., Dworkin, J., Ward, M., & Barone, D. (1990). A preliminary study of unresolved grief in families of seriously mentally ill patients. *Hospital and Community Psychiatry, 41*(12), 1321-1325.

Montgomery, J. (1985). Family compromise, members' definitions and crisis-related behavior. *Canadian Home Economics Journal, 35*, 89-93.

Moorman, M. (1988). A sister's need. *New York Time's Sunday Magazine,* 9/11/88.

Moorman, M. (1992). *My Sister's Keeper: Learning to Cope with a Sibling's Mental Illness.* New York: Norton.

Musick, J.S., Stott, F.M., Spencer, K.K., Goldman, J., & Cohler, B.J. (1987). Maternal factors related to vulnerability and resiliency in young children at risk. In E.J. Anthony & B.J. Cohler (Eds.) *The Invulnerable Child* (pp. 229-252). New York: Guilford Press.

Noh, S., & Avison, W.R. (1988). Spouses of discharged patients. Factors associated with their experience of burden. *Journal of Marriage and the Family*, 50, 377-389.

Pearlin, L., & McCail, M. (1990). Occupational stress and marital support: A description of microprocesses. In J. Eckenrode and S. Gore (Eds.), *Stress Between Work and Family* (pp. 39-60). New York: Plenum.

Prasinos, S., & Tittler, B. (1981). The family relationships of humor oriented adolescents. *Journal of Personality*, 49, 295-305.

Radke-Yarrow, M., Nottelmann, E., Martinez, P., Fox, M.G., & Belmont, B. (1992). Young children of affectively ill parents: A longitudinal study of psychosocial development. *Journal of American Academy of Child and Adolescent Psychiatry*, 31(1), 68-77.

Reid, W.H., & Morrison, H.L. (1983). Risk factors in children of depressed parents. In H.L. Morrison (Ed.) *Children of Depressed Parents*. New York: Grune & Stratton.

Riebschleger, J. (1991). Families of chronically mentally ill people: Siblings speak to social workers. *Health and Social Work*, 16(2), 94.

Rolf, J., & Garmezy, N. (1974). The school performance of children vulnerable to behavior pathology. In D.F. Ricks, A. Thomas, and M. Roff (Eds.) *Life History Research in Psychopathology: Volume 3*. Minneapolis: University of Minnesota Press.

Ross, H., & Milgram, J. (1980). Rivalry in adult sibling relationships: Its antecedents and dynamics. Paper presented at the Annual Meeting of the American Psychological Association, Montreal, Canada.

Rudolph, B., Larson, G.L., Sweeny, S., Hough, E.E., & Arorian, K. (1990). Hospitalized pregnant psychotic women: Characteristics and treatment issues. *Hospital and Community Psychiatry*, 41(2), 159-163.

Rutter, M. (1970). Sex differences in children's responses to family stress. In E.J. Anthony & C. Koupernik (Eds.), *The Child in His Family* (International Yearbook Volume I). New York: Wiley.

Rutter, M. (1987). Psychosocial resilience and protective mechanisms. *American Journal of Orthopsychiatry*, 57(3), 316-329.

Sameroff, A.J. & Seifer, R. (1981). The transmission of incompetence: The offspring of mentally ill women. In M. Lewis and L.A. Rosenblum (Eds.), *The Uncommon Child* (pp. 259-280). New York: Plenum Press.

Samuels, L. & Chase, L. (1979). The well siblings of schizophrenics. *The American Journal of Family Therapy*, 7, 24-35.

Sandmaier, M. (1994). *Original Kin: Intimacy, Choices, and Change in Adult Sibling Relationships.* New York: Dutton.

Schulz, P. M., Schulz, S. C., Dibble, E., Targum, S.D., Van Kammen, D. P. & Gershon, E. S. (1982). Patient and family attitudes about schizophrenia: Implications for genetic counseling. *Schizophrenia Bulletin,* 8(3), 504-513.

Shacnow, J. (1987). Preventive intervention with children of hospitalized psychiatric patients. *American Journal of Orthopsychiatry, 57,* 66-77.

Silverman, M. (1989). Children of psychiatrically ill parents: A prevention perspective. *Hospital and Community Psychiatry, 40* (12), 1257.

Skolnick, A. (1992). *The Intimate Environment: Exploring Marriage and the Family.* New York: Harper Collins.

Spinetta, J., & Rigler, D. (1972). The child-abusing parent: A psychological review. *Psychological Bulletin, 77*(4), 296-304.

Stiffman, A.R., Jung, K.G., & Feldman, R.A. (1988). Parental mental illness, family living arrangements, and child behavior. *Journal of Social Service Research, 11*(2/3), 2134.

Strong, M. (1988). *Mainstay: For the Well Spouse of the Chronically Ill.* New York: Penguin.

Sutton-Smith, B., & Rosenberg, B. (1970). *The Sibling.* New York: Holt, Rinehart, & Winston.

Targum, S. (1988). Genetic issues in treatment. In J.F. Clarkin, G.L. Haas, & I.D. Glick (Eds.) *Affective Disorders and the Family* (pp. 196-212). New York: Guilford Press.

Titelman, D. & Psyk, L. (1991). Grief, guilt, and identification in siblings of schizophrenic individuals. *Bulletin of the Menninger Clinic, 55*(1), 72-84.

Tyerman, A., & Humphrey, M. (1983). Life stress, family support, and adolescent disturbance. *Journal of Adolescence, 6,* 1-12.

Walker, A. (1985). Reconceptualizing family stress. *Journal of Marriage and the Family, 47,* 827-837.

Weintraub, S., Winters, K.C., & Neale, J.M. (1982). Competence and vulnerability in children with an affectively disordered parent. Paper presented at the conference on Depression and Depressive Disorders: Developmental Perspectives, Temple University, Philadelphia.

Werner, E., & Smith, R. (1982). *Vulnerable But Invincible: A Longitudinal Study of Resilient Children and Youth.* New York: McGraw-Hill.

Williams, O.B., & Corrigan, P.W. (1992). The differential effects of parental alcoholism and mental illness on their adult children. *Journal of Clinical Psychology, 48*(3), 406-414.

Winnicott, D.W. (1972). *Maturational Processes and the Facilitating Environment.* London: Hogarth Press.

Worland, J., Janes, C., Anthony, E.J., McGinnis, M., & Cass, L. (1984). St Louis Risk Research Project: Comprehensive progress report of experimental studies. In N.F. Watt, E.J. Anthony, L.C. Wynne, & J. Rolf (Eds.), *Children at Risk for Schizophrenia: A Longitudinal Perspective.* Cambridge,England: Cambridge University Press.

Wrightsman, L. (1988). *Personality Development in Adulthood.* London: Sage.

Yarrow, M., Clausen, J., & Robbins, P. (1955). The social meaning of mental illness. *The Journal of Social Issues, 11,* 33-48.

Chapter 10

FAMILIES, PATIENTS AND CLINICIANS AS PARTNERS: CLINICAL STRATEGIES AND RESEARCH OUTCOMES IN SINGLE- AND MULTIPLE-FAMILY PSYCHOEDUCATION

William R. McFarlane

THE HISTORICAL, CONCEPTUAL AND SCIENTIFIC CONTEXT OF THE APPROACH

Family psychoeducation is a clinical strategy for treating a *bona fide* disabling and chronic illness, which is best defined as a functional impairment of the brain (Weinberger, 1987). More specifically, psychoeducation is a method for training families and other natural social groups to create an interactional environment that compensates and may partially correct functional disability in one of its members. The development of this approach is a direct result of the long and tortuous search for an effective treatment for schizophrenia, a condition that continues to defy adequate, let alone simple, explanation and to evade widely varying attempts to negate its impact. While new applications of psychoeducation are being developed and tested, the focus of the most refined forms relate to schizophrenia. For that reason, the present chapter will deal primarily with theoretical issues and clinical techniques relevant to that disorder.

The rationale for developing a new therapy for schizophrenia needs little explanation. Despite widespread use of antipsychotic medication, progressive deinstitutionalization reforms of the last decade, and expanding treatment, residential, and rehabilitation services, the prognosis for patients with this illness has changed remarkably little. Between 1 and 2% of the population is afflicted; only 25% of first-episode patients recover, while the rest often are consigned to a life of increasing mental dysfunction, emotional deadness, social isolation, rejection and major disabilities in work and love (Yolles and Kramer, 1969, Bourdon et al.,

1992). Patients who take medication regularly can still expect a 40% chance of relapse during the first year after any given episode, so that for many, life consists of two alternating states and contexts: (1) psychosis and hospitalization and (2) marginal stability and dependent living with the support of others, especially the family of origin (Hogarty, et al., 1979).

It has only recently become apparent to clinicians that for the families of persons afflicted with a schizophrenic disorder, life is drastically different—more stressful and more demoralizing—than for those dealing with most psychiatric disorders and nonpsychotic family dysfunction. There has been a distressing trend in the field to ignore the devastating impact of watching one's child or sibling deteriorate into someone who is all but a stranger, and a most incapacitated one. To roughly the same degree, many clinicians have ignored the fact that families have become the *de facto* caretakers of individuals with schizophrenia, without the required knowledge, training, resources and support. Family psychoeducation can be most simply understood as an attempt to deal simultaneously with both these realities: the disappointing record of antipsychotic drugs and the complex burdens imposed on families by this illness.

It is somewhat ironic, but true nevertheless, that during the very period—the mid-1970s—in which family therapy was being abandoned in psychotic disorders, two groups were beginning to feel the effects of deinstitutionalization—community-based clinicians and families. While the original architects of the mass discharge of patients from psychiatric hospitals intended that a range of services would be provided to enhance community adjustment, budget restrictions have precluded little more than the discharge process itself. Since then, increasing numbers of families have found themselves replacing most of the functions of the state hospital: providing food, clothing, and shelter; monitoring symptoms; managing medication compliance; instituting rehabilitation efforts; and controlling dangerous and bizarre behavior. They have received some help from publicly supported clinical services, but these have been notoriously inadequate.

The Advent of Multiple-Family Groups

One relatively obscure response to families was multiple-family group therapy, in which several patients and their respective families meet together with one or two clinicians on a regular basis. Beginning about 1960, two innovators of multiple-family therapy, Laqueur (1964) and Detre (1961), assembled their groups to solve ward-management problems—rather than from a theoretical family-systems perspective—and both described immediate and surprising benefits to patients, with reference to symptoms and sociability, and to family members, with reference to morale and communication. A number of clinicians began using this approach, primarily because of practical advantages and early results that seemed unexpectedly promising.

In retrospect, one major difference between single- and multiple-family approaches was that in the latter, families were sufficiently joined to each other that messages of blame coming from therapists were usually neutralized, while direct emotional support and opportunities for trading successful techniques for managing illness-related behavior often dominated the discussions. With time, the emphasis in multiple-family groups centered on balancing the needs of patients with those of families, rather than on treating families for theoretically dysfunctional interaction patterns. Multiple-family therapy lacked the conceptual elegance of family-systems ideas, but it seemed to compensate by delivering clinical results, on the order of more recently developed psychoeducational approaches (Berman (1966), Levin (1966), Lurie (1972), Lansky et al., (1978), Falloon & Liberman (1983)). Because that efficacy was not rigorously documented, multi-family therapy remained an esoteric practice used in scattered clinics and hospitals serving the chronic mental patient. However, a few observers thought that social support for families, a major element in multiple-family groups, may be crucial in determining outcome, because, as we shall see, the social processes surrounding the relentless course of mental disability tend to leave families isolated, if not abandoned and rejected (Anderson et al., 1984; Lipton et al., 1981; Hammer, 1963; Beels, 1981). This was a compelling idea, given the growing evidence that social isolation appears to be associated with morbidity in many conditions, including depression (Lin and Ensel, 1984), ischemic heart disease (Hedblad et al., 1992) and schizophrenia (Beels, 1981). The multiple family group has emerged as a most promising vehicle within which to conduct psychoeducational treatment and rehabilitation.

The Partial Promise of Antipsychotic Medication

Maintenance medication was shown repeatedly to foster a continuation of remission at roughly twice the effectiveness of placebo. The effects of antipsychotic drugs on survival in the community are so substantial that the effects of social therapy can barely be discerned in some studies (Hogarty et al., 1974). The concept of predisposition interacting with environment—the stress-vulnerability model of Zubin and Spring (1977)—is supported further by the repeated observation that even when medication is all but guaranteed by injectable dosage, relapse rates persist in the 40% range during the first year following an acute episode, while negative symptoms persist or sometimes worsen on standard doses. This frustrating failure of drug and older psychosocial treatments has turned several clinical research teams to a search for more refined definitions of those environmental variables that might account for the residual morbidity.

Psychosocial Factors and Course of Illness

By shifting the focus of attention from etiology to determinants of course of illness, several groups of researchers have reliably and usefully clarified how social processes, including but not limited to family interaction, might influence what happens in a psychotic illness once it is established (Strauss and Carpenter, 1977; Breier and Strauss, 1984). In addition, we now have a much broader perspective on what happens to families as they attempt to cope with a member who is mentally ill. In Chapter 5, research on expressed emotion (EE) and communication deviance was reviewed. For the purpose of defining psychoeducational treatment, it is sufficient to say here that in most studies in which it has been examined, reductions in expressed emotion have accompanied improvements in course of illness (Falloon et al., 1985; Hogarty et al., 1986). Thus, reducing expressed emotion is one of the primary goals of all psychoeducational or family behavioral management approaches.

The background for psychoeducational family approaches includes two other research areas. One emphasizes the effects on the family of having an ill member; the other, the social network of the patient and family. A sizable body of literature now documents nearly devastating effects on families when faced with a mentally ill member in their midst over long periods of time. These burdens include chronic tension and fear, sleep disruption, financial drain, confusion, limitation of social contacts, interference with daily routine, deprivation of attention for siblings, marital conflict, overt depression, and exacerbation of medical conditions (Kreisman and Joy, 1974; Johnson, 1990; Lefley, 1989). Furthermore, many families complain that professionals' and friends' blaming them for the illness induces guilt, confusion, anger, and, eventually, demoralization and rejection of the patient (Hatfield, 1983).

The social networks and social supports of schizophrenic patients and their families have been studied extensively, with a singularly consistent finding: patients, particularly, and to a lesser extent families, are more isolated than their peers, even those with other psychiatric disorders.

Pattison (1979), Hammer (1963) and Garrison (1978) noted smaller network size, as did Brown (1972), who also found an association between family isolation and high EE. Patient social networks are constricted and more family-based at first admission (Tolsdorf, 1976), while the entire network decreases in size after the illness has taken hold (Lipton et al., 1981; Anderson et al., 1984). The explanation for this process includes withdrawal of contact and support by friends and extended kin as well as reduced social initiative by family members, secondary to shame and/or preoccupation with the patient. Attenuated social support leads to the loss of adaptive coping capacity for family members and exacerbates the effects of caretaking burdens.

A Core Psychological Deficit:
The Attention-Arousal Hypothesis

The studies reviewed above provided Anderson, Hogarty and Reiss (1986a) the opportunity to develop a family-based treatment that had as its principal goal the prevention of symptomatic relapse. Hogarty and Ulrich (1977) had found that the risk for relapse declined appreciably over two years, such that at the end of that period the risk was one-third the risk of relapse at the point of hospital discharge, assuming maintenance medication throughout. Combined with data from studies of natural long-term outcome, this finding suggested that a slow, natural restitution process may occur, but only when relapse does not intervene (Harding et al., 1987).

Psychophysiological research and imaging studies in schizophrenia provided a model that linked more specifically the emerging biological and drug studies with the psychosocial literature, suggesting a possible clinical strategy: to create a social environment that compensates for the vulnerabilities specifically inherent to schizophrenia and allows that natural tendency for recovery to occur in the absence of relapse, supported by maintenance antipsychotic medication.

Beginning with Kraepelin, it has appeared that individuals with schizophrenia are impaired in their capacity for controlling attention: they select irrelevant stimuli, shift attentional set inappropriately, and have difficulty remaining alert to cognitive tasks.[1] Further, many studies have found that the regulation of arousal is impaired in this disorder, leaving patients vulnerable either to nearly disabling levels of autonomic hyper-

---

1. For a comprehensive review of this complex subject, Neuchterlein and Dawson's (1984) review is highly recommended.

activity under conditions of mild stress or to under-responsivity when arousal is appropriate (van Kammen et al., 1986). Attention appears to be subject to influence by arousal, such that attention is improved at moderate levels of arousal, but begins to deteriorate rapidly at higher levels. Further, Tecce and Cole (1976) found that distraction of attention produced increases in arousal. Two methods are known to assist in the regulation of arousal and attention: antipsychotic medication and reduction of the intensity, negativity, quantity, and complexity of stimuli from the environment. It was the latter alternative that suggested a mechanism for relapse in high-EE social environments. Sturgeon et al. (1984), and Tarrier et al. (1988), had found that high EE was indeed associated with high levels of psychophysiologic arousal in the ill relative.

The Empirical Evolution of Psychoeducation

This concept suggested a clinical approach: combine antipsychotic medication with a program that helped families reduce the level of intensity and complexity in their household, and relapse could conceivably be delayed, reduced in severity, or, for the less severely ill patient perhaps eliminated entirely. Such an approach would include two major components: (1) education of family members about the details of the disorder and (2) support and guidance over a fairly prolonged period after an episode. Previous experiments in that direction seemed to have been successful (Langsley, Machotka and Flomenhaft, 1971; Beels, 1975; Goldstein et al., 1978). The psychoeducational program described below is the result. The multiple-family group version outlined here has developed as a natural extension of multiple family therapy.

Because all psychoeducational approaches developed to date are designed to address specific major psychiatric disorders, they proceed with an unusual assumption: the family is functioning normally, until clearly proven otherwise, and better outcome for the ill member is most likely when the family makes compensatory, although abnormal, adjustments to its daily life that are dictated by the specific characteristics of the disorder itself. They also assume that these disorders often tend to elicit in family members responses that are self-defeating, although understandable. Further, general family functioning varies independently of the presence of schizophrenia or other biologically based mental disorders, so that the clinician practicing family psychoeducation can expect to encounter well-functioning *and* highly dysfunctional families.

CLINICAL GOALS IN PSYCHOEDUCATIONAL TREATMENT

The ultimate goal in psychoeducation is community integration—the ability of an individual with schizophrenia to function within the normal expectations of someone who does not have the disorder. Clearly, that is a most ambitious goal. To accomplish it, two other goals must be met first: (1) prevention of relapse and (2) social and vocational rehabilitation. Psychoeducation explicitly pursues those goals in a clear sequence, assuming that preventing relapse is essential to rehabilitation and that rehabilitation is essential to community integration. This approach assumes that several types of intervention are necessary to achieve any of these goals: enhancing the family's knowledge and coping skills, establishing barriers to stimulation, adjusting communication, and establishing a special family-clinician team structure.

Knowledge and Coping Skills

Living with schizophrenia is at least as difficult and confusing as treating it. Thus, the family has to possess (1) the available knowledge about the illness itself and (2) coping skills that are specific to this or other psychiatric disorders, skills most of which are counterintuitive and still being developed. A core principle in psychoeducational work is that to expect families to understand such a mystifying condition, and to know what to do about it, is unrealistic. Thus, the adaptive family is one that has access to information, and the treatment system is a crucial source of that information. As to coping skills, many families have developed, through painful trial and error, methods of dealing with positive and negative symptoms, functional disabilities, and the desperation of their ill relatives. These successes, however, are few and far between. So, a critical need is that families have access to each other—directly via multiple-family group contact and indirectly through professionals and leaders of the family self-help movement—to develop more effective means of coping with the day-to-day challenges of managing schizophrenia at home.

Stimulus Load

Because disruption in mental functioning, especially in attention and other cognitive capacities, seems so directly related to the level of arousal being experienced, the psychoeducational approach sets the regulation of stimulus load as a primary focus. In general, the goal is to limit the amount of stimulation from the social and physical environment to that which is tolerable and rehabilitative. Anderson (1986a) has described this concept as "erecting barriers to over-stimulation." This tends to require some very fine tuning by family and clinical programs alike, because there is great variation between patients and within a given patient over time. What is overwhelming to one person may simply be entertaining to another, although some stimuli, especially criticism in men and abrupt withdrawal of affection and companionship in women, appear to be nearly universally destabilizing. On the other hand, there is a distinct danger of producing an overly calm environment that is not conducive to rehabilitation and personal growth. There is also a phasic aspect: the need for protection from environmental stimulation is greatest in the immediate postpsychosis period and diminishes with the natural course of recovery from an acute episode (Hogarty and Ulrich, 1977). The clinician's task is to gauge precisely what is excessive, find strategies for both family and clinical systems to avoid those stimuli, watch carefully for indications that resilience and resistance to stimulation is improving, and adjust demands and expectations accordingly, upward and sometimes downward again as life events intervene.

Communication

Some significant accommodations must be made to the cognitive impairments in schizophrenia. Communication, especially in the early post-hospital period, should be clear, straightforward, concrete, and moderately specific. There is abundant evidence from the EE literature that positive comments and a calm, supportive tone are crucial in getting through to, and helping stabilize, an ill relative. Requests need to be made directly and simply. In the author's experience, low-EE families tend to be markedly low-key, tentative, and nonpressuring in their communications to the patient, often waiting for the patient to take the initiative in conversation. Anderson (1986a) has recommended acknowledging the statements of others directly and taking responsibility for one's own statements, purely from a practical point of view: individuals with attentional dysfunction will find it easier to track conversations if it is clear who is saying what and why.

Structure

The family with a mentally ill member needs to have a sufficiently clear hierarchy that necessary rules can be established and respected and that the caretaking functions of the well members of the family can be carried out. A clear structure tends to allay tension; prevent nagging, criticism and excessive interaction; and induce clarity and predictability in family life. The family in which the parents are clearly in charge and which is backed by the clinical team is the calmer, more therapeutic family.

Structure and limit-setting become very important around medication compliance: parents may decide that the patient's using medication as prescribed is necessary for the *family's* well-being and may require its continuation, even if the patient does not agree. The same is true for dealing with violence and bizarre behavior: setting limits will often be the only way to extinguish these behaviors and to preserve a semblance of normality at home.

TECHNICAL OPERATIONS IN PSYCHOEDUCATION

In the remaining pages of this chapter, we will explore the concrete technical tasks that comprise family psychoeducation (PE). Techniques for two distinct formats—single-family (SFPE) and multiple-family (MFPE)—will be described separately when necessary. However, the emphasis is on a core set of phased interventions common to both. Anderson, Hogarty and Reiss (1986a) have described the single-family approach comprehensively in a very useful volume, while the author has developed and tested the multi-family version (McFarlane, 1990). Each phase of the approach has different optimal arrangements, depending on the specific needs of the patient and the treatment goals that apply during that phase. There are four sequential phases: (1) engagement with the family, usually at the time of an acute psychotic decompensation; (2) an educational workshop, in which the clinicians present information and describe key behavioral guidelines didactically; (3) a reentry period, when biweekly sessions focus on stabilizing the patient out of the hospital; and (4) a rehabilitation phase, when sessions are bent to the aim of slowly and carefully raising the patient's level of functioning. In the multiple-family version, phases 2, 3, and 4 are carried out in a group of five or six families, as is phase 2 in the single-family version. A clinician meets with one family alone during phase 1 in MFPE and during phases 1, 3 and 4 in SFPE; patients join the sessions in phases 3 and 4 in both modalities.

Assessment and Engagement of Family and Patient

A few specific tasks are critical to success in this approach. The primary one is that of building an alliance with the patient and his or her significant relatives. Both engagement and assessment should convey genuine interest in the family's experiences and reactions and the clinician's desire to help both relatives and patient. It should accomplish one major goal: the creation of a collaborative treatment system in which family members become engaged as partners and experts on the daily life of their ill relative.

During the joining phase, which usually occurs during an acute episode and hospitalization, frequent meetings, usually weekly and without the patient present, occur with a flexible duration, averaging an hour. These will allay the family's anxiety and, by diminishing intensity of communication from family to patient, contribute to more rapid recompensation of the patient. If the clinicians, usually two in number, have decided to conduct a psychoeducational multiple-family group, the usual procedure is that each engages roughly half the families, on a single-family basis, until the educational workshop occurs. Also, one single-family joint session with both clinicians is desirable during this phase.

The patient, however, is not included in these sessions unless he or she is well-compensated and capable of tolerating a discussion of his or her condition as an illness. Since the greatest advantages for successful family engagement seem to exist in the early days of an acute psychosis and hospitalization, patients rarely participate in the family meetings. The family clinician holds short and less frequent sessions with the patient to foster an alliance and acceptance of the intent and direction of treatment.

The format for the engagement and assessment process is fairly straightforward. The clinician contacts all family members with whom the patient has frequent contact and invites them to meet at a convenient time. If the family is small or if contact occurs less often with only one or two relatives, special efforts are made to involve them. Before meeting, the clinician makes sure that he or she has met or communicated with the other staff treating the patient and is aware of the latest clinical status of the patient.

Assessment can be conceived as a triad: (1) evaluating the present crisis; (2) eliciting family reactions to the illness and the treatment system; and (3) evaluating the family and social system. Each will be described in turn.

Evaluating the Present Crisis

The initial task is to determine the present state of affairs. This includes getting a clear picture from each family member of what they have observed of the patient's decompensation, what they think might be the triggers to the relapse, and what are early prodromal signs of decompensation. Further, the clinician gathers information about coincidental events that are stressful to family members and how they impact on their coping with the psychosis. The clinician also begins the contracting process at this point by asking what kinds of help the relatives would like to receive from the treatment team.

Eliciting Family Reactions to the Illness and the Treatment System

The clinician takes a history of the specific emotional effects that the patient's illness has had on each family member. The technique is straightforward, empathic inquiry: usually, families find great relief in unburdening themselves about the toll in fear, anxiety, confusion, and sense of loss that this condition exacts. It is important to be aware of the way each individual has attempted to cope with these stresses, while also assessing the personal resources in the family. The variety of responses is great. The most common include centering of attention on the patient; denial of severity; suppression of grief; sacrifice of personal pleasures and ambitions to provide protection and control; and anger and frustration with the patient and the treatment system.

Because of the last of these negative reactions, it is important to communicate to family members that the program described here will deal with family members only in a respectful, supportive, and collaborative manner.

Evaluating the Family and Social System

To prepare the way for reducing ambient stress for patient and family members, the family clinician needs to have a general sense of the interactional style, structural alliances, specific communication patterns, coping strategies, and extended-family and social network resources of the family as a whole. This will involve taking a brief family network sociogram; asking about who spends time, or tends to interact, with whom; watching for difficulties or strengths in communication; asking about contacts with friends, relatives, and outside social or community groups; asking about sources of enjoyment and distraction; and gathering information on recent life events and changes in household membership, even if these represent desirable outcomes. Pains must be taken to avoid any implication that the family's functioning is what triggers the patient's episodes.

Finally, if the intent is that the family join a multiple-family group, brief inquiry should be made into feelings about this format. Generally, at a time of crisis, most families will not be enthusiastic about sharing experiences with others. Also, it is useful to know about any previous group experiences (especially if these were negative), aspects of family life of which the members might feel ashamed, and any concurrent or past participation in self-help groups. The picture that emerges can then guide the clinician in deciding how best to frame the multiple-family group as useful to the specific needs of a given family.

Goal-setting

A salient feature of the psychoeducational model of treatment is that the goals of treatment are explicit and negotiated with all participants. Anderson's single-family and the author's multiple-family approaches have two overriding goals: the prevention of relapse and the gradual integration of the patient into the highest possible degree of community participation. For a given case, these goals are the starting point for negotiating specific goals with the patient and family. Several secondary goals apply in almost all cases:

1. Establishing a treatment team that includes key family members and that addresses the clinical goals stated above;
2. Managing the family's interaction and impinging stresses in a way that keeps family burden to a minimum;
3. Providing information about the psychiatric disorder of concern and laying out a set of clear, workable guidelines for family members to achieve the main goals;
4. Providing continuity of care for patient and family;
5. Developing an enduring social network that supports the family and clinical goals; either through resurrection or expansion of the family's natural network (in SFPE) or through the organization of a network of affected families by the clinical team (in MFPE).

Having established some general objectives, the clinician implements another process of goal-setting that follows from goal 1. above: he or she gathers from all family members, patient included, what they hope to achieve by exerting themselves on behalf of the treatment effort. Because some family goals—for example, that the patient resume working immediately, become independent of all support, be without symptoms—are unrealistic, a respectful negotiation between clinician and family members must set more attainable versions of the family's goals. Fortunately, for most families agreement about goals is readily achieved, because they usually want what the approach is designed to do: prolong remission and enhance day-to-day functioning. Other goals usually are postponed until the patient has found a functional niche in the community.

From the goal-setting process a contract emerges that establishes conditions for the patient's discharge from the hospital, agreements about frequency of sessions and membership in the meetings, an approximate length of treatment, and the agreed-on treatment goals. The clinician needs to make clear that he or she will be available to the family for crisis intervention, to represent the family's interests and concerns to the treatment system, and to act as the patient's case manager.

FAMILY GUIDELINES

Here is a list of things everyone can do to help make things run more smoothly:

1. GO SLOW. Recovery takes time. rest is important. Things will get better in their own time.
2. KEEP IT COOL. Enthusiasim is normal. Tone it down. Disagreement is normal. Tone it down too.
3. GIVE THEM SPACE. Time out is important for everyone. It's okay to offer. It's okay to refuse.
4. SET LIMITS. Everyone needs to know what the rules are. A few good rules keep things clear.
5. IGNORE WHAT YOU CAN'T CHANGE. Let some things slide. Don't ignore violence.
6. KEEP IT SIMPLE. Say what you have to say clearly, calmly, and positively.
7. FOLLOW DOCTOR'S ORDERS. Take medications as they are prescribed. Take only medications that are prescribed.
8. CARRY ON BUSINESS AS USUAL. Reestablish family routines as quickly as possible. Stay in touch with family and friends.
9. NO STREET DRUGS OR ALCOHOL. They make symptoms worse.
10. PICK UP ON EARLY SIGNS. Note changes. Consult with your family clinician.
11. SOLVE PROBLEMS STEP BY STEP. Make changes gradually. Work on one thing at a time.
12. LOWER EXPECTATIONS, TEMPORARILY. Use a personal yardstick. Compare this month to last month rather than last year or next year.

Educational Workshop

The family clinicians, after engaging a small number of families, conduct an educational workshop for them. This is preferably as a multi-family meeting, usually lasting most of a day and usually held on a weekend. The workshop is specifically for family members and friends of the patient; patients usually are not invited, unless they are exceptionally well compensated and are not delusional or denying illness. The clinicians working with the families conduct the workshop, assisted by the psychiatrist(s) treating the patients. Experience suggests that the optimal size is from four to seven families, which coincidentally seems to be the ideal range for an ongoing psychoeducational multiple-family group.

The format for these workshops differs dramatically from therapy sessions. They proceed in an informal lecture and discussion format, with a classroom seating arrangement. Audiovisual aids are used extensively, particularly to illustrate concepts of brain function, medication effects, and symptoms and signs. In the author's workshops, the biological information is presented via a professional-quality videotape with frequent breaks for questions and discussion. The family clinicians then present a number of guidelines—"Survival Skills," as Anderson (1986a) calls them—for managing schizophrenia (see Figure 1), followed by an open-ended discussion. During breaks and over lunch, there is ample opportunity for informal social contact, between families and between families and clinicians.

While some agencies have elected to have "specialists in family education" carry out the educational function, the author's experience suggests that having the actual treating clinicians conduct the workshop has enormous clinical benefits. The main advantage is that the clinicians have ample opportunity to demonstrate their authority as experts and, in multiple-family groups, because each clinician has had initial contact with but a few of the families attending, they can begin to form an alliance with the others. The value of involving the treating physicians cannot be overstated, because families continue to see them as crucial to illness management.

Reentry and Social-vocational Rehabilitation Phases

Session structure in the phases after the workshop is somewhat strictly specified. In SFPE, one clinicians meets with the family, now including the patient if at all possible. In MFPE, the same families who attended the workshop together, with the addition of patients, begin meeting with both clinicians on a regular basis. Single-family sessions usually last an hour; multiple-family group sessions are usually one and a half hours or sometimes longer. In both formats, meetings take place two weeks apart, although some multiple-family groups will need to meet weekly for four to six weeks to establish cohesion. These basic formats are continued for at least twelve months. Frequently, once the rehabilitation phase has reached a plateau, usually after eighteen to twenty-four months, frequency of sessions can be reduced to three or four week intervals. Most families, particularly those in multiple-family groups, seem to want to continue at a low level of intensity for extended periods of time. Many multiple-family groups evolve into quasi-natural social networks; "real" interpersonal relationships develop and continue through and outside the group. Increasingly, the author has seen as a central goal of the psychoeducational (PE) approach the establishment of such support networks, because they appear to be essential to pre-serving and enhancing the gains made during the active therapeutic phases.

Structure of Sessions

The internal structure of sessions in both formats has evolved in the light of experience. In general, most PE sessions proceed fairly strictly according to Figure 2.

Structure of Sessions
Conducting Psycheducational Multifamily Groups

1. Socializing with families and patients	15 m.
2. A Go-around, reviewing—	20 m.
a. The week's events	
b. Relevant biosocial information	
c. Applicable guidelines	
3. Selection of a single problem	5 m.
4. Formal Problem-solving	45 m.
a. Problem definition	
b. Generation of possible solutions	
c. Weighing pros and cons of each	
d. Selection of preferred solution	
e. Delineation of tasks and implementation	
5. Socializing with families and patients	5 m.

Figure 2

This approach is surprisingly effective in either single- or multiple-family contexts. It has become clear that a rather standardized, predictable structure is beneficial, especially during the acute episode and immediate post-hospital discharge phases, as a means for the clinician to maintain benign control over sessions and to reach consensus on a likely solution to a given critical problem. In addition, to the extent that patients and family members have difficulty controlling affect or tracking a conversation, the problem-solving approach provides an acceptable rationale for bringing errant participants back to the topic or calming overly intense participants.

While the therapeutic core of this sequence consists of steps 4-10, **steps 1-3** are essential. As **step 1**, the clinician makes an emphatic attempt to avoid beginning the session with laments from anyone about any negative events or feelings. This requires clinicians to inquire specifically about enjoyable or novel events in the family's life, even if they seem trivial; clinicians may take the lead by describing similar kinds of events in their own lives. In both single- and multiple-family group formats, it is important to hear from everyone, even if a given patient or family member can make only a brief or superficial contribution. The emphasis is on setting an optimistic, accepting, warm, and inclusive tone as preparation for what follows—direct and sometimes more stressful attention to illness-induced problems.

Steps 2 and 3 involve reviewing the success or shortcomings of the task assigned in the previous meeting. In addition, it is helpful to inquire about other intervening events as a means of assessing unforeseen stresses on the family or patient. In a psychoeducational multiple-family group, each family should have an opportunity to report progress or untoward occurrences, so that the clinicians can make an informed decision about which family may need problem-solving efforts during the present group session.

Step 4 involves placing the problem implicit in the report in a perspective that relates it to the realities of schizophrenia as an illness. This depends on the clinician's knowledge of effective strategies for managing various aspects of the recovery and rehabilitation process. In general, it involves relating psychosocial phenomena to their likely consequences for an individual with schizophrenia. Most clinician responses focus on attention and arousal or the effects of symptoms and medication on cognition and behavior.

Step 5 follows directly from 4: if a problem is present because of symptomatic or disability aspects of a disorder, then the general approach to a solution is suggested by one or more of the guidelines put forth in the educational workshop. In other words, steps 4 and 5 are closely linked: most problems occur as a result of more or less obvious effects of the disorder and can be addressed through a number of clinically reliable methods. In multiple-family groups, with time the clinicians will find that they can ask other family members to suggest which guideline is likely to be relevant. The attempt here is to induce a sense of control and clarity that sets an optimal tone for the specific problem-solving that follows.

Steps 6-10 follow well-tested problem-solving and communication skills approaches refined by Falloon and Anderson. A single problem that has been identified by any one family is selected, and the entire family or multiple family group participates in problem-solving. This problem is the focus of most of the session, during which all participants contribute suggestions and ideas. Their relative advantages and disadvantages are then reviewed by the affected family, with some input from other families and clinicians. Typically, the most attractive of the proposed solutions is reformulated as an appropriate task for trying at home and is assigned to the family. This step is then followed by another final period of socializing, which ends the session.

Maintenance Antipsychotic Medication

It is important to state explicitly that antipsychotic medication is central to the psychoeducational approaches to schizophrenia and affective disorder and therefore, to many of its procedural and technical aspects. The assumption is made and reinforced consistently throughout the course of therapy that maintenance medication is a cornerstone of recovery and successful rehabilitation. Resistance to environmental stimulation is greatly enhanced by antipsychotic medications; except in unusually calm, friendly, simple, and unpressured contexts, most patients require that protection to lead any semblance of a normal life. Because noncompliance with medication is a major cause of relapse and yet so common, a great deal of the educational material in PE methods focuses on the rationale for drug treatment, while the ongoing work involves defining compliance as facilitating specific goals of patient and family. The clinician must first convince family members to accept the value of medication and then to support the prescribed regimen. Medication issues often become the focus of problem-solving in the ongoing sessions.

PSYCHOEDUCATION IN OTHER PSYCHIATRIC DISORDERS

As is evident from the preceding, the principal application for psychoeducation has been in treating recently admitted inpatients with schizophrenia, usually in their late twenties and living with the family of origin, who are treated for a period extending well beyond discharge and through the outpatient phase. However, Glick, Haas, and their colleagues at Cornell have developed an adaptation of Goldstein's (1978) brief psychoeducational approach for use during the inpatient phase (Haas et al., 1988). They found significantly superior outcomes in the family-based treatment for well-functioning schizophrenic patients, but not for patients with affective disorders or poorly functioning patients with schizophrenia. They concluded that the sicker schizophrenic patients may be more likely to respond to the Anderson model of long-term PE treatment. Anderson and her colleagues at the University of Pittsburgh (Anderson et al., 1986b) developed and tested a one-session educational group for relatives of patients with affective disorders during an acute inpatient admission; 62% of the families were conjugal. Analysis of the data disclosed few differences in clinical outcome between the educational group and a "process-oriented" multiple-family group. Both groups seemed to induce more dyadic satisfaction in the patients than a comparison group that was denied any family involvement, while the spouses reported less marital satisfaction. The main difference was that the PE group participants reported more satisfaction with the treatment program, regardless of clinical outcome. Miklowitz, Goldstein, and their colleagues (personal communication) have preliminary data suggesting that family behavioral management in bipolar disorder induces reductions in expressed emotion and diminution in relapse frequencies. Thus, there is presently some evidence that the psychoeducational model will induce clinical change in affective disorder.

Many other diagnoses have been shown to be amenable to psychoeducational methods. These have included sexual dysfunction (Kuriansky, Sharpe and O'Connor, 1982), attention deficit disorders of childhood (Dulcan, 1985), bulimia (Connors, Johnson and Stuckey, 1984), rheumatoid arthritis (Schwartz, Marcus and Condon, 1978), myocardial infarct (Frank and Kornfeld, 1979), breast cancer (Spiegel and Yalom, 1978), senile dementia (Zarit and Zarit, 1982), childhood asthma (Abramson and Peshkin, 1979), essential hypertension (Eaustaugh and Hatcher, 1982), seizure disorders (Flora, 1977), cystic fibrosis (Johnson, 1974), and juvenile diabetes (Koukal and Parham, 1978). Note that in all such conditions, the common denominators are (1) major, chronic

Author	n	Test treatment	Control treatment	Test interval
Comparisons of family to individual treatment (annual relapse rate)				
Goldstein, et al., (1978)	49	FCT 0% (0%)	IST 17% (34%)	6 months
Leff, et al., (1982)	24	RGT 40% (20%)	IST 78% (38%)	24 months
Falloon, et al., (1985)	36	BFM IST 11% (6%)	83% (42%)	24 months
Hogarty, et al., (1986)	50	SFPE 29% (19%)	IST 69% (35%)	24 months
Tarrier, et al., (1988)	48	BFM 12% (16%)	IST 53% (71%)	9 months
Comparisons of multiple- and single-family intervention				
Leff, et al., (1989)	23	RGT 33% (17%)	BFM 36% (18%)	24 months
McFarlane, et al., (1990)	41	MFPE 50% (13%)	SFPE 72% (18%)	48 months
McFarlane, et al., (in press)	172	MFPE 16% (8%)	SFPE 28% (14%)	24 months

		Intervention	
		Family	Individual
Average rates per year	443	11%	41%

FCT = family crisis therapy; IST = individual supportive therapy; RGT = relatives' group therapy; BFM = behavioral family management; SFPE = single-family psychoeducation; MFPE = psychoeducational multiple-family group.

Table 1. Relapse outcome in family intervention trials

biological dysfunction that induces changes in social and family inter-action, and (2) some evidence that targeted intervention to alter that social interaction in a manner specific to the disorder will influence the biological and behavioral processes favorably.

OUTCOME STUDIES OF PSYCHOEDUCATIONAL TREATMENT MODELS

These approaches have been remarkably effective when rigorously evaluated in experimental outcome studies. Table 1. presents relapse rates for the studies reported in the literature to date. These outcomes are unusually consistent and point to a valid, reliable, and quite robust main effect. In fact, the main effect is equivalent to that observed in most studies that have compared maintenance antipsychotic medication to placebo. That is, family intervention, when combined with medica-tion, is as powerful as the addition of medication itself. No other psy-chosocial intervention has achieved this level of impact and consistency while retaining an outpatient, low-intensity treatment format. That there are significant rehabilitation and burden relief outcomes in the Falloon, the Hogarty-Anderson, and the author's studies confirms that sustained remission and continued clinical support to family and patient do indeed promote functional improvement, especially in the vocational domain.

Outcomes and Therapeutic Processes in Psychoeducational Multiple-Family Groups

The first attempt to experimentally assess outcome of multi-family groups and to differentiate the contributions of its various elements was a study conducted by the author and colleagues involving forty-one patients diagnosed with schizophrenia or schizoaffective disorder (McFarlane, 1990). Patients recently admitted to a county receiving hospital in Bergen County, New Jersey, were randomly assigned to one of three conditions: psychoeducational multiple-family groups, dynami-cally oriented multiple-family therapy, or psychoeducational single-fam-ily treatment. The design tested two treatment elements—psychoedu-cation and social network expansion—with the hope of distinguishing separate and possibly additive effects. Medication, set at lowest effective dose levels, was used in all cases.

At four years after discharge, the psychoeducational multiple-family groups had a significantly longer time to first relapse than did single-family treatment. Final four-year relapse rates were 50% for the psy-choeducational multiple-family group, 57.1% for the dynamically oriented multiple-family group, and 76.5% for psychoeducational single-family treatment. Six of the earliest psychoeducational multiple-family group cohort of ten patients remained in remission for five years or more. The data suggest that a specific and independent multiple-family group effect prevents or forestalls relapse in addition to the effect of psychoeducation as content

Nearly one-third, 32.5%, of all participating patients were functionally occupied at the beginning of the study. At two years, 51.6% were functionally occupied. Although the differences across treatment types were not significant, the psychoeducational multiple-family group registered the highest increase. These promising results needed replication in a larger sample.

The New York State Family Psychoeducation in Schizophrenia Study presented the opportunity to confirm these results (McFarlane, Lukens, Link et al., in press). This study of 172 patients with DSM-IIIR schizophrenic, schizophreniform, or schizoaffective disorders compared psychoeducational multiple-family and psychoeducational single-family treatment over a two-year period. The design included random assignment, full specification of the test treatments, extensive training and supervision of project staff, a standard-dose medication strategy, and wide-ranging measurement of patient and family outcomes.

Relapse rates at one year were 19.0% for multiple-family group cases and 28.6% for single-family treatment cases. At two years, the rates were 28% and 42%, respectively. For cases completing the treatment protocol (80% of the initial sample) or when controlled for medication compliance, this was a statistically significant difference. Two-year rates of clinically significant relapse were 16.3% and 25.6%, respectively. The multiple-family group result—a clinically significant relapse rate of under 10% per year—compares quite favorably to relapse rates of about 40% using medication alone or with supportive individual therapy or about 70% using placebo medication (Hogarty et al., 1979). In the highest-risk subsample—Caucasian families with high expressed emotion and with patients who only partially remitted during the index admission—multiple-family group relapse rates (9% over two years) were actually lower than in more stabilized patients and dramatically lower than in single-family treatment.

The mean number of hospitalizations during the two-year study period showed a drop to about one-third of the sample's prior two years' hospitalization rate. And, pharmacological treatment was affected positively: medication compliance averaged close to 90% for the entire sample across the two years, increasing slightly in multiple-family groups over that period—a fairly dramatic outcome that clearly contributed to the excellent overall outcome in both cohorts.

The sample as a whole increased significantly in employment from 17.3% before treatment to 29.3% at the end of the study. The multiple-family groups showed a higher rate of employment gain than single-family treatment, but the difference was not statistically significant.

These two studies indicate that multiple-family group treatment, when combined with psychoeducation and medication, not only yields better overall outcome but demonstrates a very favorable cost-benefit ratio (1:2.5 relative to single-family psychoeducation): the approach requires exactly one-half the staff time expenditure of single-family treatment, an approach that is highly effective in its own right.

With evidence in hand that psychoeducation in multiple family groups leads to better overall outcome than psychoeducation in a single-family context, the processes that might explain that result can be explored. The differences must derive from effects of the larger number of people involved in the group, that is, from an expansion of each family's social network. The most common explanation for the benefits of larger networks is that they provide more emotional support, which usually means nonspecific phenomena such as reduced tension, exasperation, or loneliness and an increased sense of validation and burden sharing. For instance, families surveyed in the New York State study reported that the most important aspects of the multiple-family groups were education, sharing of concerns, and knowledge that they were not alone in being devastated by the illness. A more specific form of emotional support comes from the realization that many of the interactions that trouble families and patients are clearly generic to having a mental illness in the family and are not the result of personal or family failure.

These affective aspects of multiple-family groups seem to be confirmed by a surprising finding in the same study. As family EE increased, relapse rates increased as expected in single-family treatment but *decreased* in multiple-family groups. A similar treatment interaction effect was observed for baseline patient symptoms: higher symptoms led to more relapses in single-family treatment but *fewer* relapses in multiple-family groups. Symptoms and EE were correlated at baseline. Thus, outcome in multiple-family groups improved the more the patient was at risk for relapse. This result suggests that the effects of EE are directly related both to the social support available to a given family and also to patient symptoms. More precisely, when the patient is especially symptomatic and the families are especially vulnerable to reacting with exasperation and criticism, the multiple-family group seems particularly effective, probably by diffusing negative affect within families among the other families in the group. Thereby, the multiple-family group may prevent or interrupt escalating cycles of negative affect precipitated by ongoing symptoms. In single-family treatment, with only the clinician for support, the family with a highly symptomatic member may need more bolstering as they wait for symptom improvement. In addition, multiple family groups, which include a great deal of casual conversation, joking, and sharing information about local events and everyday experiences, usually generate more positive affect than single-family sessions or patient-only groups. This is interesting in light of the evidence that positive family emotions, especially warmth and positive regard, predict good outcome (Spiegel and Wissler, 1986).

The social structure of multiple-family groups allows an opportunity for patients to develop relationships with members of other families, as well as with other patients. This cross-parenting process can substitute for intense relationships within families, further diffusing excess affect and anxiety. It can validate the ill members of the groups and reassure relatives that they can have a positive influence on the ill members of other families. The multiple-family group clinical approach exploits the social network inherent in these groups to enhance the illness-coping skills of family members and patients. Furthermore, the larger number of participants can generate more widely varied ideas and perspectives and thus more potential solutions. The more varied the background of the groups's participants, the more likely will novel ideas or previously successful strategies be available for sharing. The preferable and successful solution to a persistent problem in a given family commonly comes from another family member or patient. In summary, all of these factors are likely to operate in complex combinations to support families, diminish exasperation and demoralization, develop positive affect, expand personal relationships across family boundaries, generate better coping skills, and ultimately improve outcome.

CONCLUSION

It is reasonable to conclude that family psychoeducation, combined with maintenance antipsychotic medication, has become a treatment of choice for schizophrenia. The multiple family group version may be a treatment of choice for markedly or persistently symptomatic and especially distressed and isolated families. Its combination of efficacy and simplicity has potentially enormous implications for cost-effectiveness (Cardin, McGill and Falloon, 1985) and long-term course. Reducing relapse from an annual or biennial event to one that at least half the patient population may not experience for over five years could alter the expected course of the illness. The potential savings in hospitalization costs are simply staggering. It is now a matter of disseminating these outcomes to clinicians and urging that they adopt these approaches. If that succeeds, the next generation of people with schizophrenia may have a much less disabling course of illness than those who are presently afflicted.

REFERENCES

Abramson, H., & Peshkin, H. (1979) Psychosomatic group therapy with parents of children with intractable asthma: The Peters family. *J. Asthma Res.*, *16*, pp. 103-117.

Anderson, C., & Griffin, S. et al. (1986b) A comparative study of the impact of education vs. process groups for families of patients with affective disorders. *Fam. Proc.*, *25*, pp. 185-205.

Anderson, C., Hogarty, G., & Reiss, D. (1986a) *Schizophrenia and the family*. New York: Guilford Press.

Anderson, C., Hogarty, G., Bayer, T., & Needleman, R. (1984) Expressed emotion and social networks of parents of schizophrenic patients. *Br. J. Psychiatry*, *144*, pp. 247-255.

Beels, C.C. (1975) Family and social management of schizophrenia. *Schiz. Bull.*, *13*, pp. 97-118.

Beels, C. (1981) Social support and schizophrenia. *Schiz. Bull.*, *7*, pp. 58-72.

Berman, K.K. (1966) Multiple family therapy: Its possibilities in preventing readmission. *Mental Hygiene*, *50*, 367.

Bourdon, K.H., Rae, D.S., Locke, B.Z., Narrow, W.E., Regier, D.A. (1992) Estimating the prevalence of mental disorders in U.S. adults from the Epidemiologic Catchment Area Survey. *Public Health Reports*, *107*, pp. 663-668.

Breier, A., & Strauss, J.S. (1984) The role of social relationships in the recovery from psychotic disorders. *American Journal of Psychiatry*, *141*, pp 949-955.

Brown, G., Birley, J., & Wing, J. (1972) Influence of family life on the course of schizophrenic disorders: A replication. *Br. J. Psychiatry*, *121*, pp. 241-258.

Cardin, V.A., McGill, C.W., & Falloon, I.R.H. (1985) An economic analysis: Costs, benefits, and effectiveness. In I.R.H. Falloon et al. (eds.), *Family management of schizophrenia, A study of clinical, so-*

cial, family, and economic benefits. Baltimore, John Hopkins University Press.

Connors, M., Johnson, K., & Stuckey, M. (1984) Treatment of bulimia with brief psychoeducational group therapy. *American Journal of Psychiatry, 141,* pp. 1512-1516.

Detre, T., Sayer, J., Norton, A., & Lewis, H. (1961) An experimental approach to the treatment of the acutely ill psychiatric patient in the general hospital. *Connecticut Med., 25,* pp. 613-619.

Dulcan, M. (1985) Psychoeducational therapy with families of severely impaired children. *NIMH Clinical Training Human Resource Development Grant.*

Eaustaugh, S., & Hatcher, M. (1982) Improving compliance among hypertensives: A triage criterion with cost benefit implications. *Medical Care, 20,* pp. 1001-1017.

Falloon, I.R.H. & Liberman, R.P. (1983) Behavioral family intervention in the management of chronic schizophrenia. In McFarlane, W.R. (Ed), *Family Therapy in Schizophrenia,* New York: Guilford Press, pp. 117-137.

Falloon, I.R.H., Boyd, J.L., McGill, C.W., Williamson, M., Razani, J., Moss, H.B., Gilderman A.M. & Simpson, G.M. (1985) Family management in the prevention of morbidity of schizophrenia. *Archives of General Psychiatry, 42:* pp. 887-896.

Flora, G. (1977) Problem solving in diagnostics and therapeutic of neurology: The treatment of seizure disorders. *South Dakota J. Med., 30,* pp. 15-16.

Frank, K., & Kornfeld, D. (1979) Psychological intervention in coronary heart disease: A review. *Gen. Hosp. Psychiatry, 1,* pp. 18-23.

Garrison, V. (1978) Support systems of schizophrenic and nonschizophrenic Puerto Rican women in New York City. *Schiz. Bull.,* pp. 561-596.

Goldstein, M.J., Rodnick, E., Evans, J., May, P., & Steinberg, M. (1978) Drug and family therapy in the aftercare of acute schizophrenics. *Archives of General Psychiatry, 35,* pp. 1169-1177.

Haas, G., & Glick, I. et al. (1988) Inpatient family intervention: A randomized clinical trial: II Results at hospital discharge. *Archives of General Psychiatry, 45,* pp. 217-224.

Hammer, M. (1963) Influence of small social networks as factors on mental hospital admission *Human Organization, 22,* pp. 243-251.

Harding, C., Brooks, G., Ashikaga, T., Strauss, J., & Breier, A. (1987) The Vermont longitudinal study of persons with severe mental illness,

I: Methodology, study sample, and overall status 32 years later. *American Journal of Psychiatry*, *144*, pp. 718-726.

Hatfield, A. (1983) What families want of family therapists. W.R. McFarlane (Ed.), *Family Therapy in Schizophrenia* New York: Guilford Press, pp. 41-68.

Hedblad, B., Ostergren, P.O., Hanson, B.S. & Janzon L. (1992) Influence of social support on cardiac event rate in men with ischaemic type ST segment depression during ambulatory 24-h long-term ECG recording. The prospective population study "Men born in 1914", Malmo Sweden. *European Heart Journal*, *13*, pp. 433-439.

Hogarty, G., Schooler, N., & Ulrich, R. et al. (1979) Fluphenazine and social therapy in the aftercare of schizophrenic patients. *Archives of General Psychiatry*, *36*, pp. 1283-1294.

Hogarty, G.E., Goldberg, S., & Schooler, N. et al. (1974) Drugs and social therapy in the aftercare of schizophrenic patients. *Archives of General Psychiatry*, *28*, pp. 54-63.

Hogarty, G., & Ulrich, R. (1977) Temporal effects of drug and placebo in delaying relapse in schizophrenic outpatients. *Archives of General Psychiatry*, *34*, pp. 297-301.

Hogarty, G.E., Anderson, C.M., Reiss, D.J., Kornblith, S.J., Greenwald, D.P., Javna, C.D. & Madonia, M.J. (1986) Family psychoeducation, social skills training and maintenance chemotherapy in the aftercare treatment of schizophrenia. *Archives of General Psychiatry*, 43: pp. 633-642.

Johnson, D. (1990) The family's experience of living with mental illness. H.P. Lefley, & D.J. Johnson (Ed.), *Families as allies in treatment of the mentally ill*. Washington, D.C.: American Psychiatric Press, pp. 31-64.

Johnson, D. (1974) Before hospitalization: A preparation program for the child and his family. *Child Today*, *3*, pp. 18-21.

Koukal, S., & Parham, E. (1978) A family learning experience to serve the juvenile patient with diabetes. *J. Am. Diabetes Assoc.*, *72*, pp. 411-413.

Kreisman, D., & Joy, V. (1974) Family response to the mental illness of a relative: A review of the literature *Schiz. Bull.*, *10*, pp. 35-57.

Kuriansky, J., Sharp, L., & O'Connor, D. (1982) The treatment of anorgasmia: Long term effectiveness of a short term behavioral group therapy. *J. Sex Marital Ther.*, *8*, pp. 29-43.

Langsley, D.G., Machotka, P. & Flomenhaft, K. (1971) Avoiding mental hospital admission: a follow-up study. *American Journal of Psychiatry*, *127*, pp. 1391-1394.

Lansky, M.R., Bley, C.R., McVey, G.G., Botram, B. (1978) Multiple family groups as aftercare. *International Journal of Group Psychotherapy*, *29*, p. 211.

Laqueur, H., LaBurt, H., & Morong, E. (1964) Multiple family therapy: Further developments. *Int. J. Soc. Psychiatry*, *69:* Congress edition.

Leff, J.P., Kuipers, L., Berkowitz, R., Sturgeon, D. (1982) A controlled trial of social intervention in the families of schizophrenic patients: two year follow up. *Br. J. Psychiatry*, 146: pp. 594-600.

Lefley, H.P. (1989) Family burden & family stigma in major mental illness. *American Psychologist*, 44, 556-560.

Leff J, Berkowitz N, Shavit N, Strachan A, Glass I, Vaughn C. (1989) A trial of family therapy v. a relatives group for schizophrenia. *Br J Psychiatry*, 154: pp. 58-66.

Levin, E.C. (1966) Therapeutic multiple family groups. *International Journal of Psychotherapy*, *19*, p. 203.

Lin, N., & Ensel, W. (1984) Depression-mobility and its social etiology: The role of life events and social support. *Journal of Health and Social Behavior*, *25*, pp. 176-188.

Lipton, F., Cohen, C., Fischer, E., & Katz, S. (1981) Schizophrenia: A network crisis. *Schiz. Bull.*, 7, pp. 144-151.

Lurie, A. & Ron, H. (1972) Socialization program as part of aftercare planning. *General Psychiatric Association Journal*, *17*, p. 157.

McFarlane, W. (1990) Multiple family groups in the treatment of schizophrenia. H.A. Nasrallah (Ed.), *Handbook of Schizophrenia*. Amsterdam; New York; Oxford: Elsevier, pp. 167-189.

Pattison, E., Llama, R., & Hurd, G. (1979) Social network mediation of anxiety. *Psychiatry Ann.*, *9:* pp. 56-67.

Schwartz, L., Marcus, R., & Condon, R. (1978) Multidisciplinary group therapy for rheumatoid arthritis. *Psychosomatics*, *19*, pp. 289-293.

Spiegel, D., & Wissler, T. (1986) Family environment as a predictor of psychiatric rehospitalization. *American Journal of Psychiatry*, *143*(1), pp. 56-60.

Spiegel, D., & Yalom, I. (1978) A support group for dying patients. *Int. J. Gr. Psychother.*, *28*, pp. 233-245.

Strauss, J.S., & Carpenter, W. (1977) Prediction of outcome in schizophrenia. *Archives of General Psychiatry*, *34*, pp. 159-163.

Tarrier N, Barrowclough C, Vaughn C, Bamrah JS, Porceddu K, Watts S, Freeman H. (1988) The community management of schizophrenia: A controlled trial of a behavioral intervention with families to reduce relapse. *Br. J. Psychiatry*; 153: pp. 532-542.

Tecce, J., & Cole, J. (1976) The distraction-arousal hypothesis, CNV and schizophrenia. D.I. Mostofsky (Ed.), *Behavioral Control and Modification of Psychological Activity*. Englewood Cliffs, N.J.: Prentice-Hall.

Tolsdorf, C. (1976) Social networks, support and coping: An explanatory study. *Fam. Proc.*, *15*, pp. 407-417.

van Kammen, D.P., van Kammen, W.B., Mann, L.S., Seppala, T., & Linnoila, M. (1986) Dopamine metabolism in the cerebrospinal fluid of drug-free schizophrenic patients with and without cortical atrophy. *Archives of General Psychiatry, 43*, pp. 978-983.

Weinberger, D. (1987) The implications of normal brain development for the pathogenesis of schizophrenia. *Archives of General Psychiatry*, 44, pp. 660-670.

Yolles, S.F. and Kramer, M. (1969) Vital statistics. In Bellack L. and Loeb, L. (eds.), *The schizophrenic syndrome*. New York, Grune and Stratton, pp. 66-113.

Zarit, J., & Zarit, S. (1982) Families under stress: Interventions for caregivers of senile dementia patients. *Psychotherapy: Theory Res. Prac.*, *19*, pp. 461-471.

Zubin, J., & Spring, B. (1977) Vulnerability: A new view of schizophrenia. *J. Abn. Psychol.*, *86*, pp. 103-126.

Chapter 11

SERVICE NEEDS OF CULTURALLY DIVERSE PATIENTS AND FAMILIES

Harriet P. Lefley

When we speak of cultural diversity within the United States, it is difficult to differentiate the traditional values, beliefs, and practices of an ethnocultural group from socioeconomic status; minority status; migrant, immigrant or refugee status; and linguistic or acculturative status. Yet regardless of where a particular family fits into this spectrum, no family goes untouched when a member begins to suffer from mental illness. Regardless of racial or ethnic background, social or economic status, or family structure, all human beings are affected when a known person begins to act in ways that are strange, unpredictable, and negatively viewed within their own cultural system. Throughout the world, family members are impacted both by the pain and by the erratic behavior of someone to whom they are tied by kinship bonds of love and obligation.

Despite common family experiences among racial/ethnic groups in the United States, sociocultural variables affect service needs in a number of ways. They are related to epidemiologic profiles and diagnostic practices; to referral patterns and assignment of treatment modalities. They are evident in differential national statistics relating to sites, types, and duration of service delivery. Cultural factors are related both to service access and service utilization, reflecting barriers that may be institutional or self-imposed. They are manifested in the range of services available, their appropriateness for the populations served, their acceptability to patients and families, and their effectiveness.

Cultural variables are also involved in the resources available in different communities. Communities vary in the types and severity of stressors, but almost all cultural groups have strengths and adaptive strategies for dealing with illness. Families may choose to use their own indigenous healing and support networks, to use the resources of the professional mental health system, or to combine the two. Their preference for one or the other may very well depend on the history of their relations and interactions with professionals throughout the course of the illness.

In contrast to the family-professional distance historically practiced in western countries, there is evidence that in other cultures professionals have been more forthcoming in communicating with the families of their patients and involving them in the treatment process. Psychiatrists Drs. Rada Shankar and M. Sarada Menon of the Schizophrenia Research Foundation in Madras, India state that in their country the interactions of professionals and families have not been impeded by conceptual dogma:

> In contrast to those in the West, mental health professionals in India generally have not dealt with families on the basis of any etiological presupposition regarding their role in the causation of illness. Because of this, professional-family interactions have been a relatively even keel and the ideological see-saw from viewing families as schizophrenogenic in the 1950's to viewing families as equal treatment partners in the 1980's has not taken place in India. (Shankar & Menon, 1991, p. 86).

These patterns of willingness to work with families fortunately persist among some mental health professionals from developing countries currently practicing in the United States. In the main, however, most of our core of mental health professionals are of white-American middle-class background. They often find that social and cultural distance impedes their understanding of ethnically diverse patients and their family members. A substantial research literature suggests that this distance may affect diagnosis and treatment (Lefley, 1990b; Lefley & Bestman, 1991; Westermeyer, 1987). There is a need to understand the importance of cultural world view, kinship structure, and support systems as well as the role of social stressors that may erode family integration or trigger decompensation in patients. Clues to just a few of these interrelationships can be found in a brief overview of ethnic differences in the service profiles of persons with serious mental illnesses.

CULTURAL FACTORS IN EPIDEMIOLOGY
AND SERVICE UTILIZATION

The presumption is that mental disorders, particularly those that appear to be biogenic, are evenly distributed across populations. However, persons with psychophysiological vulnerability to stress may be unduly affected by socioeconomic, political, and cultural forces beyond their control. Populations suffering harsh economic and/or social pressures may have an equivalent distribution of serious mental disorders in terms of lifetime prevalence, but manifest differences in the frequency of acute psychotic episodes and in the persistence of severe disability. They may also vary in their willingness to use the mainstream mental health service delivery system.

Data on the distributions of mental disorders in the United States are derived primarily from the Epidemiological Catchment Area Survey (ECA), the largest and most scientific true prevalence study of mental disorders undertaken in this country to date. Tapping 30 of the major psychiatric disorders listed in the third edition of the *Diagnostic and Statistical Manual* (DSM-III) of the American Psychiatric Association (1980), the ECA administered standardized interviews in five states to systematic samples of almost 20,000 Americans.

The results indicated that 32% of American adults had experienced one or more of these 30 psychiatric disorders at some time in their lives and 20% had an active disorder. Although there were significant ethnic differences in prevalence rates for some of these disorders, the differences disappeared when the data were controlled for age, gender, marital status, and most importantly, socioeconomic status (Robins & Regier, 1991).

The ECA results suggest that there would be little difference among ethnic groups with respect to their needs for treatment and hospitalization, but here the picture changes dramatically. For many years government statistics have shown that admission rates to inpatient psychiatric services were significantly higher for nonwhites ("blacks and other races") than for whites, for both women and men. This pattern has never deviated and continues in the most recent data (National Institute of Mental Health, 1990). The currently reported admissions for all inpatient facilities per 100,000 population show a rate of 1074 for nonwhites versus 594 for whites, with males continuing to have higher admission rates than females in facilities that serve the most seriously disabled patients. In contrast, there is almost no racial difference in admissions for outpatient care (889 white versus 886 nonwhite, per 100,000 population).

A longitudinal study of patients served in state mental hospitals showed that for both discharged and resident patients the cohorts were largely adult(92% over age 18), predominantly male (61%), and disproportionately African-American (National Institute of Mental Health, 1987). A California study of ethnic differences among severely mentally ill recidivists found that blacks were more likely than whites to visit the psychiatric emergency room and to be hospitalized (Snowden & Holschuh, 1992).

Most National Institute of Mental Health reports have used a white/nonwhite distinction without regard to ethnic differences. However, the 1987 report gave data for other racial and ethnic groups (National Institute of Mental Health, 1987). This report showed that relative to population distributions, African Americans and American Indians had significantly higher admission rates than all other racial/ethnic groups to all inpatient facilities, including state and county mental hospitals, private psychiatric hospitals, general hospitals, and Veterans Administration hospitals. Rates per 100,000 population were: 931.8 for Blacks, 818.7 for American Indians or Alaska Natives; 550.0 for non-Hispanic whites; 451.4 for Hispanics (who could be of any race); and 268.1 for Asians. The rates for African-Americans were more than two-thirds higher than for whites, and exceeded double the rates for Hispanics and three times the rates for Asians (National Institute of Mental Health, 1987, Table 3, p. 76).

Perplexing Patterns of Service Delivery

In these national statistics there seemed to be little relation between hospital admissions and level of disability. Among inpatients, groups with the lowest admission rates (Asians, Hispanics, and whites) had considerably higher median inpatient stays than did African-American or American Indian patients (ibid., Table 3.5, p. 80). For persons diagnosed with schizophrenia, the primary diagnosis requiring hospitalization, Hispanics and Asians had median stays of 54 and 52 days respectively, considerably more than the 32 days for African Americans and 20 days for American Indians (ibid.). In fact, the rates of admission were almost directly inverse to the patients' apparent need for prolonged hospital care.

Do these paradoxical figures reflect cultural differences in service utilization? It has been suggested that perhaps Hispanic and Asian families are more likely to keep patients at home and to present them for hospitalization at an advanced stage of illness, when they might require longer hospital stays. Perhaps they are more likely to first apply to indigenous spiritual healers. Or perhaps these groups are reluctant to use the mental health service system because there are insufficient staff who speak their language. Yet these variables might also apply to American Indians or Alaska Natives, whose admissions are almost as high as those of African-Americans.

Snowden & Cheung (1990) note that data are lacking on differential access and on ethnic differences in help-seeking patterns or the use of alternatives to inpatient services. They also state that two other areas require attention from researchers: involuntary commitment proceedings, and diagnostic error. They suggest that bias in admitting practices may include a tendency to view greater psychopathology in Blacks and Native Americans, but it may also include "minimizing bias" in judging the behavior of Asian-Americans and whites (p. 354).

To what extent are these patterns artifacts of interviewing, assessment, and admitting practices that may reflect cultural bias or misunderstanding? A large research literature has indicated that certain issues may be problematic in cross-cultural diagnosis, such as assessment instruments and interviewing techniques, language and psycholinguistics, and simple misunderstanding of culturally normative behavior (Lefley & Pedersen, 1986; Rogler, 1992; Westermeyer, 1987). Research shows that when the race and sex of patient and psychiatrist vary, this can influence diagnosis even when clear-cut DSMIII criteria are used (Loring & Powell, 1988).

Diagnostic accuracy is often confounded by cultural differences in the behavioral manifestations of psychosis (Chu et al., 1985; Fabrega, Mezzich, & Ulrich, 1988). African-Americans historically have been underdiagnosed for depression; a number of studies have rediagnosed affective disorders in black patients previously diagnosed schizophrenic (Jones & Gray, 1986). There is also an emerging literature on racial/ethnic differences in response to medications, with difficulties in assessing the relative contributions of biological and cultural factors (Lin, Poland, & Lesser, 1986; Keltner & Folks, 1992). In Spring, 1991, the National Institute of Mental Health sponsored a conference of cross-cultural scholars to explore the possibility of adding a cultural axis to DSMIII-R (American Psychiatric Association, 1987). Increasing calls for a more culturally sensitive DSM-IV include proposals for a new Z code that will document psychoreligious or spiritual problems. Presumably this will allow diagnosticians to differentiate psychotic religiosity from nonpsychotic culturally-appropriate religious experiences, and hopefully "reduce iatrogenic harm from misdiagnosis" (Lukoff, Lu, & Turner, 1992, p. 673).

With respect to treatment, there is now a substantial literature questioning the cross-cultural applicability of therapeutic models developed largely in western nations with middle-class patients and focusing on individuals and individual growth. Alternative models, building on family strengths and involving kinship networks and other support systems, are deemed more culturally appropriate for traditional, family-oriented cultures (Lefley, 1990b; Shankar & Menon, 1991). In the African-American community, as noted by Griffith, Young & Smith (1984), religion has been a core social and spiritual resource. The church provides collective support, opportunities for self expression and helping others, and a reference point for meaningfulness in life. Yet these natural support systems have largely been ignored by the traditional mental health system. The system has also imposed barriers that are particularly onerous for low-income and linguistically or culturally diverse clienteles.

SYSTEMIC BARRIERS

Systemic barriers affect access to services and also may result in clients' using specific types of services when others may be more appropriate. An example of the latter is overutilization of hospital emergency rooms because of difficulties in obtaining outpatient clinic cards. Access barriers are cost-ineffective for both clients and providers and may result in underuse or misuse of expensive resources.

When community mental health centers were first started and funds came in under the jurisdiction of the National Institute of Mental Health, centers were required to provide evaluation data on availability, awareness, and accessibility of services within their catchment areas. They had to demonstrate first of all that the required services had been developed, that potential clients were aware that they existed, and that the services were accessible geographically and culturally. The latter might include the site and timing of service delivery as well as a linguistic capability for communicating with clients.

As Boyd-Franklin (1989) has indicated the many strengths of African-American families tend to be eroded by systemic barriers that often impede rather than reinforce their stabilization. The helping system itself sometimes seems designed to erode family supports and economic resources, requiring endless forms and visits to multiple agencies. Meetings are set for hours that are convenient for the agency, not the service recipient. Applying for welfare benefits or taking care of health concerns almost always involve hours of waiting. Transportation and child care must be arranged, as well as time off from one's job. Negotiating the system is time-costly, bewildering, and invariably eats into the working hours and paychecks of people on whom others depend for support.

Patients' families spend many hours negotiating the mental health, social security, and welfare systems and these issues are particularly important for lower socioeconomic families for whom time is clearly money. They also suffer from indifference or brusqueness on the part of overworked clinic staff. Minority group status often goes hand in hand with poverty, and patients from these families are unlikely to have money or insurance. Many families complain that medicaid or indigent patients are treated rudely by clinic staff; that they are shuttled around the system and often refused admission to crisis or inpatient units even when they are clearly more needful than paying patients.

Linguistic barriers are another issue. Immigrant or refugee families often find it difficult to understand the applications they must fill out or the myriad directions they must follow in acquiring services. Communications that are poorly understood may result in faulty medication regimens or poor appointment keeping.

There are several profound service needs that transcend cultural and often socioeconomic barriers. One is for institutional case managers or coordinators who can arrange for help with translators, applications, or simply explaining ambiguous admissions policies or other regulations. Another is for ombudsmen who can plead the case of patients who are denied services for reasons unrelated to their need. The third requirement is for informational materials to fill the empty waiting hours. Videotapes and reading materials can inform visitors about what to expect when patients are admitted for services. General information on mental illnesses, medications, and the like can also be offered on videotape, reaching larger audiences than is possible with standard psychoeducational interventions.

ARE THERE CULTURAL DIFFERENCES IN SERVICE NEEDS?

Research indicates that persons with major psychiatric disorders are particularly susceptible to stress, even to ordinary life stressors (Norman & Malla, 1993; Lefley, 1992). Although most minority groups tend to be less well-off economically than mainstream white-Americans, the relatively higher admission rates of African-American and American-Indian patients may reflect greater exposure to environmental stressors such as poverty, unemployment, neighborhood crime and substance abuse, loss of housing, and erosion of traditional support systems. Survival under these conditions attests to the inherent strengths of many families in these cultures. Yet, families need help in holding themselves together. The multi-systems approach advocated by Boyd-Franklin (1989) and others involves a much more comprehensive approach than typical systemic family therapy. Here, there is an effort by the therapist to enlist the larger system in providing for the economic and housing needs of the entire family, to provide a type of global family case management that aids patients by ensuring the survival of their natural support systems. For American Indian patients this may mean enlistment of supportive tribal resources or reinforcement of self-esteem by revaluing Indian cultural identity (Lefley, 1982). For immigrant or refugee groups, providing language and acculturation classes may help the patient by helping the family (Lefley, 1989).

Service providers who are oriented toward serving the needs of particular cultural groups tend to have more therapeutic successes and fewer dropout rates than are nationally reported for these clients (Lefley & Bestman, 1991). Research indicates that ethnically-oriented facilities are more acceptable and provide more culturally appropriate services than those which simply offer people of color on their staff. Takeuchi, Maku, & Chun (1992), for example, studying services for Asian Americans and Pacific Islanders, found that centers specifically serving the needs of these populations ("parallel services") were more successful than more conventional services with Asian professionals on their staff.

Common Needs Across Cultures

Studies of families of hospitalized mentally ill patients in the main show few differences among cultural groups in their assessment of specific service needs of their relatives. For example, Solomon & Marchenko (1992b), studying family members' concerns regarding community placement of their relative following hospitalization in a predominantly African-American (54%) urban sample, found that "regardless of race, sex, or age of the mentally ill relative, family concerns are consistent" (p. 345). They also found pronounced needs for case managers to be trained in social skills training, behavioral techniques, coping strategies for families, and problem-solving techniques. In a study of families' satisfaction with inpatient and outpatient treatment, the same sample of predominantly African-American families indicated that they were more satisfied with services to their relatives than for themselves. They indicated a need for family education about medications and how to motivate their mentally ill relative (Solomon & Marcenko, 1992a).

In interviews with 365 family members (51% black and 49% white) Tessler, Fisher & Gamache (1990) found that, controlling for income and education, blacks seemed to be less tolerant of disruptive and psychotic behavior while whites seemed to be less tolerant of patients who made no positive contributions to the household. However, both groups were more accepting when the behavior was seen as controlled by the illness rather than by the patient. Pickett, Vraniak, Cook, & Cohler (in press) found that white parents were less able than black parents to accommodate to the diminished life expectations and age-inappropriate behavior of their mentally ill offspring. Despite the same level of daily caregiver burden, black mothers and fathers had higher feelings of self-worth and demonstrated half the level of depression of white parents. The authors suggested that because many black parents live under greater daily life strains, they may maintain a more pragmatic view which allows them to cope with stressors without affecting their sense of self. Of great interest in this research was the finding that extended family and church networks of black parents may add to rather than mitigate family burden. Misunderstanding of mental illness, criticism, disapproval, and inappropriate advice of significant others may create friction in relationships that theoretically should be supportive.

Somewhat different findings were reported by Biegel, Milligan, Putnam, & Song (1992), who studied a lower-socioeconomic biracial sample (53% white, 47% black) of 103 family caregivers of severely mentally ill persons. They found no significant racial differences in family burden. Across cultures higher burden was related to a higher level of client behavioral symptoms and to a lower amount of perceived support from other family members. These authors also emphasized that mental health agencies need to offer families adequate information and behavioral management techniques, and may also need to include the caregiver's support system.

CULTURALLY APPROPRIATE FAMILY INTERVENTIONS

All surveys of family members, whether or not they fulfill a direct caregiving role, points to the need and desire for family education. Fowler (1992) has found family psychoeducation appropriate for families of Caribbean patients in New York City, and this approach has been pronounced culturally appropriate for Hispanics as well. Rivera (1988) has emphasized the congruence of the didactic, problem-solving approach for Hispanic families, since it does not override their authority or undermine intricate patterns of Hispanic interpersonal relationships. Both Fowler (1992) and Rivera (1988) add social events to their psychoeducational meetings, and encourage continued participation in support groups.

Yet, as Guarnaccia et al. (1992) point out, Rivera also felt that certain aspects of the psychoeducational model are problematic for application to Hispanic families. Examples are the egalitarian problem-solving technique, the problems of assessing overinvolvement in cultural terms, inadequate attention to spiritual factors, and possible misinterpretation of spiritual beliefs. Fowler (1992) was careful not to undermine families' supernatural belief systems (such as a belief in *Vodou* of a Haitian patient). Our own experience in Miami (Lefley & Bestman, 1991) is that patients may be persuaded that medication may be an important asset in enabling them to deal more effectively with their *loas*, their protective *Vodou* gods.

The work of Jenkins & Karno (1992) has indicated that Mexican-American families rarely manifest high expressed emotion (hostile criticism or emotional overinvolvement) in their interactions with mentally ill family members. Therefore one of the mainstays of psychoeducational interventions, that is, teaching families to lower expressed emotion, would be less important in this cultural context. Other research indicates that teaching families to control criticism or overinvolvement similarly may be less important than other techniques when working with families from India or other Asian countries (Lefley, 1990, 1992). Communication skills, behavior management techniques, and problem-solving strategies are needed by all families, but they must be geared to the conceptual framework of a particular culture.

Guarnaccia et al. (1992) state that other elements also make the psychoeducational paradigm problematic for Hispanic families. They argue against the ready application of the medical model. They feel that many Hispanic families view mental illness as a continuum, and their ideas permit both acceptance of current disability and hope for the future. Illness models carry value judgments and expectations for the person's future as well as the families' role as caregivers. Medical information about an illness such as schizophrenia must be given carefully, taking the families' conceptions into account. Above all, it should not convey a sense of poor prognosis.

These authors also argue that family education models assume that families are isolated and need new support networks, and that this does not apply to Hispanic families. They describe their research findings as follows:

> Many of the Hispanic families' social networks provided significant support. This suggests that family models can and need to build on these strengths of this social and cultural matrix

within Hispanic communities in designing family intervention models. Psychoeducation groups, rather than being built on groups of unrelated individuals or couples who share a similar problem, might be built on larger family networks which share ties of kinship or membership in key community institutions such as churches. At the same time, some of the poorest Hispanic families in our study experienced ruptured family networks and broken ties with others. One approach to working with these families would be to integrate them with other family networks and with community institutions, such as churches, which have resources for providing support. (Guarnaccia, et al., 1992, pp. 211-212).

In some of the AMI support groups on Indian reservations, e.g., the Colville Indian reservation in the state of Washington, "family" means the clan network, so that many more people attend a support group meeting than simply the nuclear family members. Attneave (1969) first proposed social network therapy as a culturally appropriate treatment modality for American Indian patients, since it mobilizes the extended family networks for problem-solving and conflict resolution. Social network therapy is an excellent model for all groups. It is a model that provides both psychological support and resources that may range from respite care to employment opportunities for the mentally ill family member. Involving extended family networks also does much to counteract the potentially negative influences and wrong advice of significant others by educating them about mental illness (See Pickett et al., in press).

Should Psychoeducational and Support Groups Be Monocultural or Multicultural?

My own research and experience with family support groups suggests that relatives of persons with mental illness suffer common experiences, and all will benefit from the empathic support and practical knowledge of others who have shared the same problems. However, certain variables may determine whether ethnically homogeneous support groups are essential or whether families may do better in culturally mixed groups. One factor is subcultural status. As a reminder that race and ethnicity are different concepts, it is sometimes evident that Afro-Caribbean families do not always feel culturally comfortable with African-American families, particularly if a different language is spoken. In areas where there are small ethnic enclaves with large information networks, we have been told by some clients that they do not want other clients or even staff from their own culture to hear their problems. This suggests that some families might prefer to be in a multicultural group.

Puerto Rican, Mexican-American, or Cuban family members may not view themselves as culturally homogeneous, and unless they are monolingual or clearly favor a Spanish-speaking ambiance, some may opt for an English speaking group. Socioeconomic status—primarily education—and level of acculturation are related factors in selection of a support group. All of the above researchers (Fowler, 1992; Guarnaccia et al, 1992; Rivera, 1988) have indicated that educational information must be geared to cultural concepts of mental illness, and these may often involve supernatural beliefs regarding causation and remedies. Educated middle-class families may have more extensive scientific knowledge and feel that the training level does not serve their needs.

On the other hand, scientifically sophisticated members of a particular racial/ethnic group may serve as "culture brokers," or as bilateral interpreters to less knowledgeable cultural peers and to staff from a different culture (Lefley & Bestman, 1991). Their role with cultural compatriots is one of mentor and interpreter of the mainstream culture, its concepts, values, and regulations. They also educate staff about the values, beliefs, and normative behavioral practices of their culture. This role eases the transmittal of information and makes the training more culturally appropriate, and hopefully more effective.

Cultural Themes in Support Groups

In various multi-cultural family support groups conducted over the years at the University of Miami-Jackson Memorial Medical Center, cultural differences have emerged in terms of self-blaming on the one hand and family shame on the other; the old distinctions of shame and guilt cultures have some validity in this context. Differences in world view of those raised in individualistic versus sociocentric or group-oriented settings are apparent. There is patterned variation in the emphasis on family obligations versus recognition of family members' personal rights to a peaceful or less-burdened life. Anglo relatives assert their personal rights to freedom from aversive behavior while those from more traditional cultures tend to accept the burdens of life and the duties of kinship. Black parents, particularly older ones, turn to God and church for sustenance and often have greater resources for caregiving (Lefley, 1990a).

American-born participants have been raised in a culture that transmitted messages of family culpability for mental illness. Some parents have reported years of self-blaming for obscure, Kafkaesque crimes until they were finally able to convince themselves that these accusations were groundless. In most cases indeed, so much good parenting had been invested in the mentally ill child (often to the detriment of time spent with normal siblings), that the idea of parental causation became outrageous. Such parents often report anger at the system as more and more scientific experts inform them of biogenesis. Educated families are likely to argue with and demand communication from mental health professionals, while less educated and particularly immigrant families are more likely to accept the passive roles imposed by authority figures.

In contrast to American born white and black patients, Hispanic and Asian patients usually have intact families who see it as their obligation to have disabled members live in the family home, yet suffer under this obligation. This is particularly problematic in the case of young adults with schizophrenia or other major psychotic disorders whose marriage prospects are doubtful. When the cultural expectation is that adult children remain at home as long as they are unmarried, it becomes doubly difficult to make alternative housing plans that may relieve the family and help the patient with independence.

Many Hispanic and Asian families are refugees and have experienced uprooting, loss, transplantation, and status reversal. This traumatic history is compounded and exacerbated by the deviant behavior of a child. As in any family, when the deviance is defined by authorities as an illness but is unaccompanied by any explanation, diagnosis, or prognosis, the ambiguity can become intolerable. In families that have lived with ambiguous futures for so many years and finally attained some presumed stability, one member's psychosis may invalidate the entire struggle to reach the promised land.

Erratic behavior that threatens hierarchical family relationships can be extremely unsettling to families trying to adapt to a new world. A Vietnamese father cannot deal with the disobedience and bizarre behavior of his schizophrenic elder son. The father is bewildered and ashamed for having a son who wreaks havoc and defies his authority. "I am head of family," he complains, "but he is the boss!" Family education in such cases must convince the father that old methods of punishment will not control psychotic behavior and that limit-setting requires alternative behavioral strategies. Such families must also learn to distinguish between accepting more democratic generational relationships in the new culture and tolerating arbitrary defiance of a child.

U.S. born family members tend to press for residential separation, conflicting with the cultural values of those who have profound obligations to care for disabled kin at home. Parents in all cultures have problems of ambivalence and guilt when a hospitalized adult child with a history of intolerably disruptive behavior pleads to be discharged to their home rather than to an alternative community residence which is often of inferior quality. Overall, however, the families in the group try to legitimate the option of sending an adult child to a residential program or board and care home to relieve pressure on the family. They reassure each other that this will help their patient live independently, and that this is a necessary thing in the mainstream American culture.

The role of the group facilitator in this process is to encourage a careful balance among various options, recognizing the conflicting demands of cultural world view and value systems and the realities of living with severe mental illness in the family. Kinship obligations are considered within the context of resources available in a particular area. The limitations of chronic patients to live independently and the inadequacy of most community care systems are weighed against threats to the psychological health of individual caregivers and strains on already overstressed family systems (Lefley, 1990a).

Living with severe mental illness means that many families are caught in a web of altered realities in which traditional values may become maladaptive. Under these conditions it is important to shore up defenses and provide group support for difficult choices. Sometimes decisions regarding limit-setting, hospitalization, or residential separation may be more difficult in a same-culture group with shared conceptual barriers. There may be less defensiveness in accepting advice that is culturally dystonic from cultural outsiders—particularly if they are perceived as sharing the same pain, but as having more knowledge of what is appropriate in the mainstream culture. Whether other families are of the same or different cultures, however, in this very painful situation the group becomes the therapist, and a multi-family support group may become a powerful force for change.

SUMMARY AND CONCLUSIONS

Cultural diversity in families' needs begins with a rather surrealistic picture of the service delivery system. Epidemiologic data, appropriately controlled, show minimal differences among racial/ethnic populations in the distribution of major mental disorders in the United States. Yet national statistics show great disparities in the racial/ethnic distributions of admissions to mental hospitals, and strangely inverse relationships between rates of admission and length-of-stay. These profiles may be related to cultural patterns of service utilization, or to systemic barriers that impede access or result in inappropriate uses of specific types of services. They may also be related to problems in clinical evaluation, diagnosis, referral, and treatment of clients from different cultural and socioeconomic backgrounds.

Service needs may be addressed at the societal level, or at the level of what most mental health agencies are able and willing to provide. People with major psychiatric disorders are particularly susceptible to life stressors, and these may be greater in communities where social policies have generated poverty, discrimination, and the erosion of traditional support systems. Families of such patients may need multi-system interventions, a sort of global case management to bring in needed resources and reinforce their existing adaptive structures. Neither therapy nor psychoeducation alone can shore up families who need jobs, medical care, substance abuse programs, child care, or similar survival mechanisms in order to be able to help themselves and the patient. Appropriate interventions must also be targeted toward building on the cultural strengths and human resources that continue to enrich many of these communities.

Most agencies, however, cannot offer families such multi-system interventions; their service needs must be addressed on a much more modest level. Research indicates that regardless of racial/ethnic background, families of persons with severe mental illnesses show few differences in their assessment of specific service needs for their relatives and for themselves. All families seem to want education about the illnesses and behavior management techniques.

Various clinicians have pronounced the didactic, problem-solving approach of psychoeducational interventions culturally appropriate for a particular ethnic group, and this approach would seem to be quite acceptable to traditional cultures. Some researchers have cautioned, however, against an egalitarian problem-solving model while others have emphasized that a "medical model" approach must not convey a sense of poor prognosis and counteract hope for the future. They have also cautioned clinicians to pay close attention to spiritual factors and not to undermine the explanatory models offered by cultural belief systems. Some have also suggested that many families in traditional cultures have their own support networks. In lieu of using unrelated multi-family groups, they suggest that psychoeducational interventions be built on larger kinship networks. On some American Indian reservations, "family" means a larger tribal network than first-degree relatives alone and this is manifested in attendance at support groups.

There is some research evidence that service providers who are oriented toward serving a particular cultural group have more acceptable and successful service utilization than providers who simply offer a multicultural staff. The question of unicultural versus multicultural services continues to be problematic. Unicultural support groups offer the intimacy of shared language, values, and belief systems. There are times, however, when members of subcultures or of different socioeconomic levels prefer to be in multiethnic support groups. Families from traditional cultures often find it difficult to question authority figures, to make their needs known, or to relinquish even extraordinarily burdensome caregiving roles because of obligations to disabled kin. Maintenance of traditional values sometimes becomes maladaptive in terms of family survival. Choices that defy cultural norms are often more difficult in groups that share the same conceptual boundaries. It sometimes takes a cultural outsider to convince a family member that hospitalization or residential separation is necessary for the family's successful adaptation to the mainstream American system.

Cultural Diversity and Advocacy Needs

The issue of unicultural versus multicultural approaches extends beyond support groups to issues of political advocacy and systems improvement. Both consumer organizations and the family movement, the National Alliance for the Mentally Ill (NAMI), have expended considerable efforts to attract minority group members. Conscious that their membership is primarily white middle-class, NAMI members developed an Ethnic Minority Concerns Network, now called the Multicultural Network, which has expanded its activities considerably over the years. Videos have been developed on organizing Spanish-speaking support groups and on multi-cultural AMI families. NAMI state affiliates have been active in coordinating conferences on minority mental health and in similar collaborative activities with mental health professionals.

A number of NAMI affiliates are predominantly composed of people of color, usually families of a particular minority group. Asian-American family groups are found in the San Francisco area. Los Angeles, Texas, Chicago, and New York City have Hispanic-American affiliates, and Miami has two Spanish-speaking support groups. Primarily African-American affiliates are found in Washington DC., New York, and Miami. Ohio has a People of Colors affiliate, primarily Black and Hispanic. American Indian family groups or activities are found in Washington state, New Mexico, South Dakota, and Alaska (including Alaska Native). There are AMI groups with a strong Indian presence in Oklahoma and the Pima Indian reservation in Arizona. There are also outreach programs to Native American families in the Navajo and Apache tribes.

Many AMI members are conflicted about having racially or ethnically separate groups within their organization. Most have lived through the years of the civil rights movement and the fight for equality, and many white members reject the idea of segregation in their own ranks. Yet a substantial number of minority group members appear to feel more comfortable with developing their own groups, particularly if they speak another language. Having gone through the struggle for integration, it seems as if people must now be reeducated to accept the positive aspects of cultural pluralism.

The commonalities of the needs of families of persons with severe mental illnesses far outweigh any cultural differences. For themselves, all families seem to agree on the need for education about mental illnesses and behavior management strategies. Many families benefit from support groups, whether their structure is unicultural or multicultural. For their ill relatives, families agree that the service system must have improved access and include case management, rehabilitative/vocational services, and an array of residential alternatives. Most families agree that their lives would be better if there were better services for their loved ones. To attain these ends, it is essential that regardless of cultural diversity, all families join together for political advocacy and systems improvement.

REFERENCES

American Psychiatric Association. (1980). Diagnostic and statistical manual of mental disorders (3rd ed., DSM-III). Washington DC: Author.

Attneave, C.L. (1969). Therapy in tribal settings and urban network intervention. Family Process, 8, 192-210.

Bernal, G. (1988). Latino families: Toward a progressive family therapy. The Community Psychologist, 21(2), 29-30.

Biegel, D.E., Milligan, S.E., Putnam, P.L., & Song, L-Y. (1992). Predictors of burden among lower socioeconomic status caregivers of persons with chronic mental illness. Unpublished paper. Case Western Reserve University, Mandel School of Social Sciences, Cleveland, Ohio.

Boyd-Franklin, N. (1989). Black families in therapy: A multisystems approach. New York: Guilford.

Chu, C., Sallach, H.S., Zakeria, S.A. et al. (1985). Differences in psychopathology between black and white schizophrenics. International Journal of Social Psychaitry, 31, 252-257.

Fabrega, H., Mezzich, J., & Ulrich, R.F. (1988). Black-white differences in psychopathology in an urban psychiatric popualtion. Comprehensive Psychiatry, 29, 285-297.

Fowler, L. (1992). Family psychoeducation: chronic psychiatrically ill Caribbean patients. Journal of Psychosocial Nursing, 30, 27-32.

Guarnaccia, P.J., Parra, P., Deschamps, A., Milstein, G., & Argiles, N. (1992). i dios quiere: families' experiences of caring for a seriously mentally ill family member. Culture, Medicine, & Psychiatry, 16, 187-215.

Jenkins, J.H., & Karno, M. The meaning of expressed emotion: theoretical issues raised by cross-cultural research. American Journal of Psychiatry, 149, 9-21.

Jones, B.E. & Gray, B.A. (1988). Problems in diagnosing schizophrenia and affective disorders among blacks. Hospital & Community Psychiatry, 37, 61-65.

Keltner, N.L. & Folks, D. G. (1992). Culture as a variable in drug therapy. Perspectives in Psychiatric Care, 28 (1), 33-36.

Lefley, H.P. (1982). Self-perception and primary prevention for American Indians. In S. Manson et al., New directions in prevention among American Indian and Alaska Native communities. Portland, OR: Oregon Health Sciences University.

Lefley, H.P. (1985). Families of the mentally ill in cross-cultural perspective. Psychosocial Rehabilitation Journal, 8, 57-75.

Lefley, H.P. (1989). Counseling refugees. In P.B. Pedersen, W.J. Lonner, J.E. Trimble, & J.G. Draguns (Eds.), Counseling across cultures (pp. 243-266). 3rd rev. ed. Honolulu: University P{ress of Hawaii

Lefley, H.P. (1990a).Cultural issues in training psychiatric residents to work with families of the long-term mentally ill. In E,. Sorel (Ed.), Family, culture, and psychobiology (pp. 165-180). Toronto: Legas.

Lefley, H.P. (1990b). Culture and chronic mental illness. Hospital & Community Psyschiatry, 41, 277-286.

Lefley, H.P. (1992). Expressed emotion: conceptual, clinical, and social policy issues. Hospital & Community Psychiatry, 43, 591-598.

Lefley, H.P. & Bestman, E.W. (1991). Public-academic linkages for culturally sensitive community mental health. Community Mental Health Journal, 27, 473-488.

Lefley, H.P. & Pedersen P.B. (Eds.). (1986). Cross-cultural training for mental health professionals. Springfield, IL: Charles C. Thomas.

Lin, K-M., Poland, R.E., & Lesser, I.M. (1986). Ethnicity and psycho-pharmacology. Culture, Medicine, & Psychiatry, 10, 151-165.

Loring, M. & Powell, B. (1988). Gender, race, and DSMIII: A study of the objectivity of psychiatric diagnostic behavior. Journal of Health & Social Behavior, 29, 1-22.

Lukoff, D., Lu, F., & Turner, R. (1992). Toward a more culturally sensitive DSM-IV: psychoreligious and psychospiritual problems. Journal of Nervous & Mental Disease, 180, 673-682.

National Institute of Mental Health (1987). Mental health, United States, 1987. Manderscheid, R.W. & Barrett, S.A., Eds. DHHS Pub. No., (ADM) 87-1518. Washington DC: Supt. of Docs., U.S. Govt. Print. Office.

National Institute of Mental Health (1990). Mental health, United States, 1990. Manderscheid, R.W.& Sonnenschein, M.A. eds., DHHS Pub. No. (ADM)90-1708. Washington DC: Supt. of Docs., U.S. Govt. Print. Office.

Norman, R.M.G. & Malla, A.K. (1993). Stressful life events and schizo-phrenia: I. A review of the research. British Journal of Psychiatry, 162, 161-166.

Pickett, S.A., Vraniak, D.A., Cook, J.A., & Cohler, B. J. (in press). Strength in adversity: Blacks bear burden better than whites. Profes-sional Psychology: Research and Practice.

Rivera, C., (1988). Culturally sensitive aftercare services for chronically mentally ill Hispanics: the case of the psychoeducation treatment model. Hispanic Research Center Research Bulletin, 11(1), 1-9.

Robins, L.N. & Regier, D.A. (Eds.), Psychiatric disorders in America: The Epidemiologic Catchment Area Study. New York: The Free Press.

Rogler, L.H. (1992). The role of culture in mental health disganosis: the need for programmatic research. Journal of Nervous & Mental Dis-ease, 180, 745-747.

Shankar, R.& Menon, M.S. (1991). Interventions with families of peo-ple with schizophrenia: The issues facing a community-based reha-bilitation center in India. Psychosocial Rehabilitation Journal, 15, 85-90.

Snowden, L.R. & Cheung, F.K. (1990). Use of inpatient services by members of ethnic minority groups. American Psychologist, 45, 347-355.

Snowden, L.R. & Holschuh, J. (1992). Ethnic differences in emergency psychiatric care and hospitalization in a program for the severely mentally ill. Community Mental Health Journal, 28, 281-291.

Solomon, P. & Marcenko, M.O. (1992a). Families of adults with severe mental illness: their satisfaction with inpatient and outpatient treatment. Psychosocial RehabilitationJournal, 16, 121-134.

Solomon, P. & Marcenko, M.O. (1992b). Family members' concerns regarding community placement of their mentally disabled relative: comparisons one month after release and a year later. Family Relations, 41, 341-347.

Takeuchi, D.T., Mokuau, N., Chun, C-A. (1992). Mental health services for Asians and Pacific Islanders. Journal of Mental Health Administration, 19, 237-245.

Tessler, R.C., Fisher, G.A., & Gamache, G.M. (1990). Dilemmas of Kinship: mental illness and the modern American family. Unpublished paper. University of Massachusetts Social & Demogrtaphic Research Institute, Amherst, MA.

Westermeyer, J. (1987). Clinical considerations in cross-cultural diagnosis. Hospital & Community Psychiatry, 38, 160-165.

Chapter 12

FAMILY CONCERNS ABOUT CONFIDENTIALITY AND THE SERIOUSLY MENTALLY ILL: ETHICAL IMPLICATIONS

Evelyn M. McElroy and Paul D. McElroy

Disclosure of information about the patient's condition is a common practice in many hospitals. This is particularly important when the person has a serious or catastrophic illness. Conveying status reports to members of the family waiting for such information is commonly depicted in the media. Such disclosure occurs in pediatrics, on coronary care units, and in trauma centers. Unfortunately, families who have relatives with catastrophic mental illnesses are often not treated with the same degree of concern and disclosure as those people who have relatives hospitalized in general hospital settings. This lack of disclosure by mental health professionals is often viewed as an insensitive disregard for the legitimate concern of families. The lack of critical information can elevate a health crisis to a catastrophic disaster.

It impedes the ability of families to cope with the serious illness of their relative and can create misalliances with professional caregivers.

This chapter discusses issues of confidentiality in regard to the mentally ill in treatment and research settings. Family treatments are also described with regard to confidentiality and informed consent. To underscore some of the difficulties faced by many families of the seriously mentally ill, consider the following incident involving a physician's response to the mother of an adult, who was hospitalized on a coronary care unit.

THE CORONARY CARE UNIT AND
DISCLOSURE TO A FAMILY MEMBER

The cardiologist called to Mrs. J., mother of 26 year old Janice who is hospitalized on the coronary care unit of the general hospital, to..."come over here a minute," Dr. Z said. As Mrs. J. approached the nurses station which was adjacent to Janice's room, Dr.Z. said, "Janice's EKG's are normal now. It was the lithium that was causing the arrythymia. The findings from all the other tests indicate that she has no underlying cardiac problem. We just need to make sure that she doesn't get anymore lithium in the future."

"Thanks, that's a relief off of my mind. I'm going in to see her now."[1]

This doctor was humanely sharing information about the daughter's condition without obtaining Janice's permission. The conversation does represent a violation of Janice's confidentiality with the physician. But Janice did not object because it was natural to share such information with close relatives who have an interest in the ill person's welfare. No lawsuits developed and the only side effect of such an interaction was a strong alliance among all members of the family with the treating physician. Such examples of sharing information with close relatives of patients, without their permision, abound in most areas of medicine and in most instances is helpful to the patient and the family. This type of sharing is less likely to occur in psychiatry and the failure to share has caused considerable distress for families who have a legitimate need to know some aspects of the treatment plan to help them effectively monitor and aid their mentally ill relative.

Confidential communication is defined by Webster (1968) as a "statement made in confidence to one's attorney, physician, clergyman, husband, or wife, who cannot then be compelled to divulge this in a court of law." All mental health professionals have a code of ethics that offers guidelines in these matters of patient confidentiality. The 6th U.S. Circuit Court of Appeals has ruled psychotherapists-patient communications are privileged under federal law. This ruling conflicts with rulings in

---

1.   Names of the persons described in the cases presented have been changed and other slight modifications have been made to the cases presented in this chapter to provide anonymity for the families.

other circuits, where federal appeals courts have refused to recognize a psychotherapist-patient privilege (*Mental Health Reports, 1983*).

Legally, confidentiality is described as a client privilege (Black, 1978). The *client,* not the professional, nor the facility is the holder of the privilege. With some exceptions, only at the client's discretion and with his written approval may information be imparted to other sources. Experienced mental health professionals are often adept at helping the patient to see that selected family members can be more helpful if they are informed about salient aspects of treatment (Blackwell, 1976). Since families tend to be involved with their mentally ill relative following discharge from hospitals (Goldman, 1982), they can help support the treatment and rehabilitation plan if they are informed. This usually requires the patient to waive aspects of the privileged communication rights that exist with professionals. Then, families can learn about the treatment plan and how they can augment the goals. Families are usually not interested in gaining access to information that most members of the community would deem to be private. Families are not generally interested in learning about their relative's sexual fantasies or details about psychotherapy.

How Private is Confidentiality?

Disclosure of medical care and hence, the need to keep such information confidential has importance and validity (Slovenko and Udin, 1966; Prosser and Keeton, 1985; Joseph and Onek; 1991; Appelbaum, Lidz and Meisel, 1987; Ruben and Ruben, 1972). In all states, there are provisions where the privilege protection can be overcome, based on societal interests. Suspected child abuse is one example of mandated disclosure. Civil commitment proceedings is a second area in which confidential information is disclosed. A third exception to confidentiality protection is concerned with warning potential victims to take protective action when a patient reveals serious threaths toward a potential victim (Tarassoff v. Regents of U. of California, 1976).

However, experts estimate that about 100 people learn the name of the patient, her diagnosis and other private information during the full course of treatment (Opp, 1975). Not all of these persons are health care professionals. Some may be clerks at the hospital or insurance company, auditors, or a myriad of other persons linked to the health care industry. Fleck (1986) found that in a large hospital 75 people may have a legitimate "need to know" medical information that gives them access to the patient's record. This does not include the computer data bases that track patient contacts with health providers. Computer access to such privileged information creates risks to confidentiality from a variety of sources. Hence, in reality a client or patient's communications and information about his treatment may not be truly limited to the provider/client relationship.

Invoking of Confidentiality by Mental Health Professionals

Families are affected when confidentiality is invoked by mental health professionals to keep information that is critical to the welfare of the patient from close family members, who may need to know the patient's status or other information in order to act in the best interests of the patient. In general, families of persons with serious mental illnesses want to learn about the treatment of the patient so that they can evaluate the quality of care provided; help to distinguish if the person's reactions in the community are predictive of an impending relapse, requiring them to act quickly to implement an emergency plan aimed at averting a full relapse; and help maintain the highest quality of life that is possible for their esteemed but mentally ill relative.

THE PSYCHIATRIC UNIT AND DISCLOSURE TO THE FAMILY

However, the family's interaction with a mental health professional is usually much different than that experienced by Mrs. J's interaction on the coronary care unit with Dr. Z. Consider the response to Mrs. J, one month later as she stops at the nurses station in a psychiatric unit of a general hospital.

> "Janice was admitted yesterday. How is she? I'm so concerned about her. What's wrong with her? She was hospitalized last month for her heart. I'm worried that the psychiatric medication might trigger another problem with her heart. It sometimes skips beats."
>
> The staff member replied, "I'm sorry, but I can't reveal any information to you. That is privileged. I can't even tell you if the person you identified is here."
>
> "But I'm her mother and I called her on the patient phone an hour ago. She asked me to visit. She sounded confused. I need to know how she is and what medication she is on," Mrs. J replied.
>
> "You'll have to leave. Visiting hours just ended so you'll have to leave. We can't give you any information."

Often, staff at the facility will not answer the queries of family members about whether their relative is even hospitalized at the facility, let alone provide any information about the type of treatment that is being rendered to their mentally ill son or daughter. Staff members are often unaware of the fact that the privilege regarding confidentiality belongs to the patient, not the staff member, as revealed by the above interaction. It seems likely that Janice would have allowed the type of information being requested by Mrs. J to be disclosed. Families can be valuable allies to professionals. It is obvious that knowledge about Janice's previous response to medication would have helped the new treatment team plan her care. It was doubtful that Janice could have relayed such critical information in her present state. That was why her mother was frantically attempting to determine her status and to convey critical historical information to the staff member.

Placing disclosure directives in writing, along with any limitations to disclosure, documented by Janice's attorney would possibly have helped in the situation described on the psychiatric ward. In fact, such advance directives for other types of treatment are also recommended. Interestingly, the cardiologist and the psychiatrist are both held to the same regulations concerning confidentiality; yet their response to families was drastically different. Reasons for these differences in responses are unclear.

Since the mental status of persons with serious psychiatric illnesses can show wide degrees of fluctuations over time, as revealed by Janice's case, a theme of this chapter is that additional efforts should be made by professionals to gain the patient's approval for sharing relevant treatment information with significant family members. A desirable direction for professionals to pursue with family members is to regard them as collaborators and allies, who have demonstrated abilities to act in the best interests of the patient.

Consider another example of staff's failure to disclose to the family when their 24 year old son, John, was discharged from a public psychiatric hospital.

LONG TERM EFFECTS OF FAILURE
TO DISCLOSE TO THE FAMILY

Alexis described the following events at an Alliance for the Mentally Ill (AMI) meeting. She described salient aspects of her 24 year old son, John's past. "He was always different from other children. As a six year old he would listen to classical

music and pace the room when it was on. He is very bright. He
has an IQ of over 160...and he is so handsome! Here-look at
his picture."

At the time of the meeting, Alexis had not seen her son for
the past six months. When he was discharged from the hospital,
his parents were not notified. No one has heard from him since
that time.

Alexis continued her story, "The last time I caught sight of
him was when I was on my way to work downtown and I
noticed a person who resembled him out of the corner of my
eye. He was fetching food out of a big wire trash can in downtown Baltimore. He was a beggar, wearing ragged clothes, had
long dirty hair and a long matted beard. I knew that he wasn't
taking his medication. I called out over the honking and noise,
..'John, it's me, Mom.'"

He looked at her, called her a four-letter word and ran away.
She was unable to catch him.

She continued, "Whenever I travel, I don't care if it's a country road
or a city highway and I see a hitchhiker about the height of John, I
stopped trying to match them for weight, because he had lost so much
the last time I caught sight of him, I roll down the window, slow the car
to a crawl, stick my head out the window and shout, 'John, is that you?'
It never is."

She talked about other efforts to find John. She would make rounds
at the medical examiners offices in Baltimore and the surrounding
middle Atlantic states. She checked out the accident and homicide victims who ended up at the morgue. They just might be John. If she heard
about unclaimed bodies of young men who had rolled up on the beaches
of Virginia, New Jersey, Delaware or Maryland, she would check them
out, too. She had to see if it was John. Sixteen years later, he was still
missing.

John had obviously responded well to treatment and was stabalized
at the time of his discharge. Historically, he needed encouragement to
take his medication and he was diagnosed with schizophrenia. John had
obviously decompensated and needed treatment, support and monitoring in the community. The hospital staff had discharged him to the
community without a real place to live, without the support necessary
to monitor his compliance with medication or other treatments and
with only himself to manage his financial affairs. The result was the loss

of John and the perpetual vigilance and grief exhibited by his mother and siblings.

What prompted the staff to take such drastic action regarding John's discharge and their failure to notify the family?

> Alexis had been involved in family therapy and maintained contact with the staff often when she visited John at the hospital. A review of the medical record revealed that the professionals had been discouraging John from having close contact with his mother. Some members of John's team had felt that part of John's problem was his dependance on his mother. They also viewed her as being too interested in the type of treatment he was receiving. They felt that Alexis was intrusive and highly emotionally expressive (EE). The treatment team decided to separate the two after Alexis failed to reduce her level of ex-pressed emotion. Her family therapist had used a treatment technique called, paradoxical intervention, in an attempt to reduce Alexis' anxiety about John, which took the form of inquiring about his medication, when he was to be discharged and how he was responding to hospitalization. This was the staff's definition of "high EE."

Paradoxical Interventions Paradoxical interventions are controver-sial. They are directives given to the family by the therapist which are aimed at getting the family to resist professional advice, by ordering them to perform actions that the staff already perceive them as doing. In the process of implementing this professional advice it is expected that the client will resist and hence change the maladaptive behavior. These techniques are based on the assumption that families who come for help are also resistant to the help being offered, and often become involved in power struggles with the therapist (Jones, 1984).

> In this case, the family therapist was apparently concerned that Alexis was pushing her son, John, toward a relapse because of her high levels of "EE". The assignment was telling Alexis to call the unit at least 4 times a day to ask what John was doing, how he responded to his medication and to inquire about his feelings. In effect, the family therapist was *explicitly* asking Alexis not to change her behavior because the staff perceived that Alexis already performed the tasks described in the assign-ment. However, the therapist *thought* she was sending a *covert*

message to Alexis expecting her to change her persistently inquiring behaviors. The therapist expected her to resist and to stop the assignment. However, the expectation was never made explicit. Predictably, many people do not perceive the covert message. Alexis was such a person and when she persisted in implementing her assignment (although she thought it a strange one), the staff decided that she chose not to reduce her involvement with John.

The staff then decided to act in the family's best interests and discharged John to a place other than Alexis's and purposely chose not to inform her. They wanted to help them separate and reduce their "enmeshment."

One can imagine how perplexed Alexis was to learn that although she had followed the advice of the family therapist, she continued to be viewed as a deficit to her son. The unilateral action by the team without informed consent for their family interventions had disastrous consequences for her family. It is difficult to see how Alexis could have reaped the benefits she wanted, which was to protect and care for her severely and persistently mentally ill son, under such treatment. Evidence exists that he needed it. One might speculate that the family therapist and some of the other staff had put her into a no-win situation—a double bind.

Legislation was subsequently passed in the state where Alexis lived that made it mandatory for staff to notify families of the impending discharge of their relative. Informed consent exists when the following three conditions are met: a) a reasonable disclosure to the patient of treatment risks; b) a voluntary decision is made by the patient based on this disclosure and c) the patient is competent to make such a decision (Plotkin, 1977; Appelbaum, Lidz and Meisel, 1987). All three elements of informed consent were lacking in regard to the disclosure provided to Alexis by the family therapist. No written informed consent was obtained from Alexis to participate in family therapy, nor were the use of paradoxical interventions defined nor disclosed to her in advance. It is highly recommended that a detailed written informed consent form be requested by families participating in family therapy. Actions by professionals, such as those discussed in the case of Alexis and her son, would be a violation of their ethical guidelines and pose legal problems. Several experts have written about some of the ethical and legal dilemmas encountered by families who participate in family therapy (Hare-Mustin, 1979, 1980; Margolin, 1982; Terkelsen, 1983; McElroy, 1990).

Guidelines for informed consent in family therapy were described by McElroy (1990) and specify that potential distress such as a loss of self-esteem and the development of a sense of powerlessness are possible outcomes of some forms of family therapy and should be conveyed as possible risks. Efforts of the professionals to coerce the family into compliance with this treatment modality is sometimes accomplished by specifying that hospital visits are only permitted if the family participates in family therapy (Alexis X, 1982, Personal Communication, Baltimore, Md.; McElroy, 1988; Mrs. J., Baltimore, Md., personal communication, Baltimore, Md. March 15, 1993; Mrs. X., personal communication, Denver, Colorado, January, 1993). Families have even been threatened with withdrawal of entitlements or treatment for failure to participate in family therapy (Harbin, 1982; Hsia, 1985). Families unwilling to participate in family therapy should not be forced to attend; yet, this is often a requirement of psychiatric hospitalization for children, adolescents and some adults. Too often such techniques blame parents for causing their youngsters' illnesses or relapses.

The belief system of one psychiatric nurse revealed her attitudes about families and why she thought family therapy was required for them by stating, "We know that bad apples fall close to bad trees. That's why we have 'parenting classes' in this hospital. They have to come." (Nurse X, Personal Communication, Phoenix, Arizona, June 7, 1993.)

Parents often viewed the sessions as terrorist tactics that they put up with to get their youngster treated.

Parental access to family therapy records that are a part of the medical record often requires written consent from all persons participating in the sessions (Fink, 1992). Such consensus is often hard to obtain.

DRUG EFFICACY

Findings from controlled trials suggest that the combination of drugs and psychotherapy may have beneficial additive effects in the treatment of depression (Beitman, Klerman, 1984). The psychiatric patient's right to effective treatment and the priority of treatments whose efficacy has been demonstrated over treatments whose efficacy has not been established were the emphases of the highly publicized case involving Osheroff v. Chestnut Lodge (Klerman, 1990). The patient deteriorated after being treated with psychotherapy and without medication for his psychiatric condition while hospitalized at Chestnut Lodge. Later, with different providers, the patient responded well to the addition of medication that was prescribed to treat his psychiatric condition. The case raised ethical and legal issues surrounding standards of practice concerning the rights of physicians to select treatments based on their preferences rather than relying primarily on the merit of controlled studies to offer guidelines for the treatment of specific psychiatric disorders. Klerman concluded that treatment practices required the clincian to place high priority on using findings from controlled studies.

Similarly, drug therapy and practical forms of therapy were reported to be among the most effective forms of treatments for persons diagnosed with schizophrenia (May, Tuma and Dixon, 1981). For many of the major mental illnesses effective treatments exist and most of them require some form of medication.

PSYCHIATRIC PATIENTS AS RESEARCH SUBJECTS IN DRUG STUDIES

Osheroff was not even in a research study, but during the seven months he was treated with individual psychotherapy four times a week, he lost forty pounds, experienced insomnia, agitation, and paced such that his feet became edematous and blisters developed. He received no medication during this time. After transfer to another hospital, he was treated with antidepressants and phenothiazines. His condition improved within three weeks and he was discharged within three months (Klerman, 1990). Since the later treatment reflected findings from controlled studies, it is easy to speculate what would happen to severely depressed research subjects participating in drug discontinuation studies. It becomes more difficult to understand why persons would participate in such studies when informed about the predictable responses to the lack of medication. The ethics and usefulness of most drug discontinuation studies is highly questionable. Studies of patient behavior following the withdrawal of medication sacrifice patient benefit for knowledge of the illness. The sacrifice cannot ordinarily be justified because the knowledge gained could be obtained from observation of subjects prior to beginning treatment. Furthur, when treatment ceases, the patient regresses. Resuming effective treatment is often difficult because sometimes the brain is damaged furthur by events associated with the relapse.

Similarly, it is difficult to imagine persons with schizophrenia participating in drug discontinuation studies. Most require medication to reduce symptoms. Patients often relapse when not given medication. Relapses are unpleasant, frightening experiences that are to be avoided because evidence exists that some patients never regain their previous level of functioning (Curson, et.al, 1986). Psychotic individuals require close monitoring to keep them safe and in some cases to protect others.

Consider the incident of a patient hospitalized on a hospital research unit.

> Jane was a 14 year old girl who had a diagnosis of schizophrenia. She had experienced a poor response to two different types of antipsychotic medication in the past. She was disruptive at home and in school. Her mother had learned about a research study that was designed to compare different types of medication among young persons diagnosed with schizophrenia. She wrote for information and advocated that her daughter participate. They were accepted for the study. The study paid for everthing including transportation from another state for both mother and daughter. The mother's goal was to finally get some effective medication for her daughter. If the daughter did not respond to the study medication, the doctors told her they would provide a trial with Clozaril after the study was over. This convinced the mother. How else could she know if Clozaril worked? At that time, no other doctor was willing to try Clozaril on such a young person. She couldn't have afforded it anyway.
>
> The mother readily agreed to fill out all those forms the researchers wanted about her relationship with Jane. She hated that part and wondered why she had to be researched when the focus of the study was about drugs and schizophrenia. She decided to comply with the request because she wanted help for her daughter and couldn't get it any other way. She was poor but assertive and highly committed to getting her daughter whole again. She didn't care at all about advancing scientific knowledge at her daughter's expense, but she felt the doctors would help her regardless of the procedures required in the study. After all, they were doctors, too.
>
> The protocol required "washout" periods, when no medication was provided to subjects preceeding the next phase which resulted in the use of either a placebo or an antipsychotic medication. It was necessary to have these washout periods to make sure all of the medication was out of the person's system, so that researchers could agree that the patient's subsequent responses to the placebo or antipsychotic medication was valid and not confounded. A visit to the unit during one of Jane's washout period revealed that her actions were so violent that she was required to spend long hours in seclusion and restraints.

That afternoon one of the nurses had been severely injured while attending to Jane in the seclusion room.

This case illustrates why some parents advocate that their son or daughter participate in research studies. They want help for their mentally ill relative, recognize that the researchers have distinguished reputations, prestigious universities sponsor the studies, they expect researchers to help them because they are expert clinicians and the families often can't afford other treatment. The ethics of drug discontinuation studies in schizophrenia has been challenged by experts (Chandler, 1989; Abrams and Veenhuis, 1986; Curson, 1986) the issues examined by others (Bloch and Chodoff, 1991) and advocated by others (Lieberman, et.al., 1989, 1987; Subotnik and Nuechterlein, 1988).

Witholding medication from research subjects that require drug therapy for stabilization is unethical and more stringent informed consent guidelines need to be developed for future studies. In addition, research protocols that focus on drug response of subjects *and* require that family members also receive research attention as a requirement for the mentally ill reserch subject to participate may also be unethical, if the family has no choice about participation. Many family members view such research strategies as a form of coercion. Family members will usually tolerate such tactics, as Jane's mother did, because they do not want to deny their relative a chance to succeed. The benefits of family participation in such studies is negligible.

Attention should be developed toward developing advance directives for family advocates to have legal authority for monitoring such research subjects and withdrawing them from studies, should the subjects' mental state deteriorate. It is obvious that because of the conflict of interest that researchers have in implementing their protocols as compared with treating the subjects, they cannot always be counted on to act in the best interests of their subjects.

In summary, this chapter has described some areas of concern that families of the seriously mentally ill have regarding confidentiality and informed consent in treatment, research and family therapy settings.

REFERENCES

Abrams, R.A. and Veenhuis, P. (1986) "Ethical Questions Raised by a Proposed Randomized, Double-Blind Study Involving Placebo, Standard Drug Therapy, and Experimental Antipsychotic Drug Therapy for Patients with Schizophrenia," in *Clinical Research,* Vol 34, No. 1, pp. 6-9.

American Medical Association (1954) *Principles of Medical Ethics of the American Medical Association*. Chicago, IL, American Medical Association.

Appleton, W.S. (1974) "Mistreatment of Patients' Families by Psychiatrists" in *The American Journal of Psychiatry* (22) pp. 665-667.

Appelbaum,P.S., Lidz,C.W. and Meisel,A. (1987) *Informed consent: Legal Theory and Clinical Practice*. New York: Oxford University Press.

Beitman, B.D., Klerman, G.L. (eds) (1984) *Combining Psychotherapy and Drug Therapy in Clinical Practice*. Jamaica, NY: SP Medical & Scientific Books.

Bernheim, K.F. (1990). *Patient Confidentiality and You*. Arlington, VA: NAMI, 2101 Wilson Blvd. Suite 3a, Arlington, VA 22201.

Black's Law Dictionary, 5th ed. (1978) St. Paul, Minnesota: West Publishing Co.

Blackwell, B. (1976) Treatment adherence. *British Journal of Psychiatry*, 129, 513-531.

Bloch, S. and Chodoff, P. (1991) *Psychiatric Ethics,* second edition. Oxford: Oxford University Press.

Chandler, J.D. (1989) Ethics of drug discontinuation studies in schizophrenia, *Archives of General Psychiatry,* 46, 4, p. 387.

Curson, D.A., Hirsch, S.R., Platt, S.D. Bamber, R.W. and Barnes, T.R.E. (1986) "Does short-term placebo treatment of chronic schizophrenia produce long term harm?" *British Medical Journal,* 293, pp. 726-728.

Fink,V.N. (1991) Medical Records, in *Advising Hospitals, Physicians, and Other Providers*. Baltimore, MD: MICPEL.

Fleck, L. (1986) "Confidentiality: Moral Obligation or outmoded concept?" in *Health Progress,* 61, 17-20.

Goldman, H.H. (1982) "Mental Illness and Family Burden: A Public Health Perspective", in *Hospital and Community Psychiatry,* (33) pp. 557-559.

Harbin, H. "Family treatment of the psychiatric patient," in *Psychiatric Hospital and the Family*. New York, SP Medical & Scientific Books, 1982.

Hare-Mustin, R.T. "Family therapy may be dangerous for your health" in *Professional Psychology* 11:935-938 1980.

Hare-Mustin, R.T., Marecek, J., Kaplan, A.G., et al. "Rights of clients, responsibilities of therapists" in *American Psychologist* 34:3-16, 1979.

Kane, J.M. (1991). "Obstacles to clinical research and new drug development in schizophrenia," *Schizophrenia Bulletin,* 17, 2, pp. 353-356.

Lefley, H.P. "Training professionals to work with families of chronic patients," in *Community Mental Health Journal*, 24:338-357, 1988.

Jones, S.L. (1984) Family therapy, in *The American Handbook of Psychiatric Nursing*. Edited by Suzanne Lego. Philadelphia: J.B. Lippincott Company. 230-231.

Klerman, G.L. (1990) The Psychiatric patient's right to effective treatment: Implications of Osheroff v. Chestnut Lodge, *Am. J. of Psychiatry*, 147:4, pp. 409-418.

Lieberman, J.A., Kane, J.M., et.al. (1987) Prediction of relapse in schizophrenia, *Archives of General Psychiatry*, 44 pp. 597-601.

May, P., Tuma, A. & Dixon, W.J. (1981) "Schizophrenia: A follow-up study of the results of five forms of treatment," in *Archives of General Psychiatry*, 38, pp. 776-784.

McElroy, E. (1987) "Families and mental health professionals march to the beat of a different drummer," in *Families as Care Givers*. Edited by Lefley, H., Hatfield, A. New York, Guilford, 1987.

McElroy, E. (1988) *Children and Adolescents with mental illness: A parents guide, Second Edition*. Rockville, Md. Woodbine Press.

McElroy, E. (1990) "Ethical and legal considerations for interviewing families of the seriously mentally ill" in *Familes as Allies in treatment of the Mentally Ill: New Directions for Mental Health Professionals*. Edited by Lefley,

Margolin, G. (1982) "Ethical and Legal Considerations in Marital and Family Therapy," *American Psychologist*, 37:788-801.

Mental Health Reports, "Psychotherapist-Patient Privilege," pp. 7, 19, 8.

Opp, M. (1975) "The Confidentiality Dilemma", in *Modern Healthcare*, pp. 49-54.

Plotkin, R. (1977) "Limiting the Therapeutic Orgy: Mental Patients' Right to Refuse Treatment." *Northwestern University Law Review*, (72) pp. 461-525.

Prosser, W.L. and Keeton, W.P. (1985) *The Law of Tort*, 5th Edition, St. Paul, MN, West, pp. 807-808.

Ruben, H.L. and Ruben, D. (1972) "Confidentiality and Privileged Communications: The Psychotherapeutic Relationship Revisited," *Medical Annals of the District of Columbia*, (41) pp. 364-368.

Shaw v Glickman, 45 Md App 718, 415 A2d 625 (June 13, 1980).

Slovenko, R., Udin, G.L. (1966) *Psychiatry, Confidentiality, and Privileged Communication*, Springfield, IL, Charles C. Thomas.

Subotnik, K.L. and Nuechterlein, K.H. (1988) "Prodromal Signs and Symptoms of Schizophrenic Relapse", *Journal of Abnormal Psychology*, (97) pp. 405-412.

Tarassoff v. Regents of U. of California, 529 P2d 533, Cal Rep. 14 (1976).

Terkelsen, K.G. (1988) "Schizophrenia and the Family: Adverse Effects of Family Therapy." *Family Process* (2) pp. 191-200.

Torrey E.F. (1977) "A Fantasy Trial about a Real Issue," *Psychology Today*, (10) p. 24.

*Websters' New World Dictionary of the American Language.*College Ed. (1968) Cleveland and New York: World Publishing Company.

Chapter 13

FAMILIES' VIEWS OF SERVICE DELIVERY: AN EMPIRICAL ASSESSMENT

Phyllis Solomon

Households of families have become the alternative to institutions (Goldman, 1982). Estimates have been as low as 30% to as high as 90% of discharged psychiatric patients returned to their families upon release from a psychiatric hospital (Carpentier, Lesage, Goulet, Lalonde, & Renaud, 1992; Goldman, 1982; Lamb & Goertzel, 1977; Minkoff, 1978; Tessler & Goldman, 1982). Currently, the mental health field has become more aware of the difficult and burdensome lives of families of mentally ill individuals. With the growing recognition that families are neither to blame for their relative's illness nor the consequent impairment or disability, there has been an acknowledgement of the valuable resource provided by families in the care of their ill relative. In many instances, the functional family unit is the social support system (Test, 1992) and the traditional case management system, as the family assists their members in meeting their biological, psychosocial, and economic needs (Savarese, et al, 1990).

Families report that in order to cope with their relative with serious mental illness, they need practical advice, information about the disorder, realistic expectations for their relative, and education in such areas as understanding the symptoms of the disorder, behavioral management techniques, and proper use and knowledge of psychiatric medications and their side effects (Biegel & Yamatani, 1986; Hatfield, Fierstein, &

This chapter is based on research funded by Ohio Department of Mental Health, Office of Program Evaluation and Research; Pennsylvania Department of Public Welfare, Office of Mental Health; and National Institute of Mental Health grant R18MH46082.

Johnson, 1982). Howell (1973) notes that the primary role of mental health professionals is to teach families so they can assist their ill relative rather than withdraw from their relative due to feelings of incompetence or inadequacy.

SATISFACTION WITH SERVICES

The limited research that has been conducted regarding families' views of the provision of mental health services and treatment has revealed considerable dissatisfaction with these services and feelings that these services have little value for them (Hatfield, 1979; Holden & Lewine, 1982). Spaniol and Jung (1983) compiled a list of family concerns and issues, which included families feeling left out of treatment during the relative's hospitalization and feeling abandoned by professionals when the relative returns to the community. Families desired more contact with professionals in the community than they were offered. Also, they often felt ignored and blamed, and excluded from any understanding and knowledge of the treatment plan, process, and rationale, which were rarely explained. These same criticism were recently echoed by Hanson and Rapp (1992) when they assessed families perceptions of how well community mental health programs and services meet their needs. They found that these programs did not do well at all in providing information, giving emotional support, and provision of services to their relative. The one area in which the programs did relatively well was treating them with respect.

Spaniol and Zipple (1988) surveyed 187 families regarding their satisfaction with specific mental health services. They found that 45% of family members surveyed were moderately to very dissatisfied with mental health services in general. Dissatisfaction was related to the amount of information and support available to families from mental health professionals. For example, although almost all of the disabled relatives were prescribed medications, families noted a lack of information regarding the medications and their side effects. In another survey of 192 families concerning their coping needs by the same researchers (Spaniol & Zipple, 1988), they found that approximately two-thirds of the families felt that they did not have adequate information regarding the causes and diagnosis of schizophrenia, adequate access to genetic counseling, and adequate knowledge of community resources. They also identified a need for support for themselves in developing stress management and coping skills.

Hatfield (1983) studied what families considered necessary to assist them to deal effectively with their mentally ill relatives. Knowing appropriate expectations, learning to motivate their relative, and understanding the disorder were high priorities for these families. However, Hatfield (1983) found that there was no relationship between what families wanted and what was addressed in therapy. Although families indicate dissatisfaction with mental health professionals, they continue to turn to mental health professionals for help (Holden & Lewine, 1982). This fact, combined with the recognition that families provide much of the care for their ill relative, has resulted in mental health professionals at least articulating the need for, if not attempting, to develop alliances with families. To successfully implement a good working alliance with families, there is a need for a more empirical assessment of families' perceptions of services.

In an effort to begin this empirical assessment, this chapter will present the findings from four studies conducted by the author in which views of family members were assessed regarding their concerns about their ill relatives' post hospital release, i.e., housing arrangements and discharge readiness; and their satisfaction with mental health services provided to themselves and their ill relative. The four studies involved family members of the following patient populations: 1. patients residing in a long term public psychiatric facility, 2. recently released patients from a long term state psychiatric facility that was closing, 3. children and adolescents released from a state psychiatric facility for children, and 4. ill relatives who were randomly assigned to either a consumer team of case managers or a non-consumer team of case managers. The benefit of using these four studies is that they offer findings from a range settings, inpatient and outpatient, which employed similar measures and therefore, makes for easier integration of results for purposes of implications. The implications for practice and training of mental health professionals generated from the findings of these studies will be discussed.

STUDY DESCRIPTION AND FINDINGS

Families of Hospitalized Patients: Their Views of Concerns and Services

For purposes of this study, 19 family members of hospitalized long-term patients were interviewed. They were identified by their ill relative or through their relative's hospital record. These were a relatively representative group of family members of extended care facility patients as the sample of patients was a proportional stratifed random sample of 25. The 19 family members represented 14 of these patients. The majority (69%) of family members were parent(s); many (69%) were currently married; and 44% indicated that the patient lives with them when not hospitalized. Ages ranged from 20 to 72. The interview schedule focused on concerns regarding discharge and views about how well the hospital was meeting the family's needs.

With regard to concerns relating to discharge of their ill relative, half or close to half of the family members interviewed felt that hospital discharge should be delayed due to their relatives inability to control behavior, emotions, alcohol or drug use, to stay on medication, and trouble finding a job (Solomon, Beck, & Gordon, 1988a). Approximately a third of the family respondents felt that living in an unsafe neighborhood, inability to care for themselves, and becoming a burden on their families were also reasons for delaying discharge. Two also expressed worries for their own safety. Some noted an inability to assess the patient's capabilities resulting from the hospital doing so much for the patient (Solomon, Beck, & Gordon, 1988a).

A highly structured arrangement with 24 hour supervision was most often felt to be the best placement option for their relative. For those who felt that the likely placement was not the best option, they felt that discharge should be delayed. Two commented that the hospital would be more than happy to shift the responsibility for the patient back to the family if they would accept it. Family respondents gave a clear message of wanting to be able to say that they would have their relative at home, but many felt they could not handle it. Three-quarters responded that they were relieved not to have to provide care for their relative. However, half did feel guilty that their relative was at the hospital, and most(94%) were sad that their relative was there. But only a third felt that they would rather be caring for their relative at home (Solomon, Beck, & Gordon, 1988b).

In terms of views of families regarding hospital staff, few were involved with hospital staff in talking about treatment, medication, or physical care. Much of the contacts with hospital staff occurred when families visited or called the ward; thus, they were unstructured and family initiated. Communication between family and hospital staff was relatively poor. Some family members acknowledged that they may display a lack of interest due to burnout, having been through so much before the patient was admitted to the hospital. Of those who did have contact with hospital staff, approximately half felt the hospital did not do well with regard to asking their opinion about how their relative was doing, giving them information about treatment programs, or letting them know when their relative was in some kind of trouble. About two-thirds felt the staff did not do well in keeping them informed about their relative's progress, giving them information about their relative's illness, and discussing future plans for their relative. Eighty or more per cent of the families felt that the staff did not do well in terms of giving them emotional support or practical advice on how to cope with their situation (Solomon, Beck, & Gordon, 1988b). Overall, it seems that family members did not feel that the hospital did very well in meeting their needs.

Families of Recently Released Patients: Their Views of Concerns and Services

Fifty-seven family members were interviewed face-to-face a month after their ill relative was released from a state psychiatric facility that was closing and 49 were re-interviewed a year later. The initial interview focused on such areas as their views of the hospital treatment, their relatives' readiness for discharge, and concerns regarding community placement. The second interview covered such issues as satisfaction with treatment and concerns regarding community living and adjustment.

Over three-quarters of the respondents were parents, mostly mothers. The majority were either currently married (44%) or widowed (33%). Over half were African American, and the average age was 60, with a range from 33 to 88. Thirty-seven percent of the family respondents had had their relative stay with them at some point during the year. In a number of situations this included staying for a weekend or short period of time. Only 4 of the family respondents were living with their relative at the time of the second interview, and only 6 were hospitalized. Most of their relatives were living in structured settings in the community. Their relatives had a mean age of 38 with a range from 20 to 78. Their total number of hospitalizations ranged from 2 to 25 with a mean of 8. Their most recent hospitalization was an average of 3 years in length with a range from 30 days to 24 years. Ninety-three percent were diagnosed with schizophrenia.

Although three-quarters of the family respondents felt that they had seen progress in their relative since leaving the hospital, relatively high proportions had at least some concern a year after release that their relative might have to live in an unsafe neighborhood(72%), not stay on medication (78%), would not get needed services (80%), and would not be able to take care of themselves financially (75%). Although not reaching statistical significance, a number of families had greater concerns a year after release. These included concerns that their ill relative would cause conflict in the family and not be able to control use of alcohol or drugs. The categorical areas of activities of daily living and family burden were significantly different a year later, with increase concern in these areas (Solomon & Marcenko, 1992a).

As a part of the closing process, intensive case management teams were developed. For those who were aware that their relative had an intensive case manager, over half were in regular or frequent contact with the case manager. Just over a third desired more contact, and over half were satisfied with the amount of contact. Over half were very satisfied with the case management service and 15% were moderately satisfied. In terms of families' assessment of how well case management was meeting the needs of their relative, families were most satisfied with medication assessment and monitoring, and supportive counseling, with about three-quarters rating them very well. These were followed by assistance in getting benefits, teaching their relatives to use public transportation, addressing physical health problems, teaching daily living skills, being responsive to crises, and getting rehospitalized, where about two thirds felt the case managers did very well. Families tended to be more satisfied with services provided by the case managers than with the hospital. However, they indicated a need for more job development training, more activates to occupy their ill relative's time, and more academic skill development. Another need identified by a family member was for someone to speak Spanish so she could be involved (Solomon & Marcenko, 1992b).

Families were less satisfied with the degree to which the case managers were meeting their own needs as compared to those of their relative. A third to a half were not at all satisfied with case managers in all the queried areas concerning their own needs. The areas of greatest dissatisfaction included discussing future plans for their relative, providing them with emotional support, giving practical advice, teaching them about medications and ways to motivate their relative to improve. Despite relatively high levels of dissatisfaction with case managers, families tended to feel that they met more of their needs than did the hospital. In particular they were more satisfied with case managers than with the hospital staff in providing them information (Solomon & Marcenko, 1992b).

For those with relatives who went to a mental health agency, over three-quarters were at least moderately satisfied (47%) or very satisfied (32%) with the service. Families were generally fairly satisfied with agencies' ability to meet the needs of their relative and more satisfied than with the services provided by the hospital. Three quarters or more of those who had a relative attending a mental health agency were at least fairly well satisfied in regard to medication monitoring, teaching skills, and related areas. Families were least satisfied with supportive counseling (Solomon & Marcenko, 1992b).

With regard to their own needs, about half were at least somewhat satisfied in most areas, with a quarter to a third indicating high satisfaction. Yet, approximately half felt that the agency had not met their needs at all in most areas, including teaching them about medications, keeping them informed about their relative's progress, asking their opinions about how their relative was doing, or providing them emotional support. However, families tended to be more satisfied with services of the mental health agency in terms of meeting their needs than did the hospital, but not as satisfied with mental health agencies as with case management services. With regard to the amount of contact they had with agencies, about a third (36%) had regular or frequent contact and over a third had no contact (39%). Half were satisfied with the amount of contact they had (Solomon & Marcenko, 1992b).

Family's Perceptions of Consumer and Non-Consumer Delivered Case Management Services

Fifty-five family members whose relative received either consumer or non-consumer delivered case management services were interviewed eighteen months after their relative entered the service. The families were interviewed either in-person or by telephone. Their relative had been randomly assigned to either a consumer or non-consumer team of case managers. The consumer team was predominately comprised of individuals who met the following criteria: 1. a major psychiatric diagnosis, 2. at least one psychiatric hospitalization or intensive use of emergency services, and 3. regular contact with mental health services. Of the 55 family members, 23 had a relative assigned to the consumer team and 32 to the non-consumer team. The relative or case manager identified the family member to be interviewed. The interview focused on satisfaction with services for both their relative and themselves.

Most of the family members interviewed were either parents (40%) or siblings (33%). The sample was predominately female (82%) with a mean age of 51 and a range of 28 to 85. The majority of the sample was African American (86%). Thirty-five percent of the sample were currently married, and 42% were separated, divorced, or widowed. The relatives had a mean age of 40 with a range from 20 to 75. Just over half (56%) were male and most were not currently married. They tended to live with relatives or in mental health facilities in the community. Most (85%) had a schizophrenia disorder. Almost all had prior psychiatric hospitalizations, with an average of 8 hospitalizations.

Families were generally quite satisfied with services provided by the case managers and there was no difference between the two groups in satisfaction. Forty-four percent of families were very satisfied and 27% were moderately satisfied with services. Families were asked the extent to which they felt that the case manager had been meeting the needs of their relative in such areas as medication assessment, supportive counseling, helping with housing, employment, teaching social and daily living skills, and assistance with benefits. The only area in which there was significant difference by condition was in medication assessment and monitoring, with the consumer team less likely to meet their relative's needs. Although not significantly different, there was a tendency for families to view consumer case managers as less likely to meet their relative's supportive counseling needs and teaching skills of daily living. In some areas particularly job and vocational training and teaching public transportation use, half or more of families interviewed felt that both teams were not meeting their relative's needs at all (Solomon & Draine, 1994). Families were questioned about the extent to which the case manager has been meeting their needs for information regarding their relative's problems and expectations, education about medications and their side effects, advice and emotional support, and assistance with locating resources and crisis situations. There was no difference between families by type of case management team with regard to the extent of their needs being met. In four areas, over half of the family members interviewed felt that both teams were not meeting their needs at all. These included: teaching about medications and about how to help motivate their relative, giving practical advice and emotional support (Solomon & Draine, 1994).

With regard to the amount of contact that family members had with case managers, there was no difference between the two conditions. Fifty-five percent indicated regular or frequent contact and 40% had contact only once or twice. Similarly there were no differences by condition in the satisfaction with the amount of contact and with the quality of contact. About two thirds (62%) felt the amount of contact was just right and a third would have liked more. Over half were either very (30%) or moderately (23%) satisfied with the quality of contact. With regard to specific problems, five family respondents stated that the only problem was a change in case managers (Solomon & Draine, in press).

Overall, 86% of the family members felt the case managers were well qualified for the position. In only three cases did families indicate that they knew that the case manager had a mental health problem. For the most part, families did not seem to be opposed to a consumer with the required experience and training functioning as a case manager. When families were queried as to the extent of concern they would have if their relative had a case manager who had experienced a mental illness him/her self, ll% indicated no concern, 40% were unsure, 44% would have a little concern and 3 individuals indicated a great deal of concern. The nature of concerns that family respondents indicated was whether the individual was responsible to perform the job, able to cope with the situation, able to handle stress, was under appropriate supervision, and able to do a good job for their relative. One family member said "A person's mental illness does not need to limit their ability to do a job... I would have the same concerns as with anyone who had the job" (Solomon & Draine, 1994).

Families of Children and Adolescents: Their Satisfaction with Services

Of 62 youths released to the community from a state psychiatric facility for children, not another institution, 47 parents and 7 caregivers were interviewed approximately two months after discharge. This was part of a larger study, therefore the interview covered numerous topics. This discussion will focus on assessment of service needs for the family and a rating form that contained 14 items of therapist personal and professional qualities and characteristics. The family member/caregiver was asked to complete the form for the hospital or community worker with whom they were most satisfied and least satisfied. This was adapted from Hatfield's survey (1983) which was developed for families of adult severely mentally disabled. Community agency workers, i.e., human service workers, public and private mental health workers, Juvenile Court and Family court workers, and school system personnel were also asked how they thought their primary client would rate them on each of these same items using the categories of poor, adequate, or good.

Most of the family members interviewed were biological mothers (41) and 6 were biological fathers. The ages ranged from 27 to 58 with most being in their 30's and 40's. Almost half (47%) were currently married and only 1 was never married. Over half the children were living in a one-parent household or were living in an out-of-home placement. The youths mean age was 15 with a range from 8 to 18. Fifty-two percent were male. The most common diagnoses were affective disorders (49%), adjustment disorder (27%), and identity disorder (21%), some had more than one diagnosis. The major areas of need for the family were family therapy and parent skill training, where 81% of family respondents rated these as needs (Solomon & Evans, 1992a). Families specifically expressed interest in training and education about ways to cope and manage their child, but few received these types of services (Solomon & Evans, 1992b).

For the workers with whom family's were most satisfied, two-thirds or greater of family members felt the workers were good in the majority of areas measured. Those areas in which approximately three-quarters or more of families/caregivers felt the therapist to be good included provision of information, listening, empathy, reassurance, encouragement, respect, appreciation of a difficult situation, and seeing the family as a partner in treatment. In the area of the process of treatment delivery, about two-thirds felt the worker with whom they were most satisfied was considered to be good. However, only approximately half rated these workers as good in the areas of skill teaching, such as showing ways to solve the family's problems and how to handle the child. These areas of skill teaching were the ones that the workers themselves also perceived that they would be judged poorly. Ratings of those workers whom families were least satisfied with were generally poor in all areas, i.e., treatment process, support and empathy, and skill-based teaching. It is important to note that in 74% of the situations workers regarded the child as the primary client, 18% indicated the family, 3% indicated the parent, and 5% noted other family members (Solomon, Evans, Delaney, & Malone, 1992).

SUMMARY OF FINDINGS

Based on the studies discussed, family members were most dissatisfied with the hospital providing them information about their ill relative and including them in treatment process. They were most satisfied with the provision of services by intensive case management teams to their ill relative, but they were somewhat less satisfied with the services that they themselves received from case managers. Families were more satisfied with services provided by mental health agencies than state hospitals, but not as satisfied with mental health agency services as with case management services. Families did not appear to have great concerns about case management services being delivered by qualified consumers. However, some family members appeared to have concerns regarding turnover of case managers. Areas of weakness in service provision particularly pointed out by families was in the areas of vocational rehabilitation and job training and activities to occupy their relative's time. Skill training was one area where service providers appeared to be least able to meet family needs. The workers themselves acknowledged that they felt their clients would rate them relatively poorly in this area. Some families also desired more contact with service providers.

Families also had concerns about the nature of placements for their relative post discharge. They desired places that were highly structured and provided 24 hour supervision. They desired that these places be located in safe neighborhoods. If they felt their relative was not ready due to problems controlling emotions, behaviors, or drug and alcohol use, they would prefer that their relative remain in the hospital. In many situations families felt guilty and sad that their relative was in a state hospital, but they also felt relief. They often expressed a desire to care for their relative, but did not feel that they could cope with or handle their relative. In a few situations, they were fearful for the safety of themselves and others.

Implications for Practice and Training of Mental Health Professionals

It is evident from the findings of the studies reviewed that families prefer to be allies with service workers. However, they want more information and education in methods for coping and managing their ill relative, whether the relative is an adult or child. Some families also require some help to assure their own safety. This may involve teaching them strategies for setting limits and handling problematic behaviors. But service providers appear to have the greatest deficits in the area of teaching these skills to families. Skill teaching requires specialized training in such techniques as behavior modification or parent skill training. There is also a need to better train the next generation of professionals likely to work with this population in skill-based interventions. These techniques are usually taught in psychology programs, but many case managers and other mental health workers come from social work, where these interventions are infrequently taught. In order for skill-based interventions to be operative, several strategies appear warranted. Service providers must receive adequate training in such techniques so that they are confident in their abilities to provide such services. Administrators of agencies providing services to seriously emotionally disturbed children and severely mentally disabled adults must establish such services for families as essential components to the treatment planning and service delivery (Friesen & Koroloff, 1990). They must also develop mechanisms to pay for such services, as often reimbursement systems do not pay for services to collateral. Without administrative commitment on the part of agencies even highly motivated staff will be reluctant to engage in these activities (Bernheim & Lehman, 1985; Bernheim & Switalski, 1988).

Families were also concerned with case manager turnover. Families are most satisfied with intensive case management as it provides aggressive outreach, and 24 hour, 7 day a week availability (Hanson & Rapp, 1992; Hoult et al, 1983; Stein & Test, 1980). It follows that access is also improved by the continuity of case management over time. This continuity is affected by job turnover, which is related to job status, remuneration, and the level of systemic support case managers receive. Mental health systems need to value case managers by paying them enough and providing them with appropriate support. Another concern of families was the security and the safety of their relative in terms of available community placement. Providers need to be cognizant of this and to consider housing options that are in safe and secure locations. In some instances families are concerned for their own safety and this fear may result in the use of restraining orders. Consequently, their ill relative may be arrested and enter jail when he/she violates the restraining order. Workers need to be aware of family concerns for safety and to develop appropriate options so that families do not have to resort to the use of restraining orders. Services also need to be culturally relevant and include bilingual workers so that families of other cultures are not excluded from participation.

Hospitals cannot continue to ignore the families of patients. In order for families to be effective resources for patients both while in the hospital and after discharge, hospitals need to listen to what families feel they need as well as to what they feel they can comfortably provide to their relative. Mental health providers frequently feel that the families have an obligation to care for their severely mentally ill relative and feel resentment toward them when they do not appear to be meeting their responsibility. For example, one hospital staff person interviewed in one study made the following statement about families: "They use us. They want us to keep (patient) forever. Support is flimsy at best, one out of four families may be helpful" (Solomon, Beck, & Gordon, 1988b). However, as Hatfield (1984) points out, families do not have a legal responsibility for caring for an adult mentally ill relative.

Workers serving seriously emotionally disturbed children need to understand the values of serving children in the context of their family. The system of care that is being promoted for these children is to support and assist parents in their caregiving role and to involve them in all decisions concerning service delivery. These systems are also to have a "strong and explicit commitment to preserve the integrity of the family unit whenever possible" (Stroul & Friedman, 1986). These workers need to be educated in the system of care and its values.

Although families may want to be allies in the treatment process, it cannot be achieved without the cooperation of the provider. Mental health providers state that they want to be partners with families. However, the question remains as to the extent that this has become a standard of practice (Friesen & Koroloff, 1990). The studies reported here indicate that this goal has not been adequately achieved. There were a number of families who expressed a desire for more contact with providers. Without appropriate contact, this collaboration cannot be developed. Providers often cite issues of ethical and legal mandates to maintain confidentiality. There are ways to collaborate with families in the treatment process without violating clients' confidentiality. The provision of general information about the illness and medications, practical advice on ways to cope with symptoms and difficult behaviors, and support and encouragement do not violate confidentiality mandates. Also, eliciting information from families who desire to share such material may be helpful in treatment as they have opportunities to see their ill relative in circumstances that providers do not.

CONCLUSION

Recently, there has been recognition of the needs of families and a more positive attitude toward families on the part of mental health providers. However, these attitude changes need to be accompanied by behavioral changes as well. Without a mutual working partnership between families and mental health professionals, we as mental health professionals are not most effectively serving our clients.

REFERENCES

Bernheim, K., & Lehman, A. (1985). *Working with families of the mentally ill*. New York W. W. Norton & Company.

Bernheim, K., & Switalski, T. (1988). Mental health staff and patient's relatives: How they view each other. *Hospital and Community Psychiatry. 39*, 63-68, 1988.

Biegel, D. & Yamitani, A. (1986). Self-help groups for families of the mentally ill: Research perspectives. In M. Z. Goldstein (Ed.) *Family involvement in the treatment of schizophrenia*. (pp. 58-80) Washington, D. C. American Psychiatric Association.

Carpentier, N., Lesage, A., Goulet, I., Lalonde, P., & Renaud, M. (1992). Burden of care of families not living with young schizophrenic relative. *Hospital and Community Psychiatry, 43,* 38-43.

Friesen, B. & Koroloff. N. (1990). Family-centered services. Implications for mental health administration and research. *The Journal of Mental Health Administration. 17,* 13-25.

Goldman, H. H. (1982). Mental illness and family burden: A public health perspective. *Hospital and Community Psychiatry, 33,*557-560.

Hanson, S. G. & Rapp, C. A. (1992). Families perceptions of community mental health programs for their relatives with a severe mental illness. *Community Mental Health Journal. 28,* 181-197.

Hatfield, A. (1979). Help-seeking behavior in families of the mentally ill. An exploratory study. *American Journal of Community Psychology, 7,* 563-569.

Hatfield, A. (1983). What families want of family therapy. In W. McFarlane (ed.). *Family Therapy in Schizophrenia.* New York. Guilford Press.

Hatfield, A. (1984). The family. In J. A. Talbott (ed.). *Chronic mental patient: five years later.* (pp. 307-323). Grune & Stratton.

Hatfied, A., Fierstein, R, & Johnson, D. (1982). Meeting the needs of families of psychiatrically disabled. *Psychosocial Rehabilitation Journal, 6,* 27-40.

Holden, D. & Lewine., R. (1982). How families evaluate mental health professionals, resources, and effects of illness. *Schizophrenia Bulletin, 8,* 626-633.

Hoult, J., Reynolds, I., Charbonneau-Powes, M., Weekes, P., & Briggs, J. (1983). Psychiatric hospital versus community treatment: The results of a randomized trial. *Australian and New Zealand Journal of Psychiatry, 17,* 160-167.

Howell, M. (1973). *Helping ourselves: families and the human network* Boston, Beacon.

Lamb, H. R., & Goertzel, V. (1977). The long-term patient in the era of community treatment. *Archives of General Psychiatry, 26,* 489-495.

Minkoff, K. (1978). A map of chronic mental patients. In J. A. Talbott (ed.). *The chronic mental patient.* (pp. 11-37). Washington, D. C. American Psychiatric Association.

Savarese, M., Detrano, T., Koproski, J., & Weber, M. C. (1990). Case Management. In. P. Brickner, L. K., Scharer, B., Conanan, M., Savarese, M., & Scanton, B. (ed.). *Under the safety met: The health and social welfare of the homeless in the United States.* New York, W. W. Norton.

Solomon, P., Beck, S., & Gordon, B. (1988a). A comparison of perspectives on discharge of extended care facility clients: Views of families, hospital staff, community mental health workers, and clients. *Administration in Mental Health. 15*, 166-174.

Solomon, P., Beck, S., & Gordon, B. (1988b). Family members' perspectives on psychiatric hospitalization and discharge. *Community Mental Health Journal. 24*, 108-117.

Solomon, P., & Draine, J. (1994). Family perspectives of consumers as case managers. *Community Mental Health Journal, 30*, 165-176.

Solomon, P., & Evans, D. (1992a). Service needs of youth released from a state psychiatric facility as perceived by service providers and families. *Community Mental Health Journal. 28*, 305-315.

Solomon, P. & Evans, D. (1992b). Use of aftercare services by children and adolescents discharged from a state hospital. *Hospital and Community Psychiatry. 43*, 932-934.

Solomon, P. Evans, D., Delaney, M. A., & Malone, R. (1992). Assessment of therapeutic relationship of community agency workers. *Psychiatric Quarterly 63*, 251-264.

Solomon, P. & Marcenko, M. (1992a). Family members' concerns regarding community placement of their mentally disabled relative: Comparisons one month after release and a year later. *Family Relations. 41*, 341-347.

Solomon, P. & Marcenko, M. (1992b). Families of adults with severe mental illness: Their satisfaction with inpatient and outpatient treatment. *Psychosocial Rehabilitation Journal. 16*, 121-134.

Spaniol, L. & Jung, H. (1983). *Issues and concerns of families that include a person with a severe mental illness.* Boston: Center for Psychiatric Rehabilitation, Boston University.

Spaniol, L. & Zipple, A. (1988). Family and professional perceptions of family needs and coping strengths. *Rehabilitation Psychology. 33*, 37-45.

Stein, L. & Test, M. A. (1980). Alternative to mental hospital treatment: I. A conceptual model treatment program and clinical evaluation. *Archives of General Psychiatry. 37*, 392-397.

Stroul, B. & Friedman, R. M. (1986). A system of care for severely emotionally disturbed children and youth. Washington, D.C., CASSP Technical Assistance Center.

Tessler, R. & Goldman, H. H. (1982). *The chronically mentally ill: Assessing community support programs.* Cambridge, MA., Ballinger.

Test, M. A. (1992). Training in community living. I. R. P. Liberman (ed.). *Handbook of psychiatric rehabilitation.* New York: MacMillon.

PART IV:

TRAINING AND RESEARCH

Chapter 14

TRAINING FUTURE CLINICIANS
TO WORK WITH FAMILIES

Mona Wasow

Mum: "My adult son had just been hospitalized. He spotted me as I walked in the door."

Nurse: "Look at that young man's face light up when he sees his mum."

Mum: "She understood!"

If given the opportunity, it is the people with mental illnesses and their families who provide the most important components needed by clinicians to work effectively with families. What are these components? Compassion, respect, and knowledge. There are many unknowns in the field of severe mental illness (SMI), but the need for these skills is not one of them.

It has been my privilege to have spent the past fifteen years training social work students to work with individuals with severe mental illness and their families. It has never failed: within just a few weeks of contact, students speak of their clients in terms of their bravery, good will, and fortitude. They wonder how SMI people survive with all that they are up against. They agonize when they work with people their own age and think, "There but for the grace of God go I." The same phenomenon occurs when students have their first family contact. Meeting with family members and SMI people quickly teaches students compassion and respect. Knowledge about the illnesses, treatments, deinstitutionalization, community care, and good clinical skills all take more time, and are learned from books, classes, and good supervision in direct work with clients.

Knowledge alone will not make a fine clinician. Compassions and respect without knowledge is not enough, but put them all together and you get a fine clinician who can work well with mentally ill people and their families.

GOALS

Goals and skills for working effectively in this area will vary somewhat depending upon the discipline. There are, however, some generic goals that all health care professionals should meet. Broadly speaking these are: 1) knowledge, 2) attitudes of respect and compassion, 3) clinical skills, and 4) advocacy skills. These generic goals will be briefly described, and then models from two disciplines, social work and psychiatry, will be presented. Nursing rehabilitation and occupational therapy are equally important, but less well known to this writer.

Knowledge

As mentioned above, students need to know just what is and is not known about all the severe mental illnesses and their various treatment modalities, with an emphasis on psychopharmacology, psychosocial supports, and good community care. Psychoeducational support for families is equally important. A good clinician needs to understand the deinstitutionalizational movement, both the ideals behind the movement and the realities of what has taken place. In connection with this, knowledge about legality issues and the criminalization of the severely mentally ill are important. Cross cultural perspectives help students understand that some outcomes are culture bound, and they sometimes need to question what their culture is doing. And last but not least, an emphasis on keeping abreast of research in both the social and biological sciences must be emphasized. Future clinicians should never again make the mistake of believing they know more than they do.

Attitudes

Clinicians need compassion for severely mentally ill people and their families; as close an understanding as they can possibly get to the horrendous experiences of living with severe mental illness from client and family perspectives (parents, grandparents, spouses, children, siblings, and extended family); and the ability to listen carefully to all concerned. They also need to develop a respect for themselves as clinicians, and to be proud of their difficult front-line work. It helps to develop a bifocal perspective in which one can be both realistic — and believe in miracles!

Clinical Skills

These should encompass working with a large variety of severely mentally ill people and their families—both individually and in groups—as well as working effectively with other health care providers and helping systems. The development of these skills has to be a great deal more than learning about behavior management, treatment planning, case management, and the teaching of daily living skills. This is not to put down the above, but rather as a reminder that there is so much more to working with and helping people. If you or I become disabled some-day, we probably do not want to be somebody's "case," and we will not want to be "managed" either. We must not lose sight of the heart, nor can we ignore the specific skills needed to help severely mentally ill people. There will be more about this, when the psychiatry training model is discussed.

A sense of humor, the ability to feel deeply and also to distance oneself, creativity, and above all compassion, all belong to the repertoire of good clinical skills.

Advocacy Skills

Not only do we need to know about community resources and how to advocate for people, but a good clinician also needs to be able to develop new resources and influence public policy. More coalitions are needed between legislators, mental health professionals, AMI groups, consumers, police, religious institutions, and mass media. The ability to educate others is needed, as there is so much to be overcome in the areas of stigma and prejudice.

An overall goal combining knowledge, attitude, clinical, and advocacy skills, is to at long last bring us together. Clinicians from various disciplines, families, consumers, and educators, understandably all have different agendas and biases. How could it be otherwise? On almost all issues we have different perspectives: involuntary vs. voluntary treatment, institutionalization vs. community care, medications, dependency vs. autonomy, etc. are all volatile subjects. Just to give one example of our differing perspectives: Many consumers are anti psychotropic medications, most family members are pro psychotropic medications and professionals and educators vary depending on their education and biases.

A big goal then is for all of these constituents to recognize each other's different perspectives. Given all the unknowns in the broad area of severe mental illness, we can not hope for agreement on many issues at this time. But we can aim for trying to understand and respect each other. Only then will we be able to direct our energies away from trying to convince and change each other, and towards our common goal. For we all do have a common goal, that of alleviating as much suffering as possible for mentally ill people and their families.

OBSTACLES TO TRAINING

Before getting into the specifics of training future clinicians a few obstacles will be mentioned, the better to overcome them. One problem is the curriculum lag. Many of today's educators and clinicians were trained in the 1950's and 1960's when psychodynamic models of human behavior and insight psychotherapy were in fashion. Much less was known about the genetic and biochemical components of SMI 30-40 years ago. If people do not keep abreast of current research findings—and this is all too often the case with busy, over-worked professionals—the result is an outdated curriculum (Wasow,1991: 43-49). In addition, as Gottesman noted (Gottesman, 1991: 235):

> "... 95% of what is known about brain function has been acquired in the past 10 years; There is a 10 to 15 year lag between basic science advances and their application to practical problems of illness..."

An effort is being made by the Curriculum and Training Committee of the National Alliance of the Mentally Ill to find out what text books and curriculum are being taught in professional schools of social work, psychiatry, nursing, psychology, and occupational therapy throughout the U.S. The Council on Social Work Education (Bowker [ed], 1988) is doing the same for social work, as well as offering a model of curriculum to be used. Other professional schools are doing the same. Change is slowly occurring.

Books detailing biological and genetic evidence for SMI are now prevalent in the "Decade of the Brain" (Judd, 1990). Several journals are effectively presenting the biological, genetic, and psychosocial stress theories of SMI. There is now ample literature and research out that should make dissemination of current knowledge about SMI easily available for clinicians, families, and educators. The damage done in the recent past to SMI people and their families from the curriculum lag, and the often resulting family blaming, has been horrendous. Hopefully, this era is drawing to a close, but we still need to work on updating the curriculum.

A second obstacle often mentioned is that students are not interested in working with this population, and indeed there is documentation to support this notion (Rupp, 1985; Rubin, 1984). This obstacle is easy to overcome. Students quickly pick up the attitudes and enthusiasms of their professors and agency supervisors.

> "Interestingly enough, professionals are often as unprepared as families to respond appropriately to this kind of profound crisis (SMI). In fact, we can frequently see a parallel process in the emotional and cognitive responses of the mental health professional and the family: both feel helpless, angry, despairing, and anxious." (McMillan and Spaniol, 1992: 2).

With better training of professionals, they will probably feel less despair and more enthusiasm. For 15 years I have watched reluctant, disappointed students who did not want to be placed in the SMI social work field unit, get turned around within weeks to become committed, enthusiastic champions of SMI people. Professionals play a role in this conversion process, but it is the contact with SMI people and family members that does the real job of turning students around.

The job of professionals is to make sure that our future clinicians get immediate contact with this population. The trick is an attitudinal one: that student understand the importance of learning from their clients, as opposed to thinking they have all the answers. Imparting that attitude is our job.

A third obstacle often mentioned, that makes no sense to me, is the lack of funding and time it takes for a faculty member to develop expertise in this area. It takes no funding beyond one's regular salary to sit in a library for a few hours a day, for a few months, to learn the content about SMI. The rest, as for our students, is an attitudinal one. With knowledge, commitment, and caring, wonderful programs can be developed in rapid order. Our program at the University of Wisconsin was developed over one summer, with no extra funding.

An obstacle mentioned by Faulker (Faulker *et al.*, 1989), probably exists in most of the health care professions, but especially in psychiatry: Working with this population has not been rewarded with academic recognition by department chairs and tenure committees. It is a sad commentary that care of the sickest population carries the least status.

They also mentioned that professional psychiatric organizations tend to want to preserve the status quo.

In 1988 (Factor, *et al.*) a model community psychiatry curriculum was developed for psychiatric residents at the University of Wisconsin. They mentioned as an obstacle the tension within departments between the biological and psychodynamic theories of causality that still exists among psychiatrists. Neither side pays enough attention to psychosocial rehabilitation, or to the parents. The explanation given for lack of attention paid to rehabilitation, is the reluctance on the part of psychiatrists to give up their top status. In order to give full attention to rehabilitation, or habilitation, other professionals coming from vocational rehabilitation, nursing, social work, and occupational therapy need to be seen as co-workers rather than as ancillary personnel. Doctors are not used to doing this, but the U.W. psychiatry program is working to overcome that obstacle. They also state that, "Perhaps the greatest benefit is to give legitimacy and status to working in this setting with this population." (Factor, *et al.*, 1988:318)

It is sad to note that major obstacles in the mental illness movement are conflicts and disagreements between groups. Maybe future clinicians need to be trained in conflict resolution, in addition to everything else. Chances are that agreement cannot be reached on such provocative issues as voluntary vs. involuntary treatments and commitments, medications, the differing roles of professionals and consumers, and so forth. Because of these disagreements, the emphasis should be on making the effort to stand in the shoes of the other. If we cannot agree on some big issues, let us at least aim for a respectful understanding that will enable us to stay focused on our one common agenda—the best possible care for persons with severe mental illness.

SOME TRAINING MODELS

Several models of training clinicians to work with families have developed over the past ten years. The fact that families have been involved in developing these models, and also that the models all have certain commonalties, lends credibility to the idea that we are on the right track.

In 1987 and 1988 a group of psychiatrists (Faulker *et al.*, 1989) met with representatives of AMI to develop basic curriculum for training their psychiatric residents. They wrote about the need to work with a patient's entire biopsychosocial network, and an attitude that includes both consumers and their families. Among their guiding principles they had: "the development of an effective collaborative relationship with

CMI patients, their families, and other providers..." (Faulkner, *et al*, 1989:1324)

Wasow (Wasow, 1991) writes about four basic methods used to update and achieve curriculum goals: weekly seminars for academic content and a place to discuss field issues; direct practice and supervision in the field: readings and written assignments, and cognitive and experiential assignments. Examples of assignments are attendance at AMI meetings, working at shelters for homeless people, attending workshops in town, attending consumer groups, and interviewing family members for their perspective.

Many psychiatrists (Minkoff and Stern, 1985; Nielsen, Stein, Talbott, *et al.*, 1981) have observed that professional training programs have traditionally emphasized psychotherapeutic skills appropriate to the treatment of the "worried well," or psychopharmacological skills for the stabilization of acute illness, while little attention has been paid to the psychotherapeutic need of SMI people. Minkoff (Minkoff, 1987) observed, in addition, that lack of training is BOTH A RESULT AND A CAUSE of the lack of interest in SMI people in general. Trainees who might become interested in working with SMI people are turned off when their lack of training leads them to feel incompetent and discouraged rather than capable and hopeful. This attitude is reinforced by supervisors who share the same lack of skill in working with this population (Minkoff, 1989:31) "The vicious cycle thus continues..."

In an effort to address this issue in the training of psychiatrists, several groups of community psychiatrists have proposed specific curriculum requirements for training residents in the treatment of SMI people. Nielsen *et al* (1981) emphasized the need for residents to learn to treat clients intensively, and to understand the person behind the diagnostic label. Training should emphasize biopsychosocial functional evaluation and a variety of psychotherapeutic techniques for SMI people. These include the development of motivation to attain some rehabilitative goals, collaboration with families and community caregivers, and working with other members of multidisciplinary treatment teams.

"Cutler, Bloom, and Shore (1981) described a specific training module within the University of Oregon Psychiatry Residency Training Program whose specific goal was to train residents to develop 'assertive long-term relationships' (p. 99) with long-term clients—and to become proficient in community living skills training, case management, linkage with community

providers, interdisciplinary teamwork, and ongoing supportive
therapy." (p. 31)

Faulker, Cutler, Krohn *et al.* (1989) extended these principles into
specific recommendations of a residency curriculum emphasizing not
only skill development but also the demonstration of positive attitudes
towards SMI patients and their families.

In all of these recent models the authors say that exposing residents
in working with SMI people is not enough. They also need experience
within the context of a positive clinical training experience that has
good supervision and training from people who know what they are
doing—a phenomenon that is all too rare in the SMI field. Some excellent
works, for example Lamb's 1982 book *Treating the Long Term Mentally
Ill,* have outlined general clinical principles, but case material illustrating
specific interventions or techniques is unavailable.

In 1987 the Committee on Psychiatry and the Community of the
Groups for Advancement of Psychiatry (GAP) began work on the development of a training guide for psychiatric residents in the psychosocial treatment of people with SMI. (GAP, 1993, in press) In this guide
they have tried to find a way of capturing the clinical richness of their
experiences in working with this population. In order to do this they
surveyed residents and generated a list of 32 questions the psychiatric
residents wanted answered. These questions included concerns about
safety, engagement of clients, assessments, family involvement, systems
issues and what to do when there were no resources. They also wanted
to know about treatment planning, how to provide hope, and about
special populations such as the dually diagnosed and the homeless.

In their guide GAP has tried to avoid vague and general answers. A
part of their mission was to provide a theoretical framework for working
with the client, family, and community. "We sought to involve the reader
intellectually, emotionally, and empathetically in the process of engaging
with and understanding clients and their caregivers, and providing an
ongoing program of treatment." (p. 32) Treatment options with medication, psychotherapy, family involvement and rehabilitation programs
are all described.

Under content GAP utilizes the disease model, emphasizing the biological roots of SMI, and the importance of not blaming client or family.
It emphasizes the psychosocial context in which the illness occurs, and
the importance of providing education and support to overcome denial
and stigma and to facilitate participation in treatment. Third, Gap
defines a hopeful process of rehabilitation and recovery, in which client

and family are helped to achieve stability and overcome the despair and anger attached to having an incurable illness. GAP emphasizes the need to utilize community resources. They focus on the process of engagement and assessment for the client as well as the family. Systems assessment, an area in which residents rarely have specific clinical training, is also discussed. They also include study of the legal system issues, including commitment and medication guardianship, and what happens to clients who "fall through the cracks." Treatment issues include: safety and containment, protecting the treatment alliance, control of acute symptoms, maintaining stability, and rehabilitation and growth. Specific attention is paid to compliance strategies, collaboration, education, fostering autonomy, assessing the meaning of medication for patients, assessing capacity for informed consent, and using coercive interventions.

It includes a primer for psychotherapy discussing the length and frequency of sessions, the activity of the therapist, content of the sessions, and the rehabilitative focus of treatment, as well as involving the family as collaborators, and the use of community treatment programs such as day treatment and clubhouses. They also emphasize the importance of matching programs to individual clients.

The following is a description of the model used to train clinicians, both undergraduate and graduate students, at the University of Wisconsin School of Social Work. This model works very well for social work students, where we have the advantage of a field course that devotes 16 to 20 hours a week for eight months to direct practice with clients. Not every discipline has the advantage of this much time devoted to hands on training. Also, different disciplines will want to emphasize other skills, but this model should be adaptable to various health care disciplines as well as different time frames.

Professionals need a great deal of knowledge. This is obtained through readings, weekly seminar discussions, direct work experience with SMI people and their families, and various assignments, both academic and experiential. The main content areas covered are:

    I.   The major mental illnesses, as defined by the DSM-IV. Learning what is, and is *not* known about the main mental illnesses.

   II. Different Treatment Modalities.

      1. Medications

      2. Psychosocial supports—different models of community supports.

      3. Crisis interventions.

4. Educational approaches for families.
III. Community Resources—what already exists and what needs to be developed. This includes knowledge about NAMI and local AMI groups.
IV. The Deinstitutionalization Movement—pros and cons. The criminalization of the mentally ill. The history of treating mental illnesses.
1. In the United States.
2. Cross cultural perspectives.
3. Legality issues, especially commitment laws.
V. Different Perspectives on Mental Illnesses.
1. Patient perspectives: including gender, age, sexual preferences.
2. Family perspectives.
3. Societal views in the United States.
VI. Basic Clinical Skills
1. Interviewing clients, families, both individually and in groups.
2. Team work with other disciplines and helping systems.
3. Doing assessments
4. Planning interventions and treatments.
5. Advocacy for clients and their families.
6. Understanding, influencing, and developing policy issues.
7. Educating the public; fighting stigma.
8. Creative thinking and problem solving. Because there is so much that has not worked well in the past, an emphasis is put on the need for high levels of creativity in looking for ways of helping.
VII.   Keeping Abreast of Current Research

The weekly seminars run two hours every week for the academic year. The seminars are used to discuss field concerns and theory, to brainstorm, and to problem solve. The seminar, plus a "methods of clinical practice" course, are our main vehicles for linking theory to practice. Each student is responsible for planning and running one seminar. This is an opportunity for each of them to go into depth on a topic of their choosing. We have had seminars on stigma, legality issues, medications, dual diagnosis, family issues, aging and SMI, housing problems, sexuality, criminalization of the SMI, gender issues, and many other topics. Students do best when they are covering a topic of their particular interest.

The student is totally responsible for everything: topic, methods of presentation, calling the seminar to order, keeping track of time, and soliciting feedback in the end. This is a time consuming responsibility, and tends to evoke anxiety in most students. It is the assignment they complain most about, and praise as the most helpful learning experience—after it is over!

Every student tells me about their topic of instruction two weeks prior to their presentation. I am available to assist them just as little or as much as they desire. Some people want very little help as they know exactly what they want to cover, and how they plan to do it. Others want to go through every detail. Students vary a great deal in how they work best, but going over their plans with them helps ward off poor presentations. It is important for a sense of professional accomplishment that the students do well in this assignment. It is equally important for the group as a whole that the seminar be dynamic and packed with content.

Professionals spend a lot of time teaching, trying to get ideas and information across to clients, colleagues, and community people. For this reason an emphasis is placed on learning a variety of teaching techniques including lectures, small group work, guest speakers, clients speaking to us, field trips, our field unit doing presentations in the community, working on advocacy projects, and a combination of experiential and academic exercises.

DIRECT PRACTICE IN THE FIELD

The 16 to 20 hours a week spent working directly with clients, their families, and the mental health system, are the "nuts and bolts" of the curriculum. This is where students do most of the learning. There are a large variety of field placements from which to choose, and an effort is made to match student interest and needs with available placements. Here is a partial list of placements:

- Various club houses
- Group homes
- State and county hospitals
- The YWCA and YMCA
- Shelters for homeless people
- Jail, and a jail diversionary program
- Special living arrangements for SMI People
- Model community support programs
- Adult day centers for SMI elderly people

Placements vary from highly structured, as in the group homes or hospitals, to unstructured, as in the shelter for the homeless. Since many of the placements coordinate their efforts, and clients are often involved with more than one agency, students learn the local mental health system, about community resources, and how best to use them on their clients' behalf.

Working with existing community resources and developing new resources are important components of the field experience. An example of this is a shelter for the homeless that was developed out of combined efforts of social work students, local churches, and volunteers. Our students are often the front line workers in their placements, involved in getting people who have fallen through the cracks of social services connected to desperately needed services.

SENSITIVITY TO FAMILY MEMBERS

In sensitizing students to the agonies, stresses, and needs of families, an emphasis is placed on books and articles written by family members, on attending meetings of the Alliance for the Mentally Ill, and in talking directly with family members to learn about their experiences in having a SMI relative.

We need to broaden the definition of family to include siblings, children, spouses, grandparents, and extended family members. Most of what we know to date comes from parents, and we need to know more about the rest of the family. The ripple effect of SMI on the entire family is enormous.

When students contact family members, they ask permission to learn from them what their experiences have been with having SMI in the family. An emphasis is also put on learning from them how professionals have proven helpful and/or hurtful in the past; and in what they think a good professional needs to know and do in order to be helpful. The time frame for this contact has been as little as a few hours, and as much as weekly over a period of several months, depending upon both student need and family availability. Consistently, students have declared this the most important of their educational experiences, along with client contact. After they have had family contact, they talk in terms of "loyalty, suffering, strength, courage, compassion..." and ask such questions as: "How do they manage to survive this?" This is surely a far cry from the psychopathologizing of family members that routinely took place just a generation ago.

The literature written by family members also has a strong, positive influence on student attitudes. Some recent books used for consumer perspectives are: Kytle, Elizabeth, *The Voices of Robby Wilde* (1987) and Sheehan, Susan, *Is There No Place on Earth For Me?* (1983). Some excellent books on sibling perspectives are: Swados, Elizabeth, *The Four of Us* (1991) and Moorman, Margaret *My Sister's Keeper* (1990). I have not seen any books from the spouse or grandparent perspectives. There are many fine articles on all of the above except grandparents.

Time is also spent exploring different psycho educational models used to help families cope with SMI. Today's clinicians must be prepared to fully understand that families need and want *knowledge* about the illnesses and treatments; they need help in accessing community care for their loved one; and very often their main avenue of emotional support is found in AMI and NAMI.

What clinicians should be aware of is that the majority of today's cohort of elderly parents have been through the "family bashing" era. For this reason students need to understand that they, as clinicians, may be found "guilty until proven otherwise," in the eyes of these parents. Overcoming this reaction need not be complicated. Clinicians need to express their compassion for all that the parents have been through, and to acknowledge how loyal the parents are for having hung in there with their SMI relative. That will usually diffuse the anger, and make for a good working relationship between family and clinician.

Some families with SMI members have severe emotional problems, as many other families do, and they need to be addressed. But gone are the days—or they should be gone—when automatic assumption is made of dysfunctional families when SMI exists.

There are other good models for training professionals to work with SMI people coming from social work, psychiatry, vocational rehabilitation, nursing, and occupational therapy. Before this chapter goes to print more will be developed. It is gratifying to see that a recurrent theme is the need to listen to and learn from SMI people, and likewise their families. There is also increasing recognition that families need information about the illnesses and treatments, and management skills for difficult behaviors. At long last there is recognition of the need for self-care for family members, as they cope with the unending grief and demands of caring for their loved ones.

ATTENDING TO THE MENTALLY ILL PERSON: ONE MORE THOUGHT

"The mental health center gave me training in behavior-mod skills and daily living skills, and told me to run a warm, sup-

portive foster home. Now which is it? I don't run my home and
family by rules and daily living skills. I do it with fun and love,
and sharing of jobs that need to be done."

> Kathy Schultz,
> Adult foster mother,
> Madison, Wis. 1992.

Severe mental illnesses can be such devastating illnesses; we do not know
how to cure them, and often we cannot help ill people very much. There
is a tendency when this happens to fall back on techniques of behavioral
control. As mentioned earlier, these techniques can be helpful at times,
but not when they take the place of sincere caring and common sense.

Brandon Fitch,[1] a 19 year old consumer, gave an eloquent speech
about his experiences with schizophrenia and the mental health system.
At the age of 12 he was hospitalized.

> "They seemed to have the idea that if they could make you act
> well, you *were* well. They set about trying to accomplish this
> by punishing you if you displayed any symptoms of your illness.
> They would keep tally all week of how many timeouts they had
> given you, and if it was too many you would not move to the
> next level or be allowed to have your parents visit you the next
> week or be able to make phone calls."

He went on to describe how his parents were the only thing in his life
he could hold on to, and when he knew he could not see them he just
gave up and got much sicker.

What am I saying by the above two examples? That in training a new
generation of professionals let us keep uppermost in our minds that
people with SMIs want to be treated as kindly and respectfully as all
other people.

ATTENDING TO THE FAMILY: A FEW MORE THOUGHTS

We need to remember the extended family. As all kinds of relatives are
beginning to speak up, the true magnitude of SMI on the entire family
system is coming to light. Siblings talk of their horrendous confusion,

---

1. July 6, 1992, cover story in *Time Magazine,* and plenary speaker at the
   September, 1992, NAMI Convention in Washington, D.C.

pain, guilt, loss, fear of genetic vulnerability, and the knowledge that they will one day have to take over after their parents die. Grandparents express their triple loss, with all its attending grief. They have lost their well grandchild, they agonize for what their son or daughter is going through, and for the pain their grandchild suffers. Spouses say they are being blamed and often left in the dark (under the disguise of "confidentiality"), much the same way that parents were treated 20 years ago. Cousins, nieces, uncles—they ask "What is going on?" "Can we help in any way?" There are often many family members who could use some attention. This attention, if well done, could not only spare the relatives some unnecessary pain and fear, but it also has the potential to widen the pool of support and care for all concerned.

Clinicians may need to help families learn to ask more questions and feel entitled to answers. As Mitch Snyder once said at a NAMI convention (Cincinnati, 1990), "It's time to stop being polite. You need to stand up and yell." This is often true in both the one-to-one situation (i.e., talking with a clinician), and on the macro level—political advocacy for the SMI. Many families need help in negotiating the mental health and legal systems.

REDIRECTING PAIN AND ANGER

Pain, anger, mourning with no end in sight—all of these strong, negative emotions can be destructive. Some people profit by having this negative energy redirected into positive channels. In many ways this is what AMI groups and NAMI are all about. Today's clinicians should always make sure that their families are aware of local AMI groups. There are many other ways of rechannelling negative feelings into positive actions: lecturing in local schools and colleges, political advocacy for better housing and community care, volunteering in a group home or a homeless shelter, etc. Advocacy is not everybody's cup of tea, but a professional can do a better job of exploring this as a possibility for those who would benefit from it.

SUMMARY

The future clinician needs to know about the various SMIs, their treatments, and about community care. They need a lot of knowledge, accompanied by an attitude of compassion and understanding, and the ability to get those feelings across. They must be aware of the ripple effects of SMI on the entire family, and be willing to include them.

A good clinician understands the importance of advocacy, and how pain and anger can be positively rechannelled into it. In addition, creativity and flexibility are invaluable tools. If one approach does not work, we need to look for another.

We are asking a lot from future clinicians. But think of what SMI people have to cope with. Think of their families. Then think of our rewards if we can be any part of alleviating some of that suffering.

REFERENCES

Bowker, J. (Ed.). (1988) *Services for the CMI: New Approaches for Mental Health Professionals,* (Vol. 1 & 2), Washington, D.C.: Council on Social Work Education.

Deveson, A. (1992) *Tell Me I'm Here.* Penguin Books, Australia. 487 Maroondah Hgh., P.O. Box 257, Ringwood, Victoria, Australia.

Factor, R.M., Ph.D., Stein, L.I., M.D., Diamond, R.J., M.D. "A Model Community Psychiatry Curriculum for Psychiatric Residents." *Community Mental Health Journal,* Vol. 24, No. 4, Winter, 1988. pp. 310-327.

Faulker, L.R., et al., "A Basic Residency Curriculum Concerning the Chronically Mentally Ill." *American Journal of Psychiatry,* October, 1989, 146:10, pp. 1323-1327.

Gottesman, I. I., Ph.D. (1991) *Schizophrenia Genesis. The Origins of Madness,* W.H. Freeman & Co. N.Y.

Judd, E. (1990, July). Address presented at the annual conference of NAMI, Chicago, Ill.

Kytle, E. (1987) *The Voices of Robby Wilde,* Seven Locks Press.

McMillan, L. and Spaniol, L. Ph.D. "Training Professionals in The Core Mental Health Disciplines to Work With People With A Severe Mental Illness and Their Families." Grant submitted to the Massachusetts Department of Mental Health, Dec. 1992.

Minkoff, K., M.D. "Development of a Training Guide for Psychiatric Residents in the Psychosocial Treatment of People with Long-Term Mental Illness." *Innovations and Research,* Vol. 1, No. 3, summer, 1992.

Moorman, M. (1990). *My Sister's Keeper,* W.W. Norton, N.Y., & London.

Nielsen, A.C. III, Stein, L.I., Talbott, J.A., et al. (1981) "Encouraging Psychiatarists to Work with Chronic Patients: Opportunities and Limitations of Residency Education." *Hospital and Community Psychiatry,* 32, 767-775.

Rapp, C.A. (1985), "Research the CMI: Curriculum Implications" In J. Bowker (Ed.), *Education for Practice with the CMI: What Works?*, pp. 32-49. Washington, D.C.: CSWE.

Rubin, A. (1984, Nov. 8) "Review of the Literature on CMI: What Works?" Paper presented at the CSWE Forum of CMI, Lawrence, Kansas.

Sheehan, S. (1983), *Is There No Place On Earth For Me?* Vintage Books, N.Y.

Swados, E. (1991), *The Four of Us,* Farrar, Straus, & Girous, N. Y.

Wasow, M. (1991), "They Tried Reality Therapy, But He Froze in a Cave: Curriculum Deficits," *Health & Social Work,* Feb., 1991, pp. 43-49.

Chapter 15

TRAINING PSYCHIATRY RESIDENTS AND PSYCHOLOGY INTERNS TO WORK WITH FAMILIES OF THE SERIOUSLY MENTALLY ILL

Nancy J. Warren

In recent years, professionals' attitudes toward the mentally ill and their families have begun to change. As families are more vocal about their struggles, the need for increasing family support and understanding is becoming evident. As a result there has been increasing interest and commitment to training mental health professionals to work supportively with families (Cole & Cole, 1987; Cutler, Bloom & Shore, 1981; Faulkner, et al. 1989; Group for Advancement of Psychiatry, 1993; Lefley, 1988; Lefley & Johnson, 1990; National Institute of Mental Health, 1990; Weintraub, et al., 1984).

Despite this new interest, there continue to be many obstacles to the implementation of training in family collaboration. First, clinical work with the seriously mentally ill is often not sufficiently valued by professional groups (Nielsen, et al., 1981; Wasow, 1990; Weintraub, et al., 1984) giving rise to problems such as lack of professional recognition and financial remuneration, low professional status for those who treat this population, lack of high status role models, isolation from colleagues, and demoralization and burnout. Second, training for professionals in graduate and post graduate schools typically lacks a comprehensive curriculum in serious mental illness. Experience with the seriously mentally ill may be offered but such experience is not often integrated with course work about families and family needs. Third, trainees are frequently given assignments with the seriously mentally ill early in their training, when they have the least knowledge and skill. They may avoid family contacts because of the discomfort these may engender. Fourth, trainees may be so overwhelmed with service demands in field placements with individual mentally ill clients that they do not take the time to work with families. Fifth, trainees often work alone with clients and are not given sufficient experience in collaboration, leaving them isolated from the resource network.

Finally, young professionals are frequently taught contradictory theories about the role of the family in mental illness. Psychodynamic, family systems, and communication deviance theories often fail to incorporate biological knowledge about serious mental illness (Terkelsen, 1983), while purely biological models may not take into account the impact of the illness on the family (Doll, 1976; Hatfield, 1979; Thompson & Doll, 1982). Dogmatic presentation of competing theories without integration can leave students questioning when or if a particular concept may be applicable. The resulting polarization and lack of clarity about the linkage between theory and clinical work is confusing and destructive to families.

In this chapter, I will describe a model of training professionals to work collaboratively with families with a seriously mentally ill member. I will begin by outlining the theoretical model of family crisis and transition which is used in our family training. I will then review recommendations for training of psychiatry residents and psychology interns including an outline of suggested goals and objectives, clinical experiences, and didactic topics to be covered. Methods to provide students with the opportunity to learn the attitudes, knowledge and skills outlined in this training model will then be presented. I will describe the program at Baylor College of Medicine Department of Psychiatry as a case example to illustrate some of the issues in implementing such a curriculum.

FAMILY CRISIS AND TRANSITION THEORY

In order to be successful, a curriculum designed to train practitioners to work with families of the seriously mentally ill must have a coherent theoretical base which integrates knowledge about families and family functioning with information about the experience and impact of mental illness. Coping and adaptation theory (Hatfield, 1987; 1990) and family crisis and transition theory provide a framework to understand the family's reaction to mental illness of a family member. According to Caplan (1964), a crisis is defined as a situation in which an individual or family is faced with a problem for which their usual coping resources are not adequate. An individual or family in crisis feels overwhelmed, confused, and helpless. Family members frequently feel unable to make decisions or to perform adequately in their normal roles (Hansell, 1976; Umana, et al., 1980). Attempts at coping may appear rigid and stereotyped, as families struggle unsuccessfully to problem solve using their usual coping strategies. Families also may suffer a profound sense of loss of identity and of connection with friends and extended family (Hatfield, 1990).

Early writers in crisis theory (Caplan, 1964; Hill, 1958; Lindemann, 1944; Parad & Caplan, 1956) focused on the generic features of coping with crisis. These authors had observed that the process of coping was remarkably similar in different types of crisis situations such as a natural disaster, or an unexpected death of a loved one. Several authors have described stages of coping with crisis (Caplan, 1964; Golan, 1978; Hill, 1958). When a stressful event occurs, the family first attempts to deal with the unexpected or overwhelming situation on their own, but finds that typical coping does not work. This lack of success can precipitate the actual crisis—feelings of demoralization and confusion—at which time the family may seek help or redouble their coping efforts. During the next stage, as the family struggles to find a solution that does work, they may restabilize at the level of pre-crisis functioning, or at a level lower or higher than before. During this stage, the family may settle on ways of coping which may in the long run be maladaptive. Thus, crisis can bring risk or growth to the family, depending upon their success at coping (Pittman, 1987). The period of acute reorganization from a single crisis event is fairly rapid, with a return to former levels of functioning or a movement toward some sort of equilibrium occurring within approximately four to eight weeks (Caplan, 1964; Golan, 1978; Umana, Gross, & McConville, 1980).

Crisis theory must be adapted somewhat in the case of chronic conditions such as serious mental illness. Hatfield (1987; 1990) has called mental illness "a catastrophic event". As Hatfield (1990) has so aptly described, mental illness has all the characteristics which make coping most difficult: novelty or uniqueness, pervasiveness, long duration and frequency, ambiguity or unpredictability and uncontrollability. Mental illness creates a crisis in the family, but it is not a crisis which is easily or rapidly resolved. Rather it is a prolonged state of transition (Hirshkowitz, 1976) in which family members must adapt over a long period of time, often to events which will change their family irrevocably. Divorce is another example of a transition state, in which a permanent change in family structure occurs and a prolonged adaptation process of two to three years (Hetherington, Stanley-Hagen & Anderson, 1989) ensues. Other chronic conditions also force the family into a prolonged transition process. For example several authors have written about the "chronic sorrow" (Konanc & Warren, 1984; Olshanksy, 1962; Wikler,

Wasow, & Hatfield, 1981) which parents experience when they have a mentally retarded child.

Transition states are often characterized by multiple crises, or nodal points in which change is required, and coping is stressed (Konanc & Warren, 1984). In the family with a developmentally disabled child, for example, there are multiple events such as the initial diagnosis, school decisions, yearly evaluations, changes in teachers, graduation from or leaving school, job placement, and residential decisions. Comparisons with siblings or peers can be painful and stressful. Mental illness in a family member poses a particularly difficult challenge, often with multiple crises as the disease process waxes and wanes. The almost typical uncertainty about diagnosis, prognosis, and the types of treatment and rehabilitation needed (Terkelsen, 1987) is extremely stressful for families. Other events within the family, such as family developmental stages (marriage, aging of parents) or an unanticipated event such as loss of a job, can also tax family coping, and precipitate a crisis in a family already struggling to cope with the illness.

In order to better understand a given family's response to the crisis, other information and theories of family functioning must be integrated within the context of family crisis and transition theory. Medical/biological knowledge, family systems theory, family developmental or life cycle theory (Carter & McGoldrick, 1989), theories of coping and appraisal (Hatfield, 1990; Lazarus & Folkman, 1984) and concepts from multigenerational and sociological family studies can help illuminate the family's situation. Pittman (1987) describes the clinical usefulness of understanding the "family snag point(s)", which may have their roots in any number of areas such as lack of information about mental illness, structural rules about communication, the meaning of illness in the family and subculture, intense feelings of guilt or loss, or a lack of resources for coping with such a devastating illness.

Crisis and transition theory gives rise to assumptions about families and what families need that are quite different from either traditional medical or family therapy approaches. In crisis theory, families are viewed as active coping agents who, when in crisis, are in a *temporary* state of disequilibrium. As Umana et al. (1980) note: "A common error made in the diagnosis of family problems is to characterize the family seen in the midst of crisis as normatively chaotic, disorganized and dysfunctional" (p. 4). The crisis/transition approach emphasizes family strengths, previous successful coping, and rapid mobilization of resources and information to help the family make decisions (Langsley &

Kaplan, 1968; Langsley, Pittman, Machotka & Flomenhraft 1968; Pittman, 1987; Spaniol, 1987).

Treatment goals in crisis intervention are typically focused on the resolution of the immediate situation and the return of the family to precrisis functioning (Golan, 1978; Rapoport, 1970; Umana et al., 1980). Goals in a transition intervention might include helping the family to understand and accept the change in the family and family member, education about the illness and its implications, education about the transition process (Terkelsen, 1987; Tessler, Killian & Gubman, 1987), teaching of new coping strategies, broadening support networks, and the establishment of a new equilibrium despite a permanent change in a family member. Wynne's (1983) "Phase-oriented approach" is quite similar in its emphasis on the changing needs of the family as it moves from the crisis/acute stage of the illness, to the more long term or chronic treatment of the family member. Anticipatory guidance, to help the family anticipate future stress points and plan how to cope, is another important component of work with families in transition.

If a family has communication problems, or is stuck in maladaptive coping patterns, it typically becomes evident to the family clinician in the course of a crisis or transition intervention. Pathological grief reactions, in which the family (or one member) has difficulty coming to terms with the loss of capacity of their loved one, are sometimes problematic. Such families can benefit from a combination of crisis/transition work and additional family therapy to help them work out these other problems. A non-blaming, respectful attitude is helpful in defusing guilt, and facilitating the family's entry into therapy. Within the crisis/transition model, trainees are taught to work in an open, collaborative way with the family, giving direct feedback and support.

A MODEL CURRICULUM IN FAMILY COLLABORATION

Several authors have proposed curriculum outlines for training professionals to work with the seriously mentally ill (Faulkner, et al., 1989, Group for the Advancement of Psychiatry, 1993; National Institute of Mental Health, 1990; Neilson, et al., 1981; Wasow, 1990) and for training professionals to work with families (Johnson, 1988, 1990; Lefley, 1988). Faulkner, et al. (1989) a group of specialists in community psychiatry, psychiatry training and family advocacy charged with developing curriculum, call for "education of patients and families, and collaborative treatment planning with families and other service providers" (p. 1324). Reviewing this literature, I noted common elements or key ingredients which all agree are essential in training professionals to work collaboratively with the seriously mentally ill and their families. In the next section I will review the key ingredients and describe how our program is in the process of implementing such a curriculum.

In order to work collaboratively with families, trainees need a thorough grounding in the diathesis-stress model of major mental illness, and knowledge about neurosciences, psychopharmacology, cognitive and behavioral psychology, crisis/transition theory, family systems theory, community psychiatry, cultural/ethnic issues and ethics (Cole & Cole, 1987; Faulkner, et al., 1989). Knowledge of current research in treatment outcome is critical, as is information about community resources and up-to-date treatment options. Skills are needed in crisis intervention, patient and family educational techniques (Anderson, Hogarty & Reiss, 1980; Hatfield, 1990; McFarlane, 1983), family and group psychotherapy, supportive and behavioral interventions (Bernnheim & Lehman, 1985), and collaboration with others, (GAP, 1993), both professional and non-professional.

Attitudes are shaped by teaching an understanding of the experience and needs of the patient and family (Lefley, 1988), and by modeling the value of work with seriously mentally people and their families (Wasow, 1990). Attitudes are best taught by example and experience; learning experiences should be led by well respected, committed faculty (Nielsen, et al., 1981), and emphasize collaboration, cooperation with other disciplines, and contacts with families in a both clinical and non-clinical settings, for example in Alliance for the Mentally Ill (AMI) meetings or other community settings (Lefley, 1988; Wasow, 1990). Lefley (1988) recommends "bilateral training" experiences, in which trainees learn from families in seminars and other non-clinical contacts.

Each domain—knowledge, skill and attitudes—should be taught with a combination of didactic seminars, case conferences and clinical experiential methods. Clinical experiences with families should be longitudinal, of at least 6 months to one year in duration (Faulkner et al., 1989; Lefley, 1988). Ideally, trainees should have experiences with families in both acute care settings (inpatient unit, emergency room, walk-in clinic) and continuity care settings (outpatient clinics, community placements). It is recommended that trainees work with families of one's own assigned patient (Faulkner et al., 1989) as well as with families for which there is no direct responsibility for the mentally ill member (Lefley, 1988). Trainees need experience in both family education and family therapy, so they are familiar with the different skills necessary in these quite different approaches.

IMPLEMENTATION OF THE CURRICULUM—A CASE STUDY

The challenge is to implement these recommendations within existing training programs. Johnson (1990) describes a Clinical Psychology training program in which all students have a basic exposure to concepts and knowledge and experience with basic skills, while a subgroup obtain specialty or expert training (Cohen, 1985; cited in Johnson, 1990). Because many of our graduates will be working with seriously mentally persons in the future, we decided to integrate the family training curriculum within the existing training program, rather than to develop a specialty track. Thus, all trainees receive a basic exposure to family issues and family collaboration skills.

The training curriculum in the Psychiatry Department at Baylor College of Medicine provides a case study in curriculum implementation. The Department of Psychiatry has a long history of training in community psychiatry, with a year long seminar in community and administrative psychiatry, and another on cultural and ethnic issues. As part of the community seminar, residents visit local psychosocial and clubhouse programs, and meet with representatives from consumer groups. Residents spend part of the PGY 3 year in a public community clinic setting working with the seriously mentally ill. However, despite the breadth of training in community psychiatry and a clear commitment to the seriously mentally ill, there was no systematic training in family collaboration until 1990.

We began by offering a didactic seminar to PGY 1's on the family and serious mental illness. Offered twice a year to two small groups of psychiatry residents, the seminar includes background about family—professional relationships, impact of theories of psychopathology on the family, a presentation from an AMI member about the resources of AMI and the function of family support, the experience of living with a mentally ill person, introduction to family education, and discussion of techniques to build collaboration with families. At the time of this seminar, residents are in the midst of a very challenging emergency psychiatry rotation in a public hospital. Discussion of ongoing cases allows residents to practice implementing new collaborative skills.

A second didactic seminar on family therapy is given to all third year residents and social work interns, and those psychology interns who elect the Family Transition Program rotation. Conceptualized originally as a survey course, the emphasis now integrates family coping and adaptation and crisis/transition theories. Topics include such areas as family development, crisis and transition, collaborative assessment of family needs, distinguishing family crisis from chronic maladaptive coping, systems and structural family theory, family education and family therapy techniques. The focus is on integration of concepts, and how to apply these concepts to each family's unique situation.

A key clinical component of the training in family collaboration is the Family Transition Program, a clinical rotation within the adult psychiatric outpatient clinic which was begun in 1990. Staffed by psychiatry residents (PGY 3's), social work interns and psychology interns, the family program offers short term family counseling and education to families who are in the midst of a crisis or transition. As a part of a general adult psychiatric clinic, the Family Program sees families with many different types of problems, such as parent-young adult conflict, separation or divorce, substance abuse, physical illness and aging, and in over 40% of referrals, serious mental illness. This diversity affords trainees the opportunity to learn to assess crisis responses, to help families face transitions, to become comfortable with educational interventions with families, as well as to work with families with a variety of problems. Trainees work closely with each other as cotherapists and consultants in an interdisciplinary setting, in a 6 month or one-year rotation. This fosters a deeper sense of collaboration and connection between disciplines.

In addition to the clinical experience, the Family Transition Program includes a monthly inservice training seminar, which has featured speakers from consumer groups (e.g., AMI, DMDA, Houston Council on Alcoholism), community resource programs, and experts in family therapy from other local training institutions. This series is designed to give trainees a sense of the wider context in which they work, including knowledge of community resources and of other professional collaborators.

With the success of the Family Transition Program came the realization that we needed to implement a family educational component and family collaboration training in the outpatient clinic associated with the public hospital. Not only do trainees need direct experience in family education, but this was also a service needed in our community. Both psychiatry residents and psychology interns serve in the county hospital clinic, seeing patients on follow-up from their inpatient stays. Medication management, brief crisis oriented therapy and ongoing supportive therapy are offered here. In the family training component, trainees are involved as coleaders and presenters in a multifamily educational series and receive supervision in family collaboration. Experience in an educational group clearly teaches the difference between education and therapy, and their essential interdependence in this population. Trainees in such groups invariably gain a deeper respect for the coping resources of the family and the difficulties with which they struggle. The addition of supervision in family consultation provides the integrated longitudinal family collaboration experience that is recommended by Faulkner, et al., (1989) and Lefley (1988).

Another step in the implementation of a comprehensive curriculum is to review the overall goals and objectives of the Psychiatry and Psychology training programs to ascertain if training in family collaboration is included in a comprehensive enough way. As Johnson (1990) noted, review of existing courses and clinical rotations can suggest ways to provide exposure or experience within these pre-existing experiences. For example, the emergency psychiatry rotation could be structured to include more systematic family crisis collaboration, while continuity clinic rotations could offer experience in longer term family collaboration as recommended by Faulkner, et al., (1989). Further development of the curriculum for psychology intern training, for example in the internship topic seminar and inpatient rotations would also be desirable.

As our curriculum case example illustrates we are in the process of developing a comprehensive curriculum in family collaboration in a stepwise fashion at our training site. In so doing we are gradually building the interest and commitment of the wider faculty, although we began with the commitment from those involved directly in planning curriculum. Outreach to the public sector and community groups is ongoing, as we build those linkages so important in any effective collaboration.

OBSTACLES TO CURRICULUM IMPLEMENTATION

There are a number of obstacles to implementing such a comprehensive curriculum. First among them is the already full training schedule. Seminar time is extremely full as training directors struggle to include everything that the general psychologist or psychiatrist needs in a brief period. Topics must be presented succinctly to be realistic about seminar hours. At times, all that is necessary is a shift of emphasis in existing seminars. As Johnson (1990) has noted it is helpful to meet with seminar leaders and discuss possibilities of integrating or adding mention of these topics or themes in existing courses. Integration of collaborative thinking into clinical rotations, once begun, will hopefully seem natural rather than extra.

Another obstacle to implementing a comprehensive curriculum is the fragmentation of training often experienced by social work interns, psychology interns and psychiatry residents. Clinical experiences are offered in rotations at multiple sites and courses for psychiatry residents often have multiple teachers with brief exposures to material. For the psychology interns, who come to their internship year with widely different training backgrounds, didactic materials are typically presented in topic seminars and inservice training formats rather than comprehensive courses. Social work interns typically come to the Baylor training experience with a comprehensive didactic background in family theory but with little hands on experience in clinical work with families. The challenge then is to present key ideas organized in a set of integrated cognitive and clinical experiences so that all trainees are exposed to the same ideas and then can develop or practice skills under supervision.

Two other obstacles to implementing a comprehensive curriculum are overload of trainees and isolation from other disciplines. If students have too large a caseload, they may cope by "cutting the frills". Activities such as family meetings and collaboration with community resources may be given short shrift or delegated to permanent staff in clinics and hospitals. Often young professionals under these circumstances feel that they should "handle it alone", a feeling that can block their ability to hear family input and to be able to work effectively with collaborators. It is important, therefore, that case loads be realistic enough so that trainees can learn and practice family collaboration (Neilson et al., 1981). Clinical experiences which encourage teamwork, such as our family clinic, also help trainees learn to work together.

Another problem is that of negative practice, when inexperienced trainees have unsuccessful or traumatic clinical experiences which can cement undesirable skills. Therefore, it is vital that trainees have didactic information and appropriate supervision in family collaboration early in their training to avert the development of undesirable skills, avoidance behaviors or negative attitudes toward families.

One other obstacle to implementing such training is the image of family therapy or a family clinic as associated primarily with child services. We must educate our colleagues as to the purpose and unique need for this type of family training. Family therapy experiences in a child guidance clinic or in a substance abuse program typically have a very different emphasis and the skills and attitudes learned there are frequently not applicable to the families of the seriously mentally ill.

Finally, with the cost of treatment skyrocketing, services have become increasingly compartmentalized. Patients are seen in very brief contacts, such as quarterly medication checks, for which psychiatry residents complain they are mere "medication dispensers." Family collaboration and family and patient education are time consuming and seen as expensive. Research to test the economic impact of family collaboration, over the long term, might be helpful to clarify short term and long term costs. Further, we must continue to advocate for good clinical practice, and not allow costs to completely dictate care.

SUMMARY

In summary, in this chapter I have discussed the need for training mental health professionals in a "collaborative model" (Lefley, 1988) of working with families of a seriously mentally ill member. Using the theories of coping and adaptation and family crisis and transition, we lay the groundwork for understanding what families experience when they are caring for a mentally ill member. An outline for comprehensive curriculum was suggested and specific content for didactic seminars and clinical experiences was presented. Our experience in the Psychiatry Department at Baylor College of Medicine in the development of such a curriculum, which is ongoing, was presented as a case study and some of the obstacles to implementation were discussed. It is our mission to train mental health professionals in these family collaboration skills in order to better serve both the primary consumers and the families who are beset by mental illness. We hope that we can, in years to come, put an end to the stigma and blame which families have faced as a new generation of mental health professionals is trained in collaboration.

REFERENCES

Anderson, C. M., Hogarty, G. E., & Reiss, D. J. (1980). Family treatment of adult schizophrenic patients: A psycho-educational approach. *Schizophrenia Bulletin, 6,* 490-505.

Bernheim, K. F. & Lehman, A. F. (1985). *Working with families of the mentally ill.* New York: W. W. Norton.

Carter, B. & McGoldrick, M. (Eds.) (1989). *The changing family life cycle: A framework for family therapy* (2nd ed.). Needham Heights, MA: Allyn and Bacon.

Caplan, G. (1964). *Principles of preventive psychiatry.* New York: Basic Books, pp. 38-55.

Cole, S. A. & Cole, D. S. (1987). Professionals who work with families of the chronic mentally ill: Current status and suggestions for clinical training. In A. B. Hatfield & H. P. Lefley (Eds.), *Families of the mentally ill: Coping and adaptation* (pp. 278-306). New York: Guilford Press.

Cutler, D. L., Bloom, J. D., & Shore, J. H. (1981). Training psychiatrists to work with community support systems for chronically mentally ill persons. *American Journal of Psychiatry*, *138*, 98-101.

Doll, W. (1976). Family coping with the mentally ill: An unanticipated problem of deinstitutionalization. *Hospital and Community Psychiatry*, *27*, 183-185.

Faulkner, L. R., Cutler, D. L., Krohn, D. D., Factor, R. M., Goldfinger, S. M., Goldman, C. R., Lamb, H. R., Lefley, H., Minkoff, K., Schwartz, S. R., Shore, J. H., & Tasman, A. (1989). A basic residency curriculum concerning the chronically mentally ill. *American Journal of Psychiatry*, *146*, 1323-1327.

Golan, N. (1978). *Treatment in crisis situations*. New York: Free Press.

Group for the Advancement of Psychiatry. (1993). *Resident's guide to treatment of people with chronic mental illness*. (Report No. 136). Washington, D.C.: American Psychiatric Press.

Hansell, N. (1976). Enhancing adaptational work during service. In R. G. Hirschowitz & B. Levy (Eds.) *The changing mental health scene* (pp. 93-144). New York: Spectrum Publications.

Hatfield, A. B. (1978). Psychological costs of schizophrenia to the family. *Social Work*, September, 355-359.

Hatfield, A. B. (1979). The family as partner in the treatment of mental illness. *Hospital and Community Psychiatry*, *30*, 338-340.

Hatfield, A. B. (1983). What families want of family therapists. In W. R. McFarlane (Ed.) *Family therapy in schizophrenia* (pp. 41-63). New York: Guilford Press.

Hatfield, A. B. (1987). Coping and adaptation: A conceptual framework for understanding families. In A. B. Hatfield & H. P. Lefley, (Eds.) *Families of the mentally ill: Coping and adaptation* (pp. 60-84). New York: Guilford Press.

Hatfield, A. (1990). *Family education in mental illness*. New York: Guilford Press.

Hetherington, E. M., Stanley-Hagan, M. & Anderson, E. R. (1989). Marital transitions: A child's perspective. *American Psychologist*, *44*, 303-312.

Hill, R. (1958). Social stresses on the family, *Social Casework*, *39*, 139-150.

Hirschowitz, R. (1976). Groups to help people cope with the tasks of transition. In R. G. Hirschowitz & B. Levy (Eds.) *The changing mental health scene* (pp. 171-188). New York: Spectrum Publications.

Johnson, D. L. (1990). Response to "Key issues for training in psychology for service to the seriously mentally ill." In H. P. Lefley, (Ed.),

Clinical training in serious mental illness (pp. 64-71). National Institute of Mental Health, (DHHS Pub. No. ADM 90-1679). Washington, D.C.: U.S. Government Printing Office.

Konanc, J. T., & Warren, N. J. (1984). Graduation: transitional crisis for mildly developmentally disabled adolescents and their families. *Family Relations, 33,* 135-142.

Langsley, D. G., & Kaplan, D. M. (1968). *The treatment of families in crisis.* New York: Grune and Stratton.

Langsley, D. G., Pittman, F. S., Machotka, P., & Flomenhaft, K. (1968). Family crisis therapy—results and implications. *Family Process, 7,* 145-158.

Lazarus R. S., & Folkman, S. (1984). *Stress, Appraisal, and Coping.* New York: Spring Publishing.

Lefley, H. P. (1987). Impact of mental illness in families of mental health professionals. *Journal of Nervous and Mental Disease, 175,* 613-619.

Lefley, H. P. (1988). Training professionals to work with families of chronic patients. *Community Mental Health Journal, 24,* 338-357.

Lefley, H. P. (1989). Family burden and family stigma in major mental illness. *American Psychologist. 44,* 556-560.

Lefley, H. P. & Johnson, D. (Eds.). (1990). *Families as allies in treatment of the mentally ill: New directions for mental health professionals.* Washington, D.C.: American Psychiatric Press.

Lindemann, E. (1944). Symptomatology and management of acute grief. *American Journal of Psychiatry, 101,* 141-148.

McFarlane, W. R. (1983). Multiple family therapy in schizophrenia. In. W. R. McFarlane, (Ed.) *Family therapy in schizophrenia* (pp. 141-172). New York: Guilford Press.

National Institute of Mental Health. (1990). *Clinical training in serious mental illness.* H. P. Lefley, (Ed.) (DHHS Publication. No. ADM 90-1679). Washington, D.C.: U.S. Government Printing Office.

Nielsen, A. C., III, Stein, L. I., Talbott, J. A., Lamb, H. R., Osser, D. N., & Glazer, W. M. (1981). Encouraging psychiatrists to work with chronic patients: Opportunities and limitations of residency education. *Hospital & Community Psychiatry, 32,* 767-775.

Olshansky, S. (1962). Chronic sorrow: A response to having a mentally defective child. *Social Casework, 43,* 190-193.

Parad, H. J. & Caplan, G. (1965). A framework for studying families in crisis. In H. J. Parad (Ed.), *Crisis intervention: Selected readings* (pp. 53-72). New York: Family Service Association of America.

Pittman, F. S. (1987). *Turning points: Treating families in transition and crisis.* New York: W. W. Norton.

Rapoport, L. (1970). Crisis intervention as a mode of brief treatment, In R. W. Roberts & R. H. Nee (Eds.), *Theories of social casework* (pp. 265-311). New York: University of Chicago Press.

Spaniol, L. (1987). Coping strategies of family caregivers. In A. B. Hatfield & H. P. Lefley, (Eds.) *Families of the mentally ill: Coping and adaptation* (pp. 208-222). New York: Guilford Press.

Terkelsen, K. G. (1983). Schizophrenia and the family: II. Adverse effects of family therapy. *Family Process, 22,* 191-200.

Terkelsen, K. G. (1987). The evolution of family responses to mental illness through time. In A. B. Hatfield & H. P. Lefley, (Eds.) *Families of the mentally ill: Coping and adaptation* (pp. 151-166). New York: Guilford Press.

Tessler, R. C. Killian, L. M., Gubman, G. D. (1987). Stages in family response to mental illness: An ideal type. *Psychosocial Rehabilitation Journal, 10,* 3-16.

Thompson, E. H., & Doll, W. (1982). The burden of families coping with the mentally ill: An invisible crisis. *Family Relations, 31,* 379-388.

Umana, R. F., Gross, S. J., McConville, M.T. (1980). *Crisis in the family: Three approaches.* New York: Gardner Press.

Wasow, M. (1990). A curriculum guide for fieldwork in chronic mental illness. In H. P. Lefley & D. L. Johnson (Eds.), *Families as allies in the treatment of the mentally ill: New directions for mental health professionals* (pp. 223-239). Washington, D.C.: American Psychiatric Press.

Weintraub, W., Harbin, H. T., Book, J., Nyman, G. W. Karahasan, A., Krajewski, T., & Regan, B. L. (1984). The Maryland plan for recruiting psychiatrists into public service. *American Journal of Psychiatry, 141,* 91-94.

Wikler, L., Wasow, M. & Hatfield, E. (1981). Chronic sorrow revisited: Attitudes of parents and professionals about adjustment to mental retardation. *American Journal of Orthopsychiatry, 51,* 63-70.

Wynne, L. C. (1983). A phase-oriented approach to treatment with schizophrenics and their families. In W.R. McFarlane (Ed.) *Family therapy in schizophrenia* (pp. 251-265). New York: Guilford Press.

Chapter 16

CURRENT ISSUES IN FAMILY RESEARCH: CAN THE BURDEN OF MENTAL ILLNESS BE RELIEVED?

Dale L. Johnson

That serious mental illnesses such as schizophrenia, bipolar disorder or major depression constitute a burden for those who live with or have caretaker responsibilities for the person who has the mental illness has been attested to many times by family members. Just what the burden is, what characteristics of the illness are burdensome, when burden is greatest, and how the burden affects family members are questions that call for answers from research. The research literature on burden of mental illness on the family has been reviewed several times, most comprehensively by Fadden, Bebbington and Kuipers (1987), Johnson (1990), and Maurin and Boyd (1990). This chapter will review the most recent research on burden and give additional attention to affective disorders. This review update is intended to provide a context for the extent and weight of family burden, but the main purpose of the chapter is to review interventions designed to ease burden.

TYPES OF FAMILY BURDEN

The term "burden" has been used in several ways. Serious mental illness may be seen as a burden for the person afflicted with the illness (e.g., Clayton, 1990) or as a burden on the state (e.g., Mendelewicz, 1989; Shen, Chen, Zhang, Xi, et al., 1990; Stoudemire, et al. 1986). In general, however, the burden literature has dealt with the difficulties caused by mental illness as experienced by near relatives of people who have a mental illness and who either live with the person or have a continuing responsibility for and/or emotional tie to the person.

The division of burden into two types, objective and subjective, was suggested by Hoenig and Hamilton (1966). According to Schene (1990)

309

"...objective burden..is regarded as the symptoms and behavior of mental patients within their social environment, and their consequences. Subjective burden relates to the psychological consequences for the family." (p. 289) Objective burden includes characteristics of the person with mental illness such as the presence and severity of positive or negative symptoms (Raj, Kulhara & Avasthi, 1991), but it also includes effects of mental illness on such aspects of the social environment as household routines, family relations, social relations, leisure time, work, finances, and children and siblings (Schene, 1990). There is general agreement that subjective burden includes effects upon the psychological state or physical health of the caretaking person. Thus, depression or anxiety associated with care for a person with a mental illness are considered subjective burden.

RECENT BURDEN RESEARCH

In their reviews of the family burden literature to 1990, Fadden, Bebbington and Kuipers (1987), Johnson (1990) and Maurin and Boyd (1990) are in agreement that there are many problems associated with living with mental illness, with consequences for social and leisure activities, financial standing, and personal distress. Recent research has added to those assessments (see Table 1). In a creative approach to the problem, Raj, Kulhara and Avasthi (1991) categorized patients with schizophrenia into either positive symptom or negative symptom groups. Then, the burden reported by the relatives of the two groups of patients, 30 in each, were compared at intake and follow-up. At intake, the two relatives' groups were found to be quite similar in amount of both objective and subjective burden, but at follow-up the relatives of negative symptom patients had higher levels of both types of burden.

MacCarthy, LeSage, Brewin, Brugha, Mangen and Wing (1989) in a community survey of 45 relatives of long-time users of psychiatric services found high levels of objective and subjective burden. The most common problems had to do with the patient's dependency and lack of social skills. Sixty-two percent of the caretakers reported adverse effects on their own mental health. This report also provides an unusually rich account of the types of burden experienced.

Families of patients with who had schizophrenia for not more than two years were included in research by Birchwood and Cochrane (1990). The 53 families in this sample were found to be highly stressed by the disturbed behavior of their relatives. Stress was high overall and for 38% of the respondents stress levels were in the "pathological range."

Gopinath and Chaturvedi (1992) found high levels of objective burden in their research with families in Bangalore, India. Common problems were the patient's not doing any work, not doing household tasks, poor personal hygiene, and slowness. They also found that relatives with more education were more often distressed by the behavior of the patient.

Relatives (n = 19) who had a family member ready for discharge from an extended-care facility were the subjects of research by Solomon, Beck and Gordon (1988). They found high levels of concern, chiefly about the patients not having a highly structured supervised living arrangement when released to the community. Families were prepared to provide some assistance to the patient when in the community, but did not feel they could assume a major role in providing care.

These recent reports have added to the literature on burden by including more community surveys and more representative samples of relatives of psychiatric patients. There is little evidence, however, of measurement improvement and sample sizes continue to be small. No attention has been given to changes in burden as a function of adaptation to a continuing problem, or to differential response to acute crises versus day-to-day coping.

Despite these methodological problems, the findings are consistent with the earlier literature in supporting the contention that life with a person who has a serious mental illness is burdensome for relatives of the person.

Depression

Most of the research on family burden has not provided breakdowns of results by patient diagnosis. When diagnoses are reported it is apparent that most of the patients have schizophrenia. There are a few reports of patient groups other than schizophrenia, depression being the most prevalent.

Although the study by Jacob, Frank, Kupfer and Carpenter (1987) of 112 relatives and friends of people suffering from depression and taking part in a depression treatment research project did not have a control group, it is still clear that the burden associated with depression is great. Fifty-nine percent said the depressed person's behavior was often or almost always a source of worry.

Fadden, Bebbington and Kuipers (1987) examined the burden experienced by 24 spouses of patients with one of three types of depression: bipolar, unipolar or neurotic. Loss of income associated with the illness was a major problem as was restriction of social activities. What is most striking about these results is that so many areas of married life were adversely affected by the depression. Coping with the symptoms of bipolar disorder was especially difficult. The authors note that despite a burden so great that one-third felt they could not continue the relationship, few spouses had complained to service providers or had asked for help for themselves.

Coyne, Kessler, Tal, Turnbull, Wortman and Greden (1987) conducted research with 42 near relatives of depressed people who were in an affective episode and who were compared with 23 relatives who had had similar disorders, but were not in an episode. They found that 40 percent of the people living with a person who was currently depressed were also sufficiently distressed to meet criteria for psychiatric referral. This effect was not found for the control group. The distress was attributed to annoyance about the depression, worry about recurrence, feeling fatigued, and being discouraged by the depressed person's sense of hopelessness and lack of interest in things. The choice of a control group made up of relatives of people who had been psychiatrically disturbed, but were currently in remission, and the finding that these relatives were not perturbed by behavior of the one-time patient supports the observation that it is the level of the patient's symptomatology that is important in burden assessment.

Chakrabarti, Kulhara and Verma (1992) found in a study with 90 families that burden was greater for families of patients with bipolar disorder than those whose family member had another form of affective disorder, but that nearly all families reported moderate to severe burden. They also found that the amount of dysfunction shown by the patient was correlated (r = .62) with amount of burden experienced.

Discussion of Recent Burden Research

These results are consistent in showing that affective disorders are causes of burden in family members. Although no direct comparisons of affective disorders and schizophrenia were included in these studies, it seems that the two types of disorders do not differ in amount of burden experienced. There is, of course, room for research on this matter. There is one common feature: extent and degree of burden appears to be related to the amount of patient dysfunction. On this matter, Brown, Bone, Dallison, and Wing, (1966), Chakrabarti, et al. (1992), and Pai and Kapur (1982) are in agreement.

BURDEN AMELIORATION

Many of the reports on family burden conclude by recommending that families receive education about mental illness and training in coping with difficult behaviors (e.g., Gopinath & Chaturvedi, 1992; Mac-Carthy et al., 1989). This review includes all available publications that reported attempts to relieve family burden (Table 1).

For inclusion in this review, the intervention had to include results on family burden. Attempts to help the person with mental illness without mention of family burden were not included, nor were family-focused studies if they did not include an attempt to alleviate burden.

Family Focused Interventions

The interventions in this category focused on the relatives and did not include the people with mental illness in the program. Three studies reported positive intervention effects.

Abramowitz and Coursey (1989) used a six-session educational support program based on a stress-coping framework with 24 relatives of people with schizophrenia. The relatives were trained in problem-solving skills for managing patient behavior and provided with information about how to gain access to resources. The control group (n = 24 was matched with the experimental group and assigned to a waiting list. At the end of the program, experimental group members were significantly less anxious, less distressed, and made more use of community resources. There were no differences in negative feelings toward the patient or generalized sense of efficacy. The use of a waiting list control group precluded a follow-up of the results.

Pakenham and Dadds (1987) used a supportive educational program with relatives of people with schizophrenia who were living in the home. The study used multiple measures of burden and positive results were claimed for several of the variables, but there were only 7 participants in the study and there was no control group.

The largest study of this type was conducted by researchers with the New Jersey Division of Mental Health and Hospitals (Reisser, Minsky & Schorske, 1991). Eight community programs were invited to develop packages of services for families of people with serious mental illnesses, e.g., schizophrenia or affective disorders. These services were to include individual family consultations and could also include respite services, family psychoeducation groups, family support groups or advocacy and referral consultation. During the six month study period, 376 families received services and research data were gathered on 191 of these families. The intention was to have 20 families sampled from each program or 160 families, but some programs overresponded. Several measures were used in a design that called for pre, 3-month and 6-month assessment. Unfortunately, no control group was used and there was no follow-up. Families made use of a wide range of services offered, but single family consultation was preferred by the greatest number of families (91%). The family psychoeducation group was used by 49% and the support group by 37%. Respite care was least popular (14%). Significant reductions were found for all measures of burden. However, the item receiving the highest concern score, "Worry about the ill family member's future" continued at the end of the program to be at the top of the list of concerns. Concern about crisis management was reduced substantially, but other objective burden items were not changed. Satisfaction with services improved significantly and measures of the psychiatric status of ill family members showed positive changes. The authors noted the persistence of concerns related to several issues: need for housing, stigma of mental illness, and planning for the future. The results of this study are interesting, but the lack of a control group makes it impossible to conclude that the results were a function of the program. Another problem is that the program elements were inadequately described in the report. "Psychoeduational groups" may mean different things to different people and as Lam (1991) has pointed out, different forms of family education may have different outcomes. Finally, it is unfortunate that no measures of subjective burden were included.

Three other interventions reported no effects on burden. A family education approach was used by Posner, Wilson, Kral, Lander and McIlwraith (1992) with relatives of people with schizophrenia. Fifty-five families were assigned randomly to either a family education group or a control group. At the end of the program, families in the special program had greater knowledge about schizophrenia and were more satisfied with services provided than were members of the control group. However, subjective burden, coping behavior, and family satisfaction were not affected by the program.

MacCarthy, Kuipers, Hurry, Harper and LeSage (1989) used a single home session followed by 10 monthly group sessions with families of people with mental illnesses. At the end of the program, compared to a control group of 17 families, the 13 discussion group families showed lower expressed emotion and positive changes in coping styles. The samples were small, the report of changes in coping styles lacked quantification, and there was no evidence that burden was eased.

Smith and Birchwood (1987) used a 4-session educational program that included a videotape on schizophrenia and booklets presenting information on the illness and ways of coping. Families were assigned randomly, 20 in each group, to this group or to a control group which received the printed materials by mail. Family members in the educational groups acquired more knowledge about schizophrenia than control families, but the groups did not differ in level of burden experienced at the end of the program or at the 6-month follow-up.

Reports of several other interventions were found in a PsycLIT bibliographic search, but only the abstracts of the reports were read as the journals in which they appeared could not be located in a search in four university libraries. Therefore, the results are mentioned only briefly. Orhagen and D'Elia (1992) developed an educational program for relatives of people with schizophrenia. The 6 session program resulted in changes in expressed emotion for the 47 participants, but there were no effects on subjective burden, coping methods, or patient relapse. Glick and associates (1990) reported that family burden was eased with inpatient family intervention. Rao, Barnabas and Gopinath (1988) found a decrease in financial burden and burden associated with routine activities and leisure for 19 families that made use of a day treatment center for the disturbed family member. Sidley, Smith and Howells (1991) compared two educational "packages" in a study with 18 relatives of people with schizophrenia. They concluded, "Both educational programs were associated with significant gains in knowledge per se (but not in functional knowledge) and significant positive changes in families' beliefs about their own role in the treatment process." (p. 305).

Patient and Family Focused Interventions
Smith and Birchwood (1987) found that their educational sessions did not ease burden, but that both experimental and control group reported less burden at the post-test time. The authors did not report correlates of this drop in burden. It may have resulted from changes in the severity of the patient's illness or from adaptation to the illness by the relatives. These results suggest that the key to reducing burden may be in improving the patient's condition, especially when the program provides the family with some guidance, consultation, or training.

The Wisconsin Training in Community Living program (Test & Stein, 1980) consisted of training psychiatric patients to live in the community. Training was conducted in the community and hospitalization was used minimally. The evaluation of the program included a few measures with 28 experimental group and 21 control group relatives. At 1 and 4 months after initiation of the program, objective burden on the families was assessed through interviews. There were no statistically significant differences between groups at either time. No attempt was made to measure subjective burden.

A program in Australia (Reynolds & Hoult, 1984) was based on the Stein and Test Training in Community Living model (Stein & Test, 1978). This study compared 120 patients and families who had been assigned randomly to experimental or control groups. The experimental condition consisted of community treatment and training for patients by an team of professionals. Families received guidance by the staff in home visits. The control group received conventional hospital treatment. Experimental group patients did better than controls as assessed by several measures. Families of relatives in the community living group were "very satisfied" with the treatment, and more believed their family member had "greatly improved." They were also more inclined to say they had received enough information to help them cope with the problems presented by the patient. In addition, community program relatives reported significantly less worry. Nevertheless, there were no group differences in reported objective burden such as disruption of work, social life or daily routines. These burdens declined for both groups.

Falloon and Pederson (1985) reported results of a study that goes a step further in working with families as well as the patient. The University of Southern California project (Falloon, Boyd & McGill, 1984) was designed explicitly to improve the quality of life of patients with schizophrenia and their relatives. They found decreases in subjective burden as measured by a global subjective burden scale at the end of the program and at two-year follow-up. Similar positive results were obtained for family coping behaviors. This study included only 17 families each in the experimental and control groups.

Carpentier, Lesage, Goulet, Lalonde and Renaud (1992) used a case control design to assess the impact of a comprehensive program consisting of psychoeducation elements and extensive case management. Program families were compared with conventional care for the relatives of young patients with schizophrenia. Group assignment was random after matching source groups of patients for gender, age and number of previous hospital admissions. There were 15 families in the comprehensive program and 22 families in the control group. Relatives in the comprehensive program reported feeling less burden, had more contact with professionals, and had less need for further services. These results were obtained despite lack of significant differences for patients in the two groups. There was no mention of the time of assessment in the service delivery process.

Pai and Kapur (1982) compared burden experienced by relatives of patients with schizophrenia who were treated in a hospital with those treated at home. Groups were assigned randomly (n = 27 families in each condition) and there were no pre-intervention differences. Somewhat surprisingly, the families in the home-treatment condition reported less burden at post-test. The authors attribute this result to the use of nurses as home visitors who not only attended to the needs of the patients, but provided the families with counseling and guidance on an on-going basis.

Several other treatment programs have had potential for relieving burden in that they have many features of the program reported by Falloon and Spencer (1985), but these other programs have not reported results for family burden. McFarlane (1990) commented that Psychoeducational Multifamily Groups "...can have equally positive effects on family burdens." (p. 174) and went on to say that "...both the sense and reality of burden are reduced" (p. 174). Although burden was specifically measured, in Chapter 11 of this book McFarlane suggests that the sharing and social network expansion of multi-family groups are important factors in reducing burden.

The family psychoeducational programs of Leff, Kuipers, Berkowitz and Sturgeon (1985), Tarrier and associates (1989) and Hogarty and associates (1991) found to be essentially as effective in reducing relapse in patients as Falloon's program (Falloon, Boyd & McGill, 1984), have not reported effects on family burden.

Discussion of Intervention Research

What can be made of these diverse intervention results? First, it is difficult to make direct comparisons between intervention studies because methods differ greatly. Nevertheless, the results provide something more than hints about to how to develop effective programs. Interventions that focus only on the family had mixed results. Only the intervention of Abramowitz and Coursey (1989) demonstrated positive effects with appropriate controls and adequate sample sizes. In contrast, several other investigators using equally adequate methods did not find significant effects on burden (Posner, et al., 1992; MacCarthy, et al., 1989; Smith & Birchwood, 1987) and for methodological reasons two other studies (Reisser, Minsky & Schorske, 1991; Pakenham & Dadds, 1987) did not produce convincing results.

It might be noted in passing that despite the common perception that mutual support group/advocacy organizations such as the National Alliance for the Mentally Ill (NAMI) are effective in reducing burden (e.g., Lyles, Ware & Breen, 1989) only one project (Reisser et al., 1991) even mentioned such an organization and the analyses of data from that project did not reveal whether NAMI membership had an independent effect on burden. NAMI-type organizations might be effective in reducing family burden, especially for those members who are active over the long-term, but the issue has not been tested.

Projects that focused on the family and patient together provided the best, albeit still mixed, results. The most positive outcomes for burden were obtained by Falloon and Peterson (1985), Carpentier and associates (1992), and Pai and Kapur (1982). The two Training in Community Living programs provided encouraging results, but did not alleviate burden. The difference in outcomes between the first three projects in this section and the latter two may be in amount of attention given families. Families were a major focus of attention in the Falloon and Peterson project and in all three of these successful projects families received information about the mental illness of their relative and consultation and guidance about how to cope with the relative's behaviors. These resources were also provided in the Training in Community Living projects, but judging from the reports family contacts were fewer and less intense. In contrast to the family-focused projects, the family and patient projects all provided assistance to families in their homes.

The results should not be unexpected. They are in accord with other program evaluation outcomes that deal with problems that essentially involve relationships between closely associated individuals. For example, marital therapy is more effective when both partners are treated together than when treated separately (Jacobson & Margolin, 1979) and treatment of child behavior problems is most effective when child and parent are mutually involved in treatment (e.g., Barkley, 1992; Sanders & Dadds, 1993).

PROSPECTS FOR THE REDUCTION OF BURDEN

The research reviewed provides some evidence that interventions have been successful in reducing the burden on families associated with mental illness. However, the evidence is still thin and the research does not set new standards for quality. The sample sizes tend to be small, several of the studies lacked control groups and follow-ups were seldom conducted (See Table 1). Perhaps most importantly, there continues to be uncertainty about just what constitutes burden (Maurin and Boyd, 1990; Schene, 1990). Until that issue is resolved better it is unlikely that strong intervention programs will emerge. Quite obviously, this is an immature research area.

Theory Development

An important first step for progress is that the area of burden be reconceptualized in terms of stress and stress reduction. In effect this means regarding what has been termed subjective burden as the result of stress and the object of preventive efforts. Behaviors and events considered as objective burden would be viewed as stressors. Viewed in this way, the role theory framework, the Double ABCX model, of McCubbin and Peterson (1983) may be useful in ordering components of stress. The stress and coping theory of Lazarus and Folkman (1984) provides further conceptual guidance.

The question arises as to whether the relief of burden is really prevention. In primary prevention the intervention occurs before the onset of symptoms with a population at risk for an illness or disorder. For most families, probably all, the discovery that a loved one has developed a serious mental illness is a shock that requires time for adaptation. How the patient's illness proceeds and how the family member adapts determines whether the traumatic event becomes an illness or disorder. Quite likely scores on measures of depression or demoralization would reflect that shock. Thus, prevention of disorders related to the burden of mental illness would constitute primary prevention for some people and early secondary prevention for others. In either case, the intervention would be directed at removing or minimizing stressful events associated with living with a person who has a serious mental illness.

Service Delivery

It is apparent from the research on interventions reviewed here that it is possible for professionals working from hospitals or community clinics to provide burden alleviation services. There is little evidence that this practice has become common; indeed, it continues to be unusual despite the calls for these interventions by those who have done burden research. Apparently, professionals responsible for the deployment of services are not yet convinced that these services are necessary, effective, or as important as providing services to the primary client. Making a convincing case may depend upon the stronger evidence that could result from a well-designed preventive intervention. There is little evidence that service providers see the relatives as being at risk for psychiatric disorders. They are seen only as persons who have responsibilities for a person who has a diagnosable mental illness, and their needs continue to be more or less ignored. With rare exceptions they are not seen as individuals in their own right who happen to live with the burden of mental illness. There is a training issue involved to bring this situation to the attention of providers.

Families' Participation

There is yet another service delivery problem. Most surveys of families have shown that they want more information about mental illness and help with coping. Nevertheless, their response to workshops, training sessions and the like is often poor. This raises the question of whether families want to participate and are able to participate in programs. The desire for training/education is related to the time the program is offered during the course of the illness. McCreadie and associates (1991) invited 63 relatives of patients with schizophrenia to participate in educational sessions and support groups and found that 32 (51%) declined to take part. The authors noted that these patients were living in the community and in remission. The most common reason for declining to participate was that "things are fine at the moment." Relatives who did agree to participate had a family member who had been admitted to the hospital within the past year. On the other hand, Birchwood and Cochrane (1990) had a 100% participation response with families whose relative had a fairly recent diagnosis of schizophrenia. So timing is an important factor in families' participation.

The major diagnostic focus of the interventions review in this chapter is schizophrenia. The review of the burden of depressive illness has shown that it is great, but there is no evidence at hand to indicate whether the anticipatory response to the burden associated with depressive illness should be different from that of schizophrenia. There is need for research on this matter.

Program Components

Judging from the relative success in easing burden of some programs the following program elements are prime candidates for inclusion in prevention programs:

1. Work with patient and family.
2. Individualize interventions to accommodate to differences between families in adapting to the illness.
3. Provide information about the illnesses.
4. Provide problem solving skills as needed.
5. Provide information about access to additional resources needed by the patient or family.

6. Provide consultation about decisions to be made; e.g., whether the patient should live at home or elsewhere, whether to change from a known medication to one that is new and "promising."

In addition, although not mentioned by any of the authors of the interventions reviewed, the presence of so much distress, anxiety and depression suggests the need for specific training. Using the depression training modules developed by Rehm (1984) may add to program effectiveness.

Program Evaluation

The following changes in research on burden are suggested:

1. Larger sample sizes are needed to provide adequate statistical power and carry out subgroup analyses.
2. Random assignment to groups.
3. Follow-up of at least 6 months, but preferably longer.
4. Clear description of the program and control conditions.
5. Improved assessment of subjective burden including use of multiple measures.
6. Identification of clinical levels of distress in subjective burden.
7. Family members respond for themselves on subjective burden measures.
8. Inclusion of entire concerned family in interventions.
9. Association of burden to time in the psychiatric career of the patient. Early interventions may be better, but interventions tailored for different levels of adaptation should be provided.
10. Attention must be given to service delivery issues to account for differences in participation response rates as a function of culture, social class, and adaptation to the illness.

CONCLUSIONS

The burden associated with mental illnesses continues to be great for the family members with whom the patients live or for those having caretaking responsibilities. Interventions designed to alleviate burden show some promise, especially if they are carried out with patient and family together and provide on-going consultation and education. The time is ripe for further research staged on a stress reduction model and conducted within a prevention frame of reference.

In recommending strong interventions to relieve and prevent burden of mental illness on families it is not intended to mean that other interventions should be discontinued or neglected. Professionals should provide information, families should be referred to NAMI, and so forth, but they should be aware that the research for these efforts is not only weak, it is largely lacking. Nevertheless, the burden of mental illness is so great that families need help of all reasonable kinds. With improved research best methods of helping families can be determined.

REFERENCES

Abramowitz, I. A., & Coursey, R. D. (1989). Impact of an educational support group on family participants who take care of their schizophrenic relatives. *Journal of Consulting and Clinical Psychology, 57,* 232-236.

Barkley, R. A. (1992). *Attention-deficit hyperactivity disorder.* New York: Guilford.

Birchwood, M., & Cochrane, R. (1990). Families coping with schizophrenia: coping styles, their origins and correlates. *Psychological Medicine, 20,* 857-865.

Brewin, C. R., & Wing, J. K. (1988). *MRC Needs for care assessment manual.* London: Medical Research Council.

Carpentier, N., Lesage, A., Goulet, J., Lalonde, P., & Renaud, M. (1992). Burden of care of families not living with young schizophrenic relatives. *Hospital and Community Psychiatry, 43,* 38-43.

Cochrane, R. (1980). A comparative evaluation of the Symptom Rating Test and the Langer 22-item index for use in epidemiological surveys. *Psychological Medicine, 10,* 115-124.

Derogatis, L. R., Lipman, R. S., Rickels, K. Uhlenuth, E. H., & Covi, L. (1974). The Hopkins Symptom Checklist (HSCL): A self-report symptom inventory. *Behavioral Science, 19,* 1-15.

Fadden, G., Bebbington, P., & Kuipers, L. (1987). The burden of care: The impact of functional psychiatric illness on the patient's family. *British Journal of Psychiatry, 150,* 285-292.

Falloon, I. R. H., Boyd, C., & McGill, C. (1984). *Family care of schizophrenia.* New York: Guilford.

Falloon, I. R. H., & Pederson, J. (1985). Family management in the prevention of morbidity of schizophrenia: The adjustment of the family unit. *British Journal of Psychiatry, 147,* 156-163.

Glick, I. D., Spencer, J. H., Clarkin, J. F., Haas, G. L. et al. (1990). A randomized clinical trial of inpatient family intervention: IV. Followup results for subjects with schizophrenia. *Schizophrenia Research, 3,* 187-200.

Goldberg, D. P. (1978). *Manual of the General Health Questionnaire.* Windsor, England: NFER Publishing Co.

Gopinath, P. S., & Chaturvedi, S. K. (1992). Distressing behaviour of schizophrenics at home. *Acta Psychiatrica Scandinavica*, 86, 185-188.

Gopinath, P. S., & Charurvedi, S. K. (1986). Measurement ofd distressful psychotic symptoms perceived by the family: preliminary findings. *Indian Journal of Psychiatry*, 28, 343-345.

Greene, J. G. (1982). Measuring behavioural disturbance of elderly demented patients in the community and its effects on relatives: a factor analytic study. *Age and aging*, 11, 121-126.

Henderson, S., Byrne, D. G., & Duncan-Jones, P. (1981). *Neurosis and the social environment*. Australia: Academic Press.

Hogarty, G. E., Anderson, G. M., Reiss, D. J., Kornblith, S. J., Greenwald, D. P., Ulrich, R. F., and Carter, M. (1991). Family psychoeducation, social skills training, and maintenance chemotherapy in the aftercare treatment of schizophrenia. *Archives of General Psychiatry*, 48, 340-347.

Jacob, M., Frank, E., Kupfer, D. J., & Carpenter, L. L. (1987). Recurrent depression: An assessment of family burden and family attitudes. *Journal of Clinical Psychiatry*, 48, 395-400.

Jacobson, N. S., & Margolin, G. (1979). *Marital therapy*. New York: Brunner/Mazel.

Lyles, W. B., Ware, M. R., & Breen, M. J. (1989). Family burden. *Hospital and Community Psychiatry*, 40, 855-856.

MacCarthy, B., Kuipers, L., Hurry, J., & Harper, R., et al. (1989). Counseling the relatives of the long-term mentally ill: I. Evaluation of the impact on relatives and patients. *British Journal of Psychiatry*, 154, 768-775.

Lam, D. (1991). Psychosocial family intervention in schizophrenia: a review of empirical studies. *Psychological Medicine*, 21, 423-441.

Leff, J., Kuipers, L., Berkowitz, R., & Sturgeoun, D. (1985). A controlled trial of social intervention in the families of schizophrenic patients: Two year follow-up. *British Journal of Psychiatry*, 146, 594-600.

MacCarthy, B., & Brown, R. G. (1989). Psychosocial factors in Parkinson's disease. *British Journal of Clinical Psychology*, 148, 727-731.

MacCarthy, B., Lesage, A., Brewin, C. R., Brugha, T. S., Mangen, S., & Wing, J. K. (1989). Needs for care among the relatives of long-term users of day care: A report from the Camberwell High Contact Survey. *Psychological Medicine*, 19, 725-736.

McFarlane, W. R. (1990). Multiple family groups and the treatment of schizophrenia. In M. I. Herz, S. J. Keith and J. P. Docherty (Eds.) *Handbook of schizophrenia: Vol. 4, Psychosocial treatment of schizophrenia*. New York: Elsevier.

MacCarthy, G., Kuipers, L., Hurry, J., Harper, R., & LeSage, A. (1989). Counseling the relatives of the long-term adult mentally ill. I. Evaluation of the impact on relatives and patients. *British Journal of Psychiatry*, 154, 768-775.

Maurin, J. T., & Boyd, C. B. (1990). Burden of mental illness on the family: A critical review. *Archives of Psychiatric Nursing*, 4, 99-107.

Mendlewicz, J. (1989). The social burden of depressive disorders. *Neuropsychobiology*, 22, 178-180.

Orhagen, T. & D'Elia, G. (1992). Multifamily educational intervention in schizophrenia: Does it have any effect? *Nordisk Psykiatrisk Tidsskrift*, 46, 3-12.

Pai, S. & Kapur, R. L. (1981). The burden on the family of a psychiatric patient: development of an interview schedule. *British Journal of Psychiatry*, 138, 332-335.

Pakenham, K. I., & Dadds, M. R. (1987). Family care and schizophrenia: The effects of a supportive educational program on relatives' personal and social adjustment. *Australian and New Zealand Journal of Psychiatry*, 21, 580-590.

Pasamanick, B., Scarpitti, F., & Dinitz, S. (1967). *Schizophrenia in the community*. New York: Appleton-Century-Crofts.

Platt, S. (1985). Measuring the burden of psychiatric illness on the family: An evaluation of some rating scales. *Psychological Medicine*, 15, 383-393.

Platt, S., Weyman, A., Hirsch, S., & Hewett, S. (1980). The Social Behaviour Rating Schedule (SBAS): Rationale, contents, scoring and reliability of a new interview schedule. *Social Psychiatry*, 15, 43-55.

Posner, C. M., Wilson, K. G., Kral, M. J., Lander, S., & McIlwraith, R. D. (1992). Family psychoeducational support groups in schizophrenia. *American Journal of Orthopsychiatry*, 62, 206-218.

Raj, L., Kulhara, P., & Avasthi, A. (1991). *International Journal of Social Psychiatry*, 37, 242-250.

Rao, K., Barnabas, I. P., & Gopinath, P. S. (1988). Family burden in chronic schizophrenia: The role of the day hospital. *Indian Journal of Psychological Medicine*, 11, 131-135.

Rehm, L. P. (1984). Self-management therapy for depression. *Advances in Behaviour Therapy and Research*, 6, 83-98.

Reisser, G., Minsky, S., & Schorske, B. (1991). *Intensive family support services: A cooperative evaluation*. Bureau of Research & Evaluation Report. Trenton, NJ: New Jersey Department of Human Services.

Reynolds, I., & Hoult, J. E. (1984). The relatives of the mentally ill: A comparative trial of community-oriented and hospital-oriented psychiatric care. *Journal of Nervous and Mental Disease*, 172, 480-489.

Sanders, M. R., & Dadds, M. R. (1993). *Behavioral family intervention*. New York: Longwood.

Schene, A. H. (1990). Objective and subjective dimensions of family burden: Towards an integrative framework for research. *Social Psychiatry and Psychiatric Epidemiology*, 25, 289-297.

Shen, Y., Chen, C., Zhang, W., Xi, T., et al. (1990). An example of a community-based mental health/home-care programme: Haidian District in the suburbs of Beijing, China. *Psychosocial Rehabilitation Journal*, 14, 29-34.

Schulz, P. M., Schulz, S. C., Targum, S. D., et al. (1982). Patient and family attitudes about schizophrenia: implications for genetic counseling. *Schizophrenia Bulletin*, 8, 504-513.

Sidley, G. L., Smith, J., & Howells, K. (1991). Is it ever too late to learn? Information provision to relatives of long-term schizophrenia sufferers. *Behavioural Psychotherapy*, 19, 305-320.

Smith, J. V., & Birchwood, M. J. (1987). Specific and non-specific effects of educational intervention with families living with a schizophrenic relative. *British Journal of Psychiatry*, 150, 645-652.

Spielberger, C. D., Gorsuch, R. L., & Luschene, R. E. (1970). *The State/Trait Anxiety Inventory*. Palo Alto, CA: Consulting Psychology Press.

Stein, L. I., & Test, M. A. (Eds.) (1978). *Alternatives to mental hospital treatment*. New York: Plenum.

Stoudemire, A., Frank, R., Hedemark, N., Kamlet, M., et al. (1986). The economic burden of depression. *General Hospital Psychiatry*, 8, 387-394.

Tarrier, N. Barroughclough, C., Vaughn, C., Bamrah, J. S., Porceddu, K., Watts, S., & Freeman, H. L. (1989). Community management of schizophrenia: a two year follow-up of a behavioural intervention with families. *British Journal of Psychiatry*, 154, 625-628.

Test, M. A., & Stein, L. I. (1980). Alternative to mental hospital treatment: III. Social cost. *Archives of General Psychiatry*, 37, 409-412.

Vaughn, C., & Leff, J. P. (1976). The measurement of expressed emotion in families of psychiatric patients. *British Journal of Social and Clinical Psychology*, 15, 157-165.

TABLE 1

Methodological Characteristics of Burden Survey and Intervention Studies

Report	Burden Measure	Research Sample	Size	Control	Follow Up
Survey Research					
Raj	FBIS	Hospital Clinic	60	Yes	No
MacCarthy	CFI MCRSBS 4-NS	Clinic	45	No	No
Birchwood	Coping SRT	Hospital	53	No	No
Gopinath	SAFD	Clinic	62	No	No
Solomon	Interview	Hospital	19	No	No
Jacob	FDSD	Clinic	112	No	No
Fadden	SBAS	Hospital Clinic	24	Yes	No
Coyne	Interview HSCL-25	Clinic	42:23	Yes	No
Chakrabarti	FBIS DAQ	Hospital Clinic	90	No	No

Intervention Research

Abramowitz	STAI RSS	Clinic	24:24	Yes	No
Pakenham	SBAS	Clinic	7	No	No
Reisser	Reinhard	Clinic	160	No	No
Posner	GHQ	Hospital	28:27	Yes	No
MacCarthy	CFI MRCSBS 4-NS	Clinic	13:13	Yes	No
Smith	FDS Stress	Hospital	40	No	No
Test	FBS	Hospital Community	28:21	Yes	Yes
Reynolds	Constructed	Hospital	48:46	Yes	Yes
Falloon	SBAS HSCL-25	Clinic	18:18	Yes	Yes
Carpentier	SBAS	Clinic	15:22	Yes	No
Pai & Kapur	FBIS	Clinic	27:27	Yes	No

Abbreviations:
4-NS	Four item scale (Henderson et al., 1981)
CFI	Camberwell Family Interview (Vaughn & Leff, 1976)
FBIS	Family Burden Interview Schedule (Pai & Kupur, 1982)
FBS	Family Burden Scale (Test & Stein, 1980)
FDS	Family Distress Scale (Pasamanick, et al., 1967)
GHQ	General Health Questionnaire (Goldberg, 1978)
HSCL-25	Hopkins Symptom Checklist (Derogatis et al.,1974)
MRCSBS	MRC Social Behaviour Schedule (Brewin & Wing, 1988)
Reinhard	No reference provided
RSS	Relatives' Stress Scale (Green, 1982)

SAFD   Scale for Assessment of Family Distress (Gopinath
                  Chaturvedi, 1986)
SBAS   Social Behavior Assessment Schedule (Platt et al., 1980)
SRT   Symptom Rating Test (Cochrane, 1983)
STAI   State Trait Anxiety Inventory (Spielberger, Gorsuch &
                  Lushene, 1970)
Stress   Cochrane (1980)

PART V:

FUTURE DIRECTIONS: FAMILY, CONSUMER, AND PROVIDER RELATIONS

Chapter 17

THE CONSUMER PERSPECTIVE
ON FAMILY INVOLVEMENT

Stephen M. Kersker

The world of mental illness is changing. Persons with severe and persistent mental illnesses are recovering at an increasing rate. In this process, consumers have to learn to survive the effects of a devastating illness and a treatment system that is geared toward disability and loss of function. Mental health professionals are coming to understand that different approaches and methodologies are needed to help people recover from the long-term effects of psychiatric disorders.

It is important to begin with the obvious statement that mental health consumers were not born patients. We were born as people and it is as people that we need to be seen and experienced. This perception is growing, and new attitudes toward consumers and families are beginning to change our mental health system. Healthy conflict is part of that change. Conflict arises with regard to education, treatment, and the appropriate roles of professionals, families, and consumers in the recovery process. There are conflicts over the nature of mental illness, an individual's potential for improvement, and desired outcomes. Discussion of these issues leads to ever increasing understanding, to honesty

The author wishes to acknowledge the contributions of the following consumers. The chapter was edited by Franklin Robison, and reviewed by Jimmy Webb, Stacey Pope, Carolyn Wilson, Jeff Ryan, Mike Branche, Melinda Barrett, Joyce Williams, Gary Quick, Mark Moening, KC Phelan, Jane Terrin, and Richard Phillips. The chapter is dedicated to Bobbie Lee Clement, Lee Murrill, Eloise Scott, Gilbert Riordan, Frank Burgman, Dick Bradley, and the staff of G. Piece Wood Memorial State Hospital in Arcadia, Florida.

332 Stephen M. Kersker

and partnership of all the parties who are involved in helping our recovery.

EDUCATION

Families and consumers need to be educated about rehabilitation, treatment, and recovery. Different approaches to education are needed for parents, siblings, and consumers to reflect their various roles in the recovery process. I believe that these differences require educational themes and content to be developed separately. Through specialized education, family members may understand the effects of their behaviors and learn how to detach and distance themselves from the work that their loved ones must do in order to get better. Intervention and over-involvement by other family members may produce serious impediments to progress for individuals who have a mental illness. Because of the impact of their relationships on what is happening to us and within us, families need a crash course on what mental illness means to our lives and what it means to recover.

Families also need to understand that hospitals are not the proper places for long-term treatment. The crisis care that hospitals provide is not recovery oriented. Stabilization is not recovery. Rehabilitation and recovery can start in a treatment facility, but such settings can never support the full recovery potential of any individual. Rehabilitation and effective treatment are more likely to occur in community settings, under the most normalized conditions possible. The current development of enhanced supports for community living are allowing us to live more normal lives and experience fuller rehabilitation than practitioners thought possible just a few years ago. Families need to have their expectations adjusted upward to allow greater normalization to occur.

Education will help our families understand how to resolve their conflicts over accepting a more detached role, and will help consumers break an unhealthy reliance on others. Dependency cripples the functioning of both families and consumers. Consumers need to be allowed to go their own way, as painful as this may seem to people who love them. Families must not control our lives and our activities. We have to learn the wisdom of taking our medications as prescribed, abstaining from alcohol and illegal drugs, making friends, getting proper amounts of sleep, eating balanced meals, and engaging in meaningful activities. It often takes years to figure out the wisdom and value of these simple truths.

We can only learn these truths through experience, and experience is painful. Our families must stop trying to rescue us. Our families must not give in to our ploys, demands, and manipulations. Families should work closely with mental health professionals, who are there to help us change. Consumers may see change as torture and abuse, and view the professional staff as our torturers and abusers. We then use our anguish in rejecting our need for change as a means to manipulate our families into taking us out of hospitals or treatment facilities when we really need them.

Family members do not experience the devastation of mental illness as consumers do. Even when stabilized on medications, we still may be in regressed states and suffer the effects of our illness. By regression, I mean reversion to childish approaches and responses to our environment. This is one of the reasons that we need differential education. Much is new to a person who has experienced a severe regression due to mental illness. We have to relearn how to do things that most people take for granted; to relearn how to live again. Many persons who are physically injured in serious accidents have to relearn how to walk, write, or speak. Stroke victims have to relearn how to use their mental faculties. Recovery from mental illness involves the relearning of many skills and is essentially the development of a new life. The recovery process takes years and continues as long as an individual chooses to grow and develop.

Families need to be educated that they are in no way responsible for our illnesses. Our mental illnesses are not the result of poor parenting. No one is to blame for our genetic imbalances. Our families are not culpable of some crime. They have nothing to be ashamed of. When families understand how we manipulate them into helping us avoid the reality of our changed situations and life circumstances, then they can be an integral part of our treatment process.

Families also need treatment in the sense of being educated in the normal psychological responses to any devastating illness. Our families need to learn that their responses are normal, just as their loved ones' responses to illness are normal. The role of families in our recovery is working with our treatment team, and not working directly with their loved ones. We have to learn to be dependent on ourselves and our resources, and independent from our families.

Education, like all growth and development, comes in stages of readiness. We consumers need to be educated gradually and over a long period of time. A regressed person has great difficulty in relating to other people and in meeting adult needs for safety, security, and continuity in living. Education for people in such states needs to be highly practical and concrete.

Families need to learn that relapse and regression are normal parts of recovery and not evidence of failure. Sort-term hospitalization is also part of a necessary transition to recovery. Families must learn to accept risks and changes. Risks may lead temporarily to relapse and rehospitalization, but a static environment is deadly to recovery. We need guided and directed stimulation . A person raised in a risk-free and nonstimulating environment can only stultify and regress, remaining in the perpetual throes of childhood.

Sickness is static. Recovery is change. Families and consumers must accept the lifelong challenges of impairment and change; they need to learn that recurrence of symptoms does not exclude recovery. The long-term view for persons with psychiatric disabilities is quite good if families are willing to work with mental health professionals and accept their loved one's new life. Only professionals who believe that we can recover should be allowed to work with seriously ill persons.

Family education needs to focus on a change in perspective. Persons with a mental illness need to be seen with new eyes. Instead of dysfunction, incompetency, disease, or illness, we need to be seen as persons who can function, are competent, and have capability and potential. Consumers are people who need to feel pride and self-worth, to recognize their abilities as well as their limitations. Families are our support system, our lifelines in the years of struggle, hardship, and pain. Yet families must learn that support is often times not being there, not rescuing us, and not interfering in our attempts to develop new and differently functional lives.

CONSUMERS AND FAMILY SUPPORT GROUPS

It is healthy for consumers to attend family support groups. Consumers need to learn how their illnesses impact on family members and how their families perceive their behavior and thoughts. Attendance at family support group meetings helps consumers understand why we need to change and the ways in which we need to change. We learn that many of the things we take for granted, such as our families' willingness to care for us the rest of our lives, is simply not true or possible. We come to understand that our families do love us and are concerned for us, and that their letting go is not an act of abandonment.

We learn that our families are as confused by our illnesses as we are. It is easier sometime to relate to parents other than our own. Listening to families discuss their own children, we learn about regressive behavior, thought disorders, and other symptoms of our illnesses. It also helps us to learn how to behave differently by being around people who do not have a serious mental illness.

Our families, by interacting with us, come to understand that they are watching a process or natural course of illness and recovery which only we can control. In listening to us as we participate in group discussions, family members gain insight into the types of support and encouragement that we do need to overcome the continuous hurdles that we face in adapting to our new lives.

Consumers who want to attend support groups with family members are often well along in their personal recovery process. Our recovery is further aided by our inclusion. Family members change their perspective about our potential and capabilities by working with us. Our participation also affords opportunities for some families to shift their attention from their own loved one, to transfer some of their concerns from their own family members to others outside the family.

Families have a recovery process of their own to experience as they distance themselves from our lives and our illnesses. The goal of recovery for families is the reconstruction of their own lives—lives that are not centered around the illness of their child, sibling, or other relative. Support groups are not meant to replace the lives that families had before the onset of our illnesses. By including us in their support groups, we can learn together how to build new lives.

INDEPENDENCE

People with psychiatric disabilities face a challenge in learning to balance dependency and independence. Dependency is a natural response and outgrowth of any disabling condition. Independence is self-sufficient community living with a minimum of necessary outside supports from our families and our mental health system. The conflict facing consumers and families is our natural desire and need for independence and a countervailing need for dependency as we learn the realities of our illnesses. We need to learn how to become interdependent. Interdependence is not possible in an unequal relationship, but grows out of mutual self-sufficiency. It is hard for families or professionals to accept persons with thought disorders, chemical imbalances, and regressive personalities as equals and partners. Yet we can never truly recover and lead rewarding lives until we are seen as people capable of being partners in our own recovery.

Dependency that is found in custodial care, that is, care that is directed toward maintenance, safety, and security, offers neither treatment nor rehabilitation. It is improper for families to attempt to place themselves between us and the reality of our struggle, pain, and disappointment. Our families can not struggle for us. If they want us to live independently in the community they must accept that learning to be independent means risks and chances for injury. Our families feel they have to insure our safety and security at any cost, yet this emphasis on safety and security is a custodial response to disability. The cost for such an approach is that consumers cannot assume responsibility for their lives and therefore cannot recover.

Some families will rush to rescue us from treatment and rehabilitative programs because we don't like them. Rehabilitation means change and consumers, like most people, fight change. People with mental illnesses simply wish to remain insulated from the realities of their need to meet new demands. Mental illness can be overwhelming and we do need appropriately protective, nurturing, and sustaining environments that help us as we recover and learn to lead lives of our own. But desires not to change must not be encouraged by overzealous family protection.

Our families do need to be there in supportive roles as we flounder, grow, and develop. Families need outside help in being there for us. They need to work closely with mental health professionals who understand supportive roles and the recovery process.

Families have to let go of their "children." We are not children, but adults. Yes, we do have emotional illnesses that mimic child-like responses to reality, nonetheless, we have to learn to live on our own. It takes true strength for families to accept that our agony and misery are part of the growth process. Families should not get caught up in our pain as we face the reality of accepting responsibility for our own lives. Consumers want to remain immured in a changeless world. Our families have to help us leave that world.

TREATMENT PLANNING

The role of families in the actual treatment process is minimal, so treatment planning should be defined by the individual receiving services. Therapists need to understand that treatment planning is actually a process of encouragement. Consumers are often discouraged or depressed over their apparent limitations, the symptoms of their illnesses, and the side effects of their medications. Treatment planning revolves around stimulating positive action; hence treatment planning should not be directed primarily at solving behavioral problems.

Treatment planning is a process that involves professionals and consumers working together. The family's role in the process of developing goals is one of supportive and distant observer. Since one day families will be gone and we will be alone, dependent on ourselves, we must learn to do things on our own.

The treatment plan must take into account that it is unhealthy for adults to live with their parents. Independence is not typically developed at home. A treatment system operating on a system of "chronic" disability with families as agents of custodial care is disempowering. Families often desire (as do many unprogressive professionals) that their loved ones be compliant, tractable, and accepting of family requests. But custodial treatment planning is in opposition to recovery, which involves feeling in control of one's own life.

RECOVERY

The concept of recovery is changing our mental health system from a perspective of disability and pessimism to one that fosters capability and hope. Recovery is not remission, nor is it a return to a pre-existing state. The idea that we can be "cured" is counterproductive to recovery. When people with mental illness believe that they are cured they often believe that they no longer need their medications. Thus relapse is frequently the consequence of our thinking that we are well.

Recovery is a lifelong process, connoting the long-term nature of our illnesses. Some persons reject the concept of recovery, based on a denial of the reality that they have a mental illness. Recovery is rejected because the term implies that something was wrong in the first place. Recovery also involves change, which is extremely frightening to many consumers. Sometimes we think we will die if we change, or we may tell ourselves that a person cannot become different than before. Also, many consumers believe that they do not deserve to succeed so they reject or undermine the processes of growth.

Recovery is the development of new ego and identity structures to replace those damaged by our illnesses. The process starts by accepting the simple fact that our lives have been irrevocably changed by our illness. Recovery is about wellness, that is, it is the redevelopment of a new and healthier personality and lifestyle; an independent personality that is strong enough to stand on its own. Recovery takes place through creation of a new life and new patterns of behavior that make our lives more satisfying and productive. People in recovery like themselves as they are, accept their disability, and enjoy the life they have. Acceptance of one's disability can lead to greater appreciation of one's own strengths and new levels of self-esteem.

The Stages of Recovery

Recovery is a continuing process, which, just like childhood, is experienced in a progression of stages. As we grow, our wishes and desires for the future mature and change. Stages of recovery revolve around denial, awareness, rebellion, resistance, understanding, acceptance, hope, motivation, and gratitude. We can become stuck or blocked at any stage: we can regress, regain, and improve. So relapse, vigilance, and perseverance are also part of the process. It is the job of our mental health system to create enriched environments in which we can successfully traverse these stages of developing ego strength. Enriched environments can be created in hospitals, provider agencies, day activity programs, residential programs, sheltered workshops, community case management units, self-help groups, and especially in consumer run drop-in centers. An enhanced environment is one of positive regard, encouragement, opportunities, and choices. Enriched environments give us feelings of control and power.

Recovery is often threatening to other family members since it means change for them too. When their loved one changes, the established patterns of the family are disrupted. Recovery usually requires a breaking away from parental control and care-taking. We need a life of our own apart from, and yet in healthy relationship with, our families. Recovery is based on personal choice, responsibility, self-determination, and self-esteem. These can only come from action. A person who has no way of creating or becoming involved in meaningful activity can only live a life of despair and low self-esteem. These qualities are symptoms of our cultural environment and frequently nontherapeutic, over-restrictive life situations. We suffer from being treated with discrimination that magnifies the underlying symptomatology of our illness, To have hope we must have a future. To stare into the future and see nothing is an unimaginable terror for person with serious psychiatric disabilities.

Role Models and Advocacy

Successful recovery is based on hope and motivation, which comes from a variety of positive role models to whom we can relate and to whose level we can aspire. We need to see how others have changed. We need role models of survivors who have struggled with and successfully developed capacities to overcome and cope with their illness. Our suffering becomes bearable and then begins to disappear as we begin to follow the example of others who have moved successfully through this process.

Role models are the cornerstone of recovery as we begin to observe persons with disabilities engaged in various types of meaningful activities. We encourage persons with mental illnesses to serve on boards, councils, and other important volunteer activities. Anything that actively involves our minds is recovery-oriented. That is one of the reasons that consumer advocates are so adamant about our mental health system involving and including consumers in our treatment and in planning the delivery of services. Recovery is active, not passive. We need a mental health system that we can buy into. Noncompetitive job positions in the mental health system are requirements within all treatment settings for enhanced work opportunities. Traditional consumer jobs, such as dishwasher or janitor, reflect the traditional perceptions of mental health professionals that we could not learn to accommodate to the residual effects of our illnesses. The critical characteristics of any job are that the work be suitable to the worker, that the illness is understood and accepted, and that the individual is supported and reasonably accommodated.

Our involvement as decision makers and advocates in our mental health system and our need to learn to speak up and speak out, are areas of conflict between consumers and families. Families want to advocate for us but do not always know our true concerns, so it is best if we advocate for our own issues and think for ourselves. Advocacy is a form of rehabilitative activity that leads to recovery; it induces and supports growth and builds pride. The challenge for both consumers and families is to learn to work together in their advocacy efforts as equal partners. This is the promise and hope of recovery.

RELATIONSHIPS WITH THERAPISTS AND FAMILIES

Many therapists do not understand that they often create or support unnecessary dependency in those persons with whom they work. In unhealthy relationships, therapists make decisions for and take control over the lives of the people they seek to serve. When this happens, the therapeutic relationship becomes one of conflict. Consumers will try to manipulate their therapists in order to regain control.

Frequently, similar conflicts are found in relations with family members over who will control the consumer's life and life style. Will the family or therapist assume control and make decisions? It is not uncommon to find the family and therapist fighting for control while the involvement of the person is thwarted along with her or his recovery. As the individuals with the disability try to express and act on their choices, their efforts are labeled as manipulative. This is because their wishes and desires are often at odds with those of other parties, who wish them to change. Normally people choose rehabilitation as a last resort. The predominant interest of most people is not to change. Consumers are no exception.

Most professionals and families are still unwilling to accept the normal processes of recovery in which rebellion against authority figures is an integral, healthy, and normal part. Independence comes through assertion. Professionals and families are not comfortable with assertiveness and often mislabel people as aggressive when they assert themselves in the dynamics of conflict.

Any long-term dependency relationship that intervenes against the natural recovery process leads to conflict. Relationships have to be future-oriented with overall goals of self-sufficiency and self-determination. Persons receiving treatment must be involved as the decision makers. Their choices must be elicited and become the driving force of their treatment and recovery.

Our illnesses at first do impair our thoughts and behaviors. We still have to learn to think and act for ourselves. We have to learn through trial and error. Because someone, be it parent or therapist, thinks better or faster than we do because of our illness, does not mean that we are incapable of learning to think for ourselves. When the process of our growth and development is impeded through misdirected kindness and concern, we are locked into a regressed condition. As we learn to think and care for ourselves, make responsible choices, and live independently, we are no longer "patients," "clients," or "consumers." We simply are persons who need help relearning some of the skills that most people take for granted.

NEW INDENTITIES AND ALTERNATIVE CONSUMER SERVICES

One of the most tragic and common outcomes of mental illness is the development of an identity that is defined by that illness. Persons with mental illness need new ways of looking at themselves rather than being stigmatized as "mental patients." In the minds of consumers, patients are not viewed as people. Patients are dysfunctional, incompetent, helplessly passive and dependent, or hopelessly noncompliant with medical advice. People have jobs and work. Patients are disabled and seldom work. Stereotypes lead to discrimination and lack of opportunity. Consumers and our progressive professional and family friends are advocating for a major departure from the traditional perspective of permanent and delimiting "patienthood."

Alternative consumer services offer one way of attaining new identities. These can be seen as services in which consumers are in charge of the environment in which services are being delivered, for example, a drop-in center. Another way of looking at alternative consumer services involves using consumers in new roles in our mental health system, that is, in roles other than that of "patient." There have to be more opportunities for us to grow and develop than an endless array of mind-numbing day care programs, sheltered workshops, and supported employment.

New roles are opening up to us or being created for us in innovative programs. These include positions as peer counselors, case managers, outreach workers, consumer liaisons, consumer advocates, day activity program workers, discharge planning assistants, drivers, receptionists, secretaries, group leaders, drop-in center workers, and program directors. Persons diagnosed with a serious mental illness are already filling these paid jobs in a number of programs. We can be rehabilitated to do numerous existing jobs in the mental health field.

Alternative job opportunities enable us to think of ourselves in terms of competency, pride, and capability. We need to accept that we do have long-term illnesses, but also to see that persistence or chronicity of illness is not the end of the world. Families and mental health practitioners need to learn to view us as persons who have talents, abilities, and potentials, not as perpetual patients. Helping consumers learn to be workers sends powerful and positive messages to families, mental health professionals, society, and most importantly, to consumers themselves. The creation of more innovative alternative job opportunities will revolutionize the field of psychiatric rehabilitation. We salute our progressive friends and families who are helping us create these new realities and positive outcomes for our often shattered lives.

Chapter 18

FUTURE DIRECTIONS AND SOCIAL POLICY IMPLICATIONS OF FAMILY ROLES

Harriet P. Lefley

In this final chapter, we address the direction that the mental health system is taking and its impact on families. The future of families' relations with professionals, the mental health system, and consumer-run services, and the fulfillment of families' needs within the context of quality care for patients, are related to a range of interactive variables. These include fiscal issues, political orientations, research findings, and the shape and form of a managed health care system. The state of the national budget will obviously affect the monies available for all health care, as will the political inclinations of the legislators with respect to provision and prioritization of federally mandated services. Research findings—biologic, pharmacologic, and services research—may have an impact on the course of major psychiatric illnesses and/or their treatment. Discovery of more effective psychopharmacologic agents will affect service delivery to long-term clients. States may even be willing to pay for unusually expensive medications, such as clozapine, if they prove effective in returning dysfunctional persons to independent lives and tax-paying productivity. Research on the cost-effectiveness of various treatment and rehabilitation models will affect the scope, direction, and distribution of state investments in mental health services.

Above all, we anticipate that families' needs and roles will be affected by health care reform—probably in more ways than can currently be predicted. Will the era of managed care, with its emphasis on cost controls, restrict payments to direct services for patients, and thereby militate against any help for caregivers? Will family education be viewed as an ancillary or secondary service need of little importance to managed care providers? Will volunteer services that are developed and administered by consumer and family groups be favored as substitutes for more costly professional services? Or, on a more positive note, will managed care systems be wise enough to incorporate consumer-providers, at adequate salaries, in a comprehensive system? Will they be prescient enough to make available to families public resources and/or specialized services that will lighten or prevent the stressors indicated in the research findings cited in this book?

Our basic premise is that the best cure for family burden is a well-ordered mental health system that assures acceptable housing, treatment, supportive resources, and economic benefits for their loved ones. In this connection, we review some of the issues in mental health law which appear to families to favor rights to refuse treatment over rights to survival. We discuss some proposed solutions whereby persons with severe and persistent mental illnesses may be served by a system that does not threaten their sense of autonomy, but on the contrary, enhances their self-concept as persons of value and competence.

The preceding chapter on the consumer viewpoint makes it clear that many persons with mental illness want a recovery focus and look to themselves, rather than their families, to solve their problems of community reintegration. This goal is in everyone's best interest, and many clinicians have begun to realize that families, too, desperately want their loved ones to live their own lives as autonomous human beings. Any seeming overprotectiveness stems from families' fears (many of them well-grounded in experience) that failure and decompensation of a loved one may result in increased dependency, rather than from a pathological need for that dependency. There are both psychodynamic and practical issues to be addressed in balancing the various needs of families to offer maximum help, maintain realistic expectations, sustain hope, and at the same time cope with the existential realities of living with recurrent episodes of psychotic behavior. It is apparent that families need ongoing help in dealing with the diminished lives and behavioral problems that are consistent features of chronic mental illnesses. But families also need a message of hope and belief that rehabilitative interventions and a well-balanced service system may offer their ill relatives the potential for a better quality of life and a higher level of functioning.

In this connection, we address the rise of the consumer movement and consumer-operated services, and their meaning for new directions in service delivery. Role differences between family and consumer movements with respect to developing and operating new mental health resources are discussed. Some service models are presented that may bring families and consumers closer together and at the same time offer cost-effective alternatives to current modes of working with families.

Finally, we anticipate the major advocacy roles that families are likely to fulfill in the coming years.

A CHANGING SERVICE DELIVERY SYSTEM: IMPACT ON FAMILIES

Recent years have seen dramatic changes in the conceptualization, shape, and delivery of services to persons with chronic mental illnesses. With an increasing focus on community care, access to long-term hospitalization has been severely curtailed. Many community mental health centers have expanded their crisis stabilization units (CSUs), which presumably can return decompensated individuals to the community after less than a week's stay. Many systems, however, report that these CSUs are always at capacity or overcapacity. Some stays extend up to six months for persons who need a type of long term sheltered care that is no longer easily available. Other patients continue to go through the revolving door of psychiatric emergency rooms, a process costly to the system in terms of dollars and to the patients in terms of constantly destabilized lives.

Few systems have been able to resolve the dilemma of maintaining a state hospital system that may consume two-thirds of the state dollars for mental health, and their ability to provide adequate substitutes for the total care environment of the state hospitals in the community. State hospital beds continue to be closed, currently at an accelerating rate. The Center for Mental Health Services (1993) reports a current annual reduction of 9% in state and county public sector hospital beds, as compared with a 2.5% reduction in the preceding five-year period. Meanwhile, the psychiatric units of private general hospitals expand. Public sector hospital beds, however, are free to indigent patients, while private hospital beds are subject to insurance and Medicaid caps for inpatient care. Both families and psychiatric staff report that as a result, many very sick patients are prematurely discharged as soon as their insurance limits are reached.

In the patchwork of most local mental health systems, families are still frantically seeking meaningful services for relatives suffering severe psychotic episodes. Patients are frequently not admitted even to emergency rooms unless dangerousness can be demonstrated. Even when patients are admitted on court order they may be discharged within 72 hours, often to resume the same old pattern of a short period of temporary stabilization followed by decompensation and renewed need for crisis or inpatient care. Other persons experiencing psychosis end up in jail. A large collection of data indicates that in many locales the criminal justice system is clearly becoming an alternative to mental hospitals for persons with serious psychiatric disorders (Torrey et al., 1992).

There are formidable systemic barriers to a rational long-term treatment plan for the individual who is chronically mentally ill. There are legal barriers to involuntary treatment; regulatory barriers to ongoing treatment in a hospital setting; and a dollar-driven inpatient system that fails to penalize and in fact may encourage early discharge of symptomatic people, even to the street. Community rehabilitation programs erect barriers against admission or maintenance of some of the sickest people of all—those who are belligerent, disruptive, or who exacerbate their psychosis with substance abuse. Community mental health centers have frequent turnover of their psychiatric and case management staff, disrupting continuity of care. Programs for persons with dual diagnoses or for forensic patients are few and far between.

Families also continue a desperate search for appropriate housing for their ill relatives. This means housing that does not expose vulnerable mentally ill persons to crime or drugs; housing without undue restrictions on mobility; and housing managements that will not evict tenants for manifesting symptoms of mental illness.

Although the system imposes barriers, corresponding barriers are erected by the patients themselves. Noncompliance with medication typically means sporadic psychotic episodes, grossly impaired judgment, inability to manage money, acting out, and gross self-neglect. Persistent psychotic behavior leads to termination from programs, eviction from housing, and potential homelessness. There may be constant badgering of the family for money or a place to stay; stealing or nonpayment of bills in restaurants and stores; and jail time for misdemeanors (Backlar, 1993; Group for the Advancement of Psychiatry, 1986). Families are often faced with the dilemma of whether to allow mentally ill loved ones to remain in jail, facing possible beatings, exploitation, or sexual abuse from criminal inmates, or to bail them out with no available treatment resource. The dilemma is that in jail they may receive treatment, while posting bond may permit an impaired loved one to slip back to a life on the streets.

SOCIAL POLICY AND MENTAL HEALTH LAW

Mental health law advocates have focused on protection of the rights of mentally ill persons. Many efforts have been directed toward protecting patients from abuse in treatment or residential settings, resulting in saluatory regulations insuring that such abuse is stopped and prevented from recurring. Each state has a federally funded Protection and

Advocacy (P&A) Center to protect disabled persons from abuses in institutional settings; this has now been extended, under Public Law l02-173, to community care facilities as well, including jails and prisons. Lawsuits have been directed toward institutions requiring physical amenities and proof that they are providing treatment rather than custodial care alone. Primarily, however, mental health law has focused on protection of patients' civil liberties. This includes their carefully delineated rights to refuse treatment.

The conceptual framework of mental health law does not deal with the survival of mentally ill persons as an intrinsic right. Unless they are adjudicated incompetent in a court of law, mentally ill persons are presumed to be of sound enough judgment to order their own lives. For families grappling with psychotic loved ones who may gradually be losing their health and physical capacity through gross self-neglect, survival rights take precedence over the right to refuse treatment (see Hatfield's chapter in this book). Families have been involved in a series of conferences on involuntary treatment sponsored by the Community Support Program of the National Institute of Mental Health (later Center for Mental Health Services) thrashing out many of these difficult issues with consumers, psychiatrists, and legal advocates. A special section of the Winter, 1993 issue of Innovations and Research, a journal co-sponsored by the National Alliance for the Mentally Ill (NAMI) and Boston's University's Center for Psychiatric Rehabilitation, addressed involuntary treatment from these multiple viewpoints. The issue of involuntary treatment continues to plague us as a philosophical, legal, and social issue.

ATTEMPTS TO FIND SOLUTIONS

Proposed solutions range from shifts in the locus of decision-making, to attempts to control program policy, to new resource development. Civil liberties are the cornerstone of a free society, and the rights of persons to control their own bodies and destinies is a core issue in the management of patients in a psychotic state. It is also a core issue in the recovery of persons who must learn to revalue themselves and take control of their lives.

One way of returning control to the patient is through advance directives—either a "living will" or a health proxy selected by the patient to fulfill his or her desires in the event of later incapacity. Some family advocates and consumers have proposed utilization of a "Ulysses contract," so named because Ulysses ordered his crew to bind him to the mast and ignore his pleas for release in order to keep from being lured to destruction by the sirens. This is an advance directive in which a stabilized individual may voluntarily contract for enforced medication and other required treatment if he or she should later become too psychotic to be capable of rational informed consent. Rosenson and Kasten (1991, p. 1) suggested that "the most authentic expression of autonomy may be the decision by a patient whose psychiatric symptoms are in remission to plan for treatment in the event of a crisis." Although the principle of giving a mentally ill person advance control of later contingencies seemed generally acceptable to the community of consumers, a rebuttal by former patients Rogers and Centifanti (1991, p. 10) accentuated "the right to say no as well as yes to any and all treatment." In lieu of the "self-paternalism" of the Ulysses contract, these consumers advocated a "Mill's will," based on John Stuart Mill's philosophy that individuals do not have the right to relinquish their liberties in advance, and that states can exercise power only to protect others, not to protect individuals from themselves. The Mill's will would include treatment history and reasoned arguments for and against a range of treatment choices. This would preserve autonomy, with satisfaction of society's needs for prearranged mental health treatment completely under the consumer's direction and control.

Other mechanisms are preventive attempts to keep people from decompensating and requiring involuntary treatment. In areas that attempt to coordinate mental health functions, some systems have mandated a no eject/no reject policy, requiring constituent agencies to resolve behavioral problems through counseling or behavior modification techniques. However, this sometimes means that programs are unable to fulfill their obligations to their other clients. Disrupters can interfere with program effectiveness, and belligerent or predatory clients can have a highly disturbing impact on more vulnerable peers. Other systems require only that clients cannot be totally ejected from a system; they must be offered alternatives to their current placement. Unfortunately, in many cases, the family is asked to step in both as a first and last resort to take the problem off the hands of the mental health system.

Respite houses, mobile crisis teams, and consumer-operated programs are other mechanisms proposed to treat incipient crises and thereby avert the need for involuntary treatment. As yet these are few and experimental, with data lacking on their effectiveness in attaining this goal.

Homelessness

When decompensation and acting-out lead to ejection from programs or eviction from board and care homes, clients may end up on the streets. Premature discharge from inpatient units and lack of long-term sheltered care are also factors that may lead to homelessness for mentally ill persons. Families are often unable to track psychotic, unmedicated loved ones who are unable or unwilling to return home (Lefley, Nuehring, & Bestman, 1992). Social policy dictates that an increasing array of supportive housing resources be made available for all homeless people, including the homeless mentally ill. Research has shown that mentally ill street people will accept and use housing and treatment resources, providing few restrictions are applied (Lipton, Nutt, & Sabatini, 1988). Programs must be required to adapt to the culture of street people. This means minimal regulations for persons who have learned to treasure their autonomy; acceptance and warmth for persons who have lived in an openly hostile environment; and protection against exploitation from predators.

There is now an empirical data base for programs that work for the homeless mentally ill (Lamb, Bachrach, & Kass, 1992; National Institute of Mental Health, 1991). Advocacy efforts should be focused on legislative support and funding for housing initiatives and supportive treatment programs that may take a substantial number of mentally ill persons off the street and lighten the burden of their grieving families. Meanwhile, the NAMI Network on Homeless and Missing Mentally Ill Persons continues to expend efforts, through nationwide contacts with police, families, and homeless shelters, to find homeless persons who are mentally ill, link them with services, and whenever possible, reunite them with their families (see Lefley, Nuehring, & Bestman, 1992).

SOCIAL POLICY AND ECONOMIC SURVIVAL OF LOVED ONES

Families have major role conflicts in making decisions about the economic future of their mentally ill relatives. Many parents have been afraid to leave money for mentally ill offspring because this will jeopardize their entitlement benefits, and even more importantly, their accompanying access to Medicaid or Medicare. Aging parents may put off making final wills because they are conflicted about not being able to leave money directly to their mentally ill child and are afraid that this may be perceived as rejection. Spouses of persons with schizophrenia or bipolar disorder similarly may be reluctant to have joint accounts or sign over assets. In family support groups of the Depressive/Manic

Depressive Association I have heard many a spouse of a bipolar patient reporting wild spending sprees, egregiously bad investments, and even family impoverishment as the result of one manic episode.

Discussions of parents with their offspring about the rationale for omitting them from the will are unlikely to be comprehended and may generate anger and resentment. Attorneys interested in mental health law have generally focused on legal aid to patients who have been abused or discriminated against. There is also a need to develop creative legal avenues for persons to benefit from whatever financial aid or monies their families are able to give them. Pooled trusts and other joint efforts have been one effort of AMI families. However, many patients do not have families, or families with resources. Social policy mandates against a two-tiered system of economic benefits for disabled people. Plans should also be developed that offer supplemental resources to persons regardless of socioeconomic level or kinship ties, and indeed some AMI families are trying to do this (see Lefley, 1987).

PROMOTING INDEPENDENT LIVING

A major source of conflict between members of family and consumer movements involves different expectations regarding the capabilities of severely mentally ill persons for independent living. This is not surprising inasmuch as NAMI members generally view members of consumer movements as much more high-functioning than their own relatives. Many have commented on the patent differences between the articulate, rational consumers they see at meetings, whose well-phrased presentations belie any sort of cognitive deficit, and the disoriented, hallucinating, and grossly impaired individuals they know at home. Indeed, a scientific survey by Johns Hopkins University confirmed that NAMI members represent a severely impaired population. Their relatives are persons with grave functional disabilities, multiple hospitalizations, a primary diagnosis of schizophrenia (59%), excessive involvement in the legal system, and need for long-term care (Skinner, Steinwachs, & Kasper, 1992). There is no comparable analysis of a national sample of persons in the consumer movement, so it is difficult to assess whether, as some NAMI members contend, they represent a more functional, non-chronic population.

Regardless of their level of disability, there is no question that most persons with a history of mental illness have endured humiliation, pain, and social stigmatization. Some consumers perceive the mental health system as hurting rather than helping them because of dehumanizing treatment, infantilization, and reinforcement of dependency roles (Hatfield & Lefley, 1993). They feel that service providers have also given them a message of poor prognosis and eternal reliance on the system. The recovery focus discussed in Steve Kersker's chapter is therefore important symbolically as well as pragmatically. Consumers promote a recovery focus for even the most severely impaired people. Rehabilitation specialists similarly suggest that regardless of level of functioning, most people who are mentally ill can improve given appropriate help, guidance, and examples from role models (Anthony et al., 1990).

Regardless of differences in expectations, consumers and family members have a common interest in supporting independent living. Consumers believe this is a means of self-determination and confirmation of the capacity for recovery from mental illness. Many family members support this viewpoint. Even those who do not, fervently hope that their relatives may be able to reduce their dependency on their families. Both movements have a vested interest in developing separate housing and employment opportunities. And both want to insure that social security and other entitlement benefits will not be jeopardized as people progress toward recovery.

CONSUMER AND FAMILY ROLES IN SERVICES

It is probably in the area of services that the greatest differences—not disagreements—occur between consumers and families. In the early years of NAMI, families developed multiple housing, employment, and rehabilitative resources to fill gaps in the service system. But there are conflicting views about resource development. Many NAMI members feel that volunteer efforts will relieve local governments of their responsibilities to provide for disabled persons, and may result in a two-tier system of resources for people with and without family support. Others feel also that resource development absorbs time and effort that would better be devoted to legislative advocacy for expanded services. Today, family members wonder if they should accept the offer of agencies to train them as their relative's case manager, thereby relieving overburdened staff (Intagliata, Willer, & Egri, 1988). Many fear that a volunteer capability may help with short-term needs and keep budgets in check, but in the long run strip the system of needed staffing power and erode its basic armature of services.

The consumer movements, however, have a totally different view of their role in services. Their focus is on utilizing experiences and skills of former psychiatric patients in the treatment process, whether as staff members within the system, or as operators of consumer-run alternatives. Community Support Program initiatives have been devoted to precisely that end; the funding of research demonstration grants to involve consumers as staff members or directors of a range of services. Consumer-operated programs are also funded by state and local agencies throughout the United States. They include residential facilities, case-management programs, crisis services, consumer-run businesses, peer companion programs, and social centers.

Process evaluations are now beginning to appear in the literature (Nikkel et al., 1992; Sherman & Porter, 1991). Outcome evaluations require only that consumers do as well as non-consumers doing the same work. Given the state of the art, this may not be difficult to demonstrate. Most families applaud affirmative action efforts to hire and train consumers as service providers, and many AMI groups have written support letters for consumer-run services. Nevertheless, there continue to be concerns, on the part of professionals and families, about the ability of untrained consumers to control psychotic behavior, handle violence, deal with substance abuse, and otherwise manage the range of problems posed by severe mental illnesses.

There are a number of university initiatives to enroll consumers and family members in clinical training programs. An example is the MSW specialized Mental Heath Training Program in the School of Social Work, University of Cincinnati (Paulson, 1991). By training persons who can bring both personal experience and clinical skills to their roles as service providers, such programs may help bridge the gap between professionalism and mutual self-help.

Families of persons with severe impairments in functioning are concerned about the apparent erosion of the old service system, both in the reduction of long-term beds and the inadequacy of community alternatives. Some fear that states' main motivation in funding consumer-operated services is not because they offer a valuable resource, but because they are viewed as money-saving substitutes for professional services. Similarly, an emphasis on supported housing in scattered site apartments is feared as a replacement for program-affiliated residential care. Placement of severely dysfunctional persons in scattered site apartments, without intensive case management and other appropriate supports, is feared as reinforcing loneliness and alienation. Indeed, research data indicate that mentally ill people in congregate living situations have more social networks and greater opportunities for social interaction and learning (Holschuh & Segal, 1993, 1993).

Overall, families would like a system with a continuum of resources and services tailored to individual needs. This ranges from consumer-operated programs to inpatient care; from housing that includes not only independent living units and supported housing, but group homes and even state hospital beds for persons who cannot be accommodated in the community. Despite the attractiveness of the recovery focus, many families feel that those people with severe mental illnesses who need restricted environments, whether in the hospital or community, are both stigmatized and ignored by a mental health system that tailors its services to those who can meet programmatic demands and expectations in open community settings.

Nevertheless, families would also like to see more resources available for high functioning clients who can benefit from peer socialization outside of the mental health system, and from roles as consumer advocates. In sum, families agree with consumers on many issues, including the all-important emphasis on personhood and person-first language. In studies of family satisfaction with services, the respondents' major emphasis is on the need of providers to treat clients with respect (Solomon & Marcenko, 1992). Families ally with consumers on anti-stigma campaigns, support their grants, and have helped them develop consumer-run enterprises. They recognize the importance of mutual self-help, and urge their relatives to join consumer groups.

THE IMPACT OF MANAGED CARE

Families are concerned about the impact of health care reform on services for their loved ones and for themselves. Under the Clinton health care plan, mental health services will be included in the standard benefits package. At this writing, the plans for coverage include 30 days of inpatient care per episode, with an annual limit of 60 days (rather than the 90 days originally proposed); and 30 psychotherapy sessions per years, with 50% co-payment, rather than the 20 session, 20% co-payment originally proposed. Many persons with severe mental illness can benefit from ongoing supportive psychotherapy, but this model scarcely needs their needs. Since most are on limited entitlements, they would be hard-pressed to pay even the 20%. And there are great concerns about what will happen when their 60 days are up and they need further inpatient care, particularly in view of the disappearing beds in state and county mental hospitals.

In several states, community mental health centers are being urged to contract with health maintenance organizations (HMOs) with capitated Medicaid funding. This is an acute care model that adversely affects persons with chronic conditions. Psychiatrists are already doing battle with managed care firms who restrict hospitalization and may demand discharge of even severely psychotic patients. In our medical center, psychiatric residents are particularly incensed when they must share privileged information on the patient with managed care staff whose explicit interest is in saving money, while they are forbidden to share the same information with the patient's family or caregiver in the interest of patient care.

Managed care requirements undoubtedly will have an impact on the extent to which services, if any, are offered to families. At present, systems can be reimbursed for family therapy or counseling as long as these services are justified as necessary for patient care and are offered within the framework of the individual case. Family care is an extremely fragile service, however, in managed care systems that continue to focus on the individual patient within a medical model of treatment.

These medical model precedents also extend to rehabilitation. Although psychiatric rehabilitation may be far more effective than individual psychotherapy, the latter is reimbursed at a considerably higher level and many third party payors do not honor psychiatric rehabilitation as a reimbursable service. Families understandably are concerned with the skill building and resocialization needs of chronic patients, as well as strengthening their self-esteem and coping skills through supportive individual or group counseling. The relative value of psychodynamic therapies for persons with serious mental illness has been called into question (Drake & Sederer, 1986). As yet, third party payors are unlikely to distinguish among these approaches in terms of their cost-effectiveness for individual patients, and in fact should not do so until a firm empirical basis is established.

Meanwhile, however, managed care systems are unlikely to reimburse for family psychoeducation unless it is presented under the rubric of family therapy. This places families in a double bind. It is clear throughout the many chapters in this book that although some families may need and want therapy, most want to be considered support systems rather than patients. Managed care systems, however, may be prevailed upon to offer psychoeducation to caregivers by stressing the cost-benefit aspects of deterring patients' rehospitalization (Hogarty et al, 1986).

One resolution of this issue would be for state systems to mandate that all mental health agencies and institutions receiving public funds offer families education on mental illnesses, psychotropic medications, and illness management strategies as a required service. This can be done on an individual basis, in group sessions, or as periodic seminars for the general public. As suggested in chapter 11, this type of education can be offered on videotape or in reading materials in waiting rooms.

Family services then become driven by quality assurance rather than by dollar reimbursement.

Provision of education to caregivers, and involvement of caregivers in treatment and discharge planning indeed is an issue of quality assurance. In our training of psychiatric residents at the University of Miami School of Medicine, second year residents in outpatient rotation have been assigned to work with families in several capacities. Some have followed several patients longitudinally, working with their families in a collaborative role of mutual information exchange, with the patient's active participation; others have been assigned to help local AMI support groups as resource persons (Lefley, 1988). Their role is to provide the type of medical and psychiatric information that is eagerly sought by families, rather than to lead the groups as facilitators. In AMI support groups, leadership is typically provided by one of the members. In some locales, however, AMI group leaders have benefited from being trained as facilitators by professionals. Training trainers is a cost-effective measure for managed care systems wise enough to realize that the knowledge levels and psychological wellbeing of caregivers are important in patient care. Consumer-operated services similarly may be cost-effective—not because their staff are paid considerably less than professionals, but because the role modeling and group support may indeed reduce recidivism and provide viable alternatives to hospitalization.

At present, the mental health system is changing under our very eyes, stimulated by an unlikely conjunction of consumerism, family advocacy, civil libertarianism, the fiscal needs of states, and now health care reform. Service delivery systems are being dismantled and only partially rebuilt in curious and unplanned ways. It is unclear at this point whether and to what extent governments will continue to support the needs of persons with serious mental illness, and how the attrition of many current programs may impact on a very heterogeneous group of service recipients and their families. It is unclear whether some states are using consumer-providers as a rationale for dismantling parts of the system, and whether consumers will continue to be awarded the roles, respect, and salaries they should rightly command as service providers.

Family advocates will continue to engage in productive collaborative efforts with mental health professional groups, service providers, sympathetic legislators, researchers, systems planners, and primary consumers. It is evident that in the various NAMI groups, families will continue to provide legislative and human rights advocacy, work hard for basic research funding and funding for services, promote public education, and monitor clinical training programs to make sure they provide state-of-the-art education, from etiological theory to rehabilitation technology. Families will continue to press vigorously for resources that will increase the potential for independent living of capable clients. They will also work to ensure that the system does not devalue its most disabled clients by eliminating any of the basic services needed for survival, treatment, and rehabilitation. As concerned advocates, they undoubtedly will monitor health care reform to insure quality care for persons with severe and persistent mental illnesses, including help for their families and other caregivers.

REFERENCES

Anthony, W., Cohen, M., & Farkas, M. (1990). Psychiatric rehabilitation. Boston: Boston University Center for Psychiatric Rehabilitation.

Backlar, P. (1993). The family face of schizophrenia. Los Angeles: Jeremy P. Tarcher.

Center for Mental Health Services (1993). Additions and resident patients at end of year, state and county mental hospitals, by age and diagnosis, by state, United States, 1990. Washington DC: U.S. Government. Printing Office.

Drake, R.E. & Sederer, L.L. (1986). The adverse effect of intensive treatment of chronic schizophrenia. Comprehensive Psychiatry, 27, 313-326.

Group for the Advancement of Psychiatry (1986). A family affair-helping families cope with mental illness: a guide for the professions (Report No. 119). New York: Brunner/Mazel.

Hatfield, A.B. & Lefley, H.P. (1993). Surviving mental illness: Stress, coping, and adaptation. New York: Guilford.

Holschuh, J. & Segal, S.P. (1993). The role of residential services in establishing multiplexity in support networks of persons with psychaitric disabilities. Paper presented at the 88th Annual Meeting of the American Sociological Association, August 13-17, 1993.

Intagliata, J., Willer, B., & Egri, G. (1988). The role of the family in delivering case management services. In M. Harris & L.L. Bachrach (Eds.), Clinical case management (pp. 39-50). New Directions for Mental Health Services, No. 40. San Francisco: Jossey-Bass.

Lamb, H.R., Bachrach, L.L., & Kass, F.I. (1992). Treating the homeless mentally ill. Washington DC: American Psychiatric Association.

Lefley, H. P. (1987). Aging parents as caregivers of mentally ill adult children: an emerging social problem. Hospital & Community Psychiatry, 38, 10631070.

Lefley, H.P. (1988). Training professionals to work with families of chronic patients. Community Mental Health Journal, 24, 338-357.

Lefley, H.P., Nuehring, E., & Bestman, E.W. (1992). Homelessness and mentsal illness: A transcultural family perspective. In H.R. Lamb et al. (Eds.), Treating the homeless mentally ill. Washington DC: Americn Psychiatric Association.

Hogarty, G.E., Anderson, C.M., Reiss, D. et al. (1986). Family psychoeducation, social skills training, and maintenance chemotheraoy in the aftercare treatment of schizophrenia. Archives of General Psychiatry, 43, 633-642.

Lipton, F.R., Nutt, S., & Sabatini, A. (1988). Housing the homeless mentally ill: A longitudinal study of a treatment approach. Hospital & Community Psychiatry 39, 40-45.

National Institute of Mental Health (1991). Two generations of NIMH-funded research on homelessness and mental illness: 1982-1990. Rockville, MD: Office of Programs for the Homeless Mentally Ill, NIMH.

Nikkel, R.E., Smith, G., & Edwards, D. (1992). A consumer-perated case management poject. Hospital & Cmmunity Psychiatry, 43, 577-579.

Paulson, R.I. (1991). Professional training for consumers and family members: One road to empowerment. Psychosocial Rehabilitation Journal, 14, 69-80.

Rogers, J.A. & Centifanti, J.B. (1991). Beyond "self-paternalism": Response to Rosenson and Kasten. Schizophrenia Bulletin, 17, 9-14.

Rosenson, M.K. & Kasten, A.M. (1991). Another view of autonomy: Arranging consent in advance. Schizophrenia Bulletin, 17, 1-7.

Sherman, P.S. & Porter, R. (1991). Mental health consumers as case management aides. Hospital & Com,munity Psychiatry, 42, 494-498.

Skinner, E.A., Steinwachs, D.M., & Kasper, J.A. (1992). Family perspectives on the service needs of people with serious and persistent mental illness. Part I: Characteristics of families and consumers. Innovations and Research,1(3),23-30.

Solomon, P. & Marcenko, M.O. (1992). Families of adults with severe mental illness: their satisfaction wth inpatient and outpatient treatment. Psychosocial Rehabilitation Journal, 16, 121-134.

Torrey, E.F., Wolfe, S.M., & Flynn, L.M. (1992). Criminalizing the seriously mentally ill: The abuse of jails as mental hospitals. Arlington, VA: Public Citizens Health Research Group and the National Alliance for the Mentally Ill.

Index

for children of the mentally
ill, 167
for grieving people, 29-30
Social withdrawal by the mentally ill, 139-140
Social workers, 157
Somatic treatment of mental illness, 8
Span of Apprehension Task, 86
Spouses of the mentally ill, 163,
176-182
St. John's Wort, 5
State hospitals, 7-9, 345
Stigma
and families of the mentally
ill, 11-12, 124
and siblings of the mentally
ill, 173, 176
and spouses of the mentally
ill, 179
Stimulus load, regulation of,
201-202
Stress
in children of the mentally ill,
164-167
and ethnicity, 229-230
family, 161, 310
and family burden, 43, 319
management by families of
the mentally ill, 141-143
and mental illness, 10
Stress-vulnerability model, 197-
198
Stressor, 131
Structure within family of
schizophrenic person, 202-
203
Subjective burden, 120, 121-
122, 175, 309-310, 316
Suicidal behavior of the mentally ill, 138-139

Suicide and children of the mentally ill, 165
Support groups, 48, 72, 186
for adult children of the mentally ill, 170-171
cultural content of, 233-236
for families, 48
professional-facilitated, 48
Supportive family counseling, 18
Supportive Family Training, 73
Surgical treatment of mental illness, 8
Survival skills for the patient, 17
Survivor's guilt, 124-125, 172,
175
Symptom management strategies, 136
Systems assessment by mental
health professionals, 285
Systems theory of mental illness, 52, 79-98

Technical eclecticism of mental
illness treatment, 52, 53
Theology and mental illness, 5
Therapeutic alliance, 110, 112,
151-152
Therapeutic foci, 120-127
Therapeutic models
and cultural differences, 228
Therapists
relationship with the mentally
ill, 339-340
Therapy
brief, 54
long-term psychotherapy, 54
Thorazine, 10
Thought disorder and communi-
cation deviance, 86
Threshold Thrift Shop, 71

For information on national and local
resources and support groups, contact

The National Alliance for the Mentally Ill at
2101 Wilson Boulevard
Arlington, VA 22201
(703) 524-7600